THE MGH PRIMER OF OUTPATIENT MEDICINE

THE MGH PRIMER OF OUTPATIENT MEDICINE

Chief Editors

ETHAN M. BASCH, MD

Instructor in Medicine
Harvard Medical School;
Assistant
Department of Medicine
Massachusetts General Hospital
Boston, Massachusetts

SHANA L. BIRNBAUM, MD

Clinical Fellow
Harvard Medical School;
Senior Resident
Department of Medicine
Massachusetts General Hospital
Boston, Massachusetts

CELINA GARZA, MD

Clinical Fellow
Harvard Medical School;
Senior Resident
Department of Internal Medicine
Massachusetts General Hospital
Boston, Massachusetts

WELLS A. MESSERSMITH, MD

Fellow
Department of Oncology
Johns Hopkins School of Medicine;
Fellow
Department of Medical Oncology
Johns Hopkins Cancer Center
Baltimore, Maryland

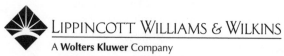

LIPPINCOTT WILLIAMS & WILKINS
A **Wolters Kluwer** Company
Philadelphia • Baltimore • New York • London
Buenos Aires • Hong Kong • Sydney • Tokyo

Acquisitions Editor: Richard Winters
Developmental Editor: Delois Patterson
Production Editor: Emmeline Parker
Manufacturing Manager: Timothy Reynolds
Cover Designer: Christine Jenny
Compositor: Maryland Composition
Printer: Quebecor Dubuque

© 2002 by LIPPINCOTT WILLIAMS & WILKINS
530 Walnut Street
Philadelphia, PA 19106 USA
LWW.com

Printed in the USA

Library of Congress Cataloging-in-Publication Data
0781740118

Care has been taken to confirm the accuracy of the information presented and to describe generally accepted practices. However, the authors, editors, and publisher are not responsible for errors or omissions or for any consequences from application of the information in this book and make no warranty, expressed or implied, with respect to the currency, completeness, or accuracy of the contents of the publication. Application of this information in a particular situation remains the professional responsibility of the practitioner.

The authors, editors, and publisher have exerted every effort to ensure that drug selection and dosage set forth in this text are in accordance with current recommendations and practice at the time of publication. However, in view of ongoing research, changes in government regulations, and the constant flow of information relating to drug therapy and drug reactions, the reader is urged to check the package insert for each drug for any change in indications and dosage and for added warnings and precautions. This is particularly important when the recommended agent is a new or infrequently employed drug.

Some drugs and medical devices presented in this publication have Food and Drug Administration (FDA) clearance for limited use in restricted research settings. It is the responsibility of the health care provider to ascertain the FDA status of each drug or device planned for use in their clinical practice.

10 9 8 7 6 5 4 3 2 1

CONTENTS

SECTION IX: MUSCULOSKELETAL

SECTION X: DERMATOLOGY

SECTION XI: NEUROLOGY/OPHTHALMOLOGY

SECTION XII: PSYCHOSOCIAL

CONTRIBUTORS

CHIEF EDITORS
Ethan M. Basch, MD
Shana L. Birnbaum, MD
Celina Garza, MD
Wells A. Messersmith, MD

EDITORS EMERITUS
Todd Gorman, MD
Arthur Kim, MD
Sheri-Ann Burnett, MD

FACULTY ADVISOR AND EDITORIAL MENTOR
Allan H. Goroll, MD

CONTRIBUTORS

Chapter	Contributors
Foundations of Evidence-Based Medicine	Gregory Abel, MD Meg Doherty, MD, MPH, PhD Carl Pallais, MD
Health Maintenance and Screening	Paula Dygert, MD Barna Tugwell, MD Francine Weist, MD Kristian Olson, MD Richard Grant, MD
Hypertension	Philip Peters, MD Steven Servoss, MD Julie Servoss, MD Jeffrey Schnipper, MD, MPH
Hyperlipidemia	Sahil A. Parikh, MD Steven Servoss, MD Richard Grant, MD Todd Gorman, MD Rocio Hurtado, MD
Coronary Artery Disease and Angina	James Beckerman, MD David Spragg, MD Arthur Kim, MD Amy Wheeler, MD
Congestive Heart Failure	Gregory Lewis, MD Steven Servoss, MD

Atrial Fibrillation	Jim Cheung, MD Zoltan Arany, MD
Lower Extremity Edema	Cynthia Cooper, MD Monty Tew, MD
Surgical Consultation	Salvatore Cilmi, MD Richard Grant, MD Todd Gorman, MD Jill Banatowski, MD
Chronic Cough	Roderick Tung, MD Vinicio Dejesus-Perez, MD Ronald Dixon, MD Arhur Kim, MD
Allergic Rhinitis	Anshul M. Patel, MD Ronald Dixon, MD Arthur Kim, MD Todd Gorman, MD
Asthma	Caroline Birks, MD Ronald Dixon, MD Evan Dellon, MD Michael Fessler, MD
COPD	Vinicio Dejesus Perez, MD Ronald Dixon, MD Seema Baranwal, MD Michael Fessler, MD
Upper Respiratory Infections	Shana Birnbaum, MD Todd Gorman, MD
Bronchitis/Pneumonia	Charles Holmes, MD, MPH Sekar Kathiresan, MD
Management of Latent Tuberculosis	Peter Crompton, MD Charles Holmes, MD, MPH Diana Brainard, MD
Urinary Tract Infections	Dan Barouch, MD, PhD Diana Brainard, MD Rocio Hurtado, MD
Sexually Transmitted Diseases	Melissa Bender, MD Laura Kehoe MD, MPH Charles Holmes, MD Arthur Kim, MD Emma Fortney, MD
HIV Management	Peter Crompton, MD Louise Ivers, MD Arthur Kim, MD Salvatore Cilmi, MD Sonia Nagy, MD

Endocarditis	Nina Aldrich-Wolfe, MD Ethan Basch, MD Amanda Peppercorn, MD John Fangman, MD
Travel Medicine	Elizabeth Price, MD Louise Ivers, MD
Obesity	Gregory Ruhnke, MD Richard Grant, MD Todd Gorman, MD
Diabetes	Brendan Everett, MD Gregory Ruhnke, MD Natasha Tiffany, MD Sherri-Ann Burnett, MD Kristin Walters, MD
Thyroid Disease	Deborah Wexler, MD Gregory Ruhnke, MD Ateev Mehrotra, MD Sherri-Ann Burnett, MD
Osteoporosis	Annabel Chen, MD Gregory Ruhnke, MD Sherri-Ann Burnett, MD Wesley Fairfield, MD
Menopause/Hormone Replacement Therapy	Naomi Hamburg, MD Gregory Ruhnke, MD Wells Messersmith, MD Rajani LaRocca, MD
Amenorrhea	Nakela Cook, MD Gregory Ruhnke, MD Rajani LaRocca, MD
Contraception	Lauren Dias, MD Anuradha Chaddah, MD Shana Birnbaum, MD Sherri-Ann Burnett, MD Rajani LaRocca, MD
Abnormal PAP Smear	Cindy Lai, MD Anuradha Chaddah, MD Arthur Kim, MD Ann Celi, MD
Abnormal Vaginal Bleeding	Caroline Birks, MD Shana Birnbaum, MD
Breast Cancer and Benign Breast Disease	Garth Graham, MD Shana Birnbaum, MD
Urinary Incontinence	Cynthia Cooper, MD Diana Brainard, MD

Benign Prostatic Hyperplasia	Elizabeth Price, MD Wells Messersmith, MD Erica Brownfield, MD
Erectile Dysfunction	Cindy Lai, MD Laura Kehoe, MD, MPH Sherri-Ann Burnett, MD Lisa Cosimi, MD
Abnormal Urinalysis	Danuta King, MD Reshma Kewalramani, MD Arthur Kim, MD Emma Fortney, MD
Chronic Renal Failure	Danuta King, MD Richard Grant, MD Reshma Kewalramani, MD Herbert Lin, MD
Gastrointestinal Complaints: Dyspepsia/ GERD/PUD	Edwin Choy, MD Laura Kehoe, MD, MPH David Forcione, MD Francine Weist, MD Nicholas Fleming, MD
Liver Function Tests	Cindy Lai, MD David Forcione, MD
Chronic Viral Hepatitis	Cindy Lai, MD Celina Garza, MD
Chronic Diarrhea	David Forcione, MD Cindy Lai, MD Ethan Basch, MD Adam Cohen, MD
Irritable Bowel Syndrome	Andrew Ross, MD Cindy Lai, MD Sherri-Ann Burnett, MD Thomas Roberts, MD
Anemia	Jennifer Brown, MD, PhD Natasha Tiffany, MD Richard Grant, MD
Anticoagulation	Andrew Yee, MD Jennifer Brown, MD, PhD Andrew Chan, MD
Musculoskeletal Exam	Celina Garza, MD Karen Costenbader, MD
Arthritis: Gout/OA/RA	Ateev Mehrotra, MD Celina Garza, MD Gregory Ruhnke, MD Karen Costenbader, MD

Low Back Pain	Celina Garza, MD Ethan Basch, MD Wells Messersmith, MD Katrina Kretsinger, MD
Benign Skin Conditions	Naomi R. L. Rice, MD, MPH Barna Tugwell, MD Rushika Fernandopulle, MD
Skin Cancers	Seema Baranwal, MD Laura Kehoe, MD, MPH Lisa Cosimi, MD
Headache	Jose Florez, MD, PhD
Dementia	John Wylie, MD Jose Florez, MD, PhD Roy Perlis, MD
Dizziness	Jose Florez, MD, PhD
Common Eye Problems	Fina Barouch, MD George Papaliodis, MD Reshma Kewalramani, MD Richard Grant, MD
Tobacco	Celina Garza, MD Ethan Basch, MD David McCarty, MD
Alcohol Abuse	Caroline Birks, MD Ethan Basch, MD David McCarty, MD
Depression	Donald Hass, MD Shana Birnbaum, MD
Sleep Disorders	Vinicio Dejesus-Perez, MD Celina Garza, MD
Domestic Violence	Seema Baranwal, MD Cinnamon Bradley, MD Richard Grant, MD Sonia Nagy, MD
Chronic Nonmalignant Pain	David O'Halloran, MD Francine Wiest, MD Todd Gorman, MD

FACULTY ADVISORS

The MGH housestaff gratefully acknowledges the mentorship and guidance of our faculty advisors:

HEALTH MAINTENANCE AND SCREENING

William Kormos MD, MPH
General Medicine Division, MGH

Michael Barry MD
Chief, General Medicine Division, MGH

Jeffrey Schnipper MD, MPH
General Medicine Division, BWH

CARDIOLOGY

Katharine Treadway MD
General Medicine Division, MGH

G. Sherry Haydock MD
General Medicine Division, MGH

Donald Lloyd-Jones MD
Cardiology Division , MGH

G. William Dec MD
Cardiology Division, MGH

Brian McGovern MD
Cardiology Division, MGH

Blair Fosburgh MD
General Medicine Division, MGH

Elaine Hylek MD, MPH
General Medicine Division, MGH

William Kormos MD, MPH
General Medicine Division, MGH

PULMONARY

Barbara Cockrill MD
Pulmonary Unit, MGH
Director, Partners Asthma Center

Gregory Randolph MD
Massachusetts Eye and Ear Infirmary

Harvey Simon MD
General Medicine Division, MGH
Infectious Disease Unit, MGH

Burton W. Lee MD
Pulmonary/Critical Care, St. Joseph, MI

INFECTIOUS DISEASE

Nesli Basgoz MD
Chief, Albright Firm
Division of Infectious Diseases, MGH
Director, Infectious Disease Associates

Mark Eisenberg MD
General Medicine Division, MGH
Co-Director of Primary Care Program, MGH

Donna Felsenstein MD
Division of Infectious Diseases, MGH
Director, GID/STD Unit

Stephen Calderwood MD
Chief, Division of Infectious Diseases, MGH

Edward T. Ryan MD, DTM&H
Division of Infectious Diseases, MGH
Director, Tropical & Geographic Medicine Center
Director, Travelers' Advice & Immunization Center

ENDOCRINE

Suzanne J. Koven MD
Bulfinch Medical Group, MGH

Lee M. Kaplan MD
Gastrointestinal Unit, MGH
Director, MGH Weight Center

James B Meigs MD, MPH
General Medicine Division, MGH

Douglas S. Ross MD
Thyroid Unit, MGH

Joel Finkelstein MD
Endocrine Unit, MGH

Karen Carlson MD
General Medicine Division, MGH
Director, Women's Health Associates

Karen O'Brien MD
Women's Health Associates, MGH

GYNECOLOGY AND GENITOURINARY

Annekathryn Goodman MD
Vincent Obstetrics and Gynecology, MGH

Janey Pratt MD
Department of General Surgery, MGH

Claus Hamann MD, MS
Geriatric Medicine Unit, MGH

Michael Barry MD
Chief, General Medicine Division, MGH

Joseph A. Grocela MD
Urology Unit, MGH

Leslie Fang MD
Renal Unit, MGH

Winfred Williams MD
Renal Unit, MGH

Hasan Bazari MD
Renal Unit, MGH
Director of Housestaff Training, MGH

GASTROENTEROLOGY

Lawrence S. Friedman MD
Chief, Walter Bauer Firm
Gastrointestinal Unit, MGH

Raymond Chung MD
Gastrointestinal Unit, MGH
Director, Liver Transplantation Unit

Bruce Sands MD
Gastrointestinal Unit, MGH
Director, Clinical IBD Research

HEMATOLOGY

David Kuter MD
Hematology/Oncology Unit, MGH

Saha Sadoughi MD
Department of General Medicine, BWH

Elaine Hylek MD, MPH
General Medicine Division, MGH

MUSCULOSKELETAL AND RHEUMATOLOGY

Celeste Robb-Nicholson MD
General Medicine Division, MGH

Karen Atkinson MD
Rheumatology Unit, MGH

Steven Atlas MD, MPH
General Medicine Division, MGH

DERMATOLOGY

Bonnie T Mackool MD, MSPH
Director, Dermatology Consultation and Inpatient Service, MGH

Charles Taylor MD
Department of Dermatology, MGH
Director of Phototherapy Unit

NEUROLOGY

F. Michael Cutrer MD
Department of Neurology, Mayo Clinic
Rochester, Minnesota

Claus Hamann MD
Geriatric Unit, MGH

Stephen W. Parker MD
Department of Neurology, MGH
Director, Otoneurology and Gait and Balance Disorders Unit

Nagagopal Venna MD, MRCP
Department of Neurology, MGH
Director, Neurology Clinic

OPHTHALMOLOGY

Claudia Richter MD
Massachusetts Eye and Ear Infirmary

MENTAL HEALTH AND PSYCHOSOCIAL

Michael Bierer MD
Director, Health Care for the Homeless, MGH

Stephanie Eisenstat MD
Women's Health Associates, MGH

Nancy Rigotti MD
General Medicine Division, MGH
Director, Tobacco Research and Treatment Center

Theodore A. Stern MD
Chief, Psychiatric Consultation Service, MGH

Kenneth C. Sassower MD
Department of Neurology, MGH
Sleep Disorders Unit

Todd E. Gorman MD
Assistant Professor of Clinical Medicine
University of Vermont College of Medicine

FOREWORD

The recognition of the increasingly important role of outpatient care to the practice of internal medicine has resulted in a major revamping of residency training over the past decade. Whereas devotion of substantial time to ambulatory care rotations was once reserved for those in primary care tracks, now all internal medicine residents are required to have one-third of their training in the outpatient setting. An annual 4-week block rotation in the ambulatory setting is a common feature of most modern internal medicine residency training programs, providing concentrated time for a variety of clinical experiences and directed reading.

The MGH Primer of Outpatient Medicine was conceptualized and written to provide a succinct summary of the basic medical knowledge pertinent to the practice of internal medicine in the outpatient setting. It grew out of a resident-initiated project at the Massachusetts General Hospital (MGH) to develop an evidence-based learning resource that trainees could read cover-to-cover during their ambulatory care block rotation. Its local popularity and usefulness as an educational tool stimulated interest in refining it to serve as a standard primer of outpatient internal medicine.

With the continued rise in the importance of outpatient care to medical practice, it is essential that all learners master the knowledge base critical to functioning effectively in the ambulatory setting. The revision of board and licensure examinations to include outpatient medicine reflects this realization. The housestaff and their faculty consultants at the MGH have done a masterful job of defining the essentials and presenting them in literate, intelligent fashion. The editors and their colleagues have produced a book by residents for residents that reflects the best in scholarship and editorial skill. It is our intent that this will become an established and regularly updated contribution by the residents of the MGH to learners everywhere. It was a pleasure and privilege to mentor the editors in this project as they make this valuable contribution to the growing literature of outpatient medicine.

Allan H. Goroll, MD, FACP
Boston, Massachusetts
January 2002

PREFACE

The evidence-based approach to the practice of medicine has become standard in both the United States and abroad. Its adoption was the result of interactions in the inpatient setting. Inquiry, reflection, and critique became the hallmarks of all good academic health centers, and the training of residents was accomplished in an environment in which learning and the delivery of quality care were properly paced.

The environment for medical care and medical education has changed significantly, causing concern among medical educators. Two of the most dramatic differences are the increasing acuity and pace of health care delivery that has, in many instances, outstripped the opportunity for conscientious, reflective education, and the shift of medical education from the inpatient environment to the ambulatory setting.

Given these changes, it is extraordinarily important that we reexamine the educational environment and recommit to the evidence-based approach in ambulatory practice. *The MGH Primer of Outpatient Medicine* attempts to meld thoughtful, reflective, and critical examination of medical care with the busy ambulatory care setting. This syllabus standardizes ambulatory training, reflecting the data at hand, and provides for constant evolution as new information allows us to change the standards of practice. It is meant to be a companion, not a bible. We hope that its users will find its utility, not only in the data it provides in a timely manner, but also in the opportunity to reflect upon the critical literature that led to the information provided. We at the MGH are proud of our ambulatory care educational program, and we are extremely pleased to have the opportunity to share this approach with our medical colleagues around the world.

Dennis A. Ausiello, MD
Jackson Professor of Clinical Medicine
Physician-in-Chief
Medical Services
Massachusetts General Hospital
Boston, Massachusetts

ACKNOWLEDGMENT

This text represents the collective efforts of more than 100 MGH house officers and faculty advisors over the past five years. We thank the Internal Medicine residency classes of 1997 through the present, and the staff members who have generously donated their time to educate and inspire us.

MGH has provided us with a rich environment in which to study medicine. We are grateful to our Chief of Medicine, Dennis Ausiello, who has instilled us with the excitement of scientific exploration—a sensibility which underlies the spirit of this text. Our Residency Program Director, Hasan Bazari, has been a role model as caring physician and scholar, and has guided us throughout our training. Our Firm Chiefs, Lloyd Axelrod, Lawrence Friedman, and Morton Schwartz, have supported housestaff career development and have reminded us of the importance of balancing professional activities with private life. This book would not have been possible without the thoughtful and caring mentorship of Allan Goroll, our chief faculty advisor.

Tanya Milosh has brought enthusiasm to the residency program's organization, and she provided invaluable help in putting together this text. The work would not have been possible without the initiative of Todd Gorman, who founded the project and initially edited it, and without the subsequent editorial efforts of Sheri-Ann Burnett and Arthur Kim. Special thanks are due to Rich Winters, our publisher and colleague at Lippincott Williams & Wilkins, who encouraged this effort and was instrumental in bringing the project forward.

Finally, we thank the individuals who provided the four of us with support and encouragement during the preparation of this manuscript: Patrick Ellinor, Vaughn Mankey, Catherine Ulbricht, and Natalie Vona Messersmith.

Ethan M. Basch, MD
Shana L. Birnbaum, MD
Celina Garza, MD
Wells A. Messersmith, MD

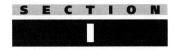

FOUNDATIONS OF
AMBULATORY MEDICINE

1

BASIC TOOLS OF EVIDENCE-BASED MEDICINE

INTRODUCTION

- Evidence-based medicine is "the conscientious, explicit and judicious use of current best evidence in making decisions about the care of individual patients. . . integrating individual clinical expertise with the best available external clinical evidence from systematic research" (Sackett et al., 1996).
- Epidemiology is the study of the distribution and determinants of health-related events in specific populations, and the application of this study to the control of health problems (Last et al., 2001).
- Biostatistics is the application of statistics to biological problems (Last et al., 2001).

EVALUATION OF STUDIES

Approach

- Evaluate systematically the study hypothesis, design, bias and/or confounding, possible effect modification, measures of association, measures of statistical significance and power, and generalizability. Note that epidemiologic studies aim to reject the null hypothesis.
  ⇒ Null hypothesis (H_0): There is no association between exposure and outcome/disease.
  ⇒ Alternative hypothesis (HA): There is an association between exposure and outcome/disease.
- Consider study design and sources of bias common to that design (see Table 1.1).

TABLE 1.1 CLASSIC STUDY DESIGNS

Type of Study/Descripton	Measure of Effect	Advantages	Disadvantages	Principle Problem/ Source of Bias
Ecologic: Compares rates of disease in populations to rates of exposures in populations.	Correlation coefficient (Pearson's r).	Easy, inexpensive; fast. Can be done in library,	Population rather than individual level; hypothesis generating only. Limited to census-type data.	Ecologic fallacy.
Cross-sectional: Disease and exposure status are assessed at same point in time; represents "snapshot."	Prevalence; relative A prevalence; estimate of relative risk.	Easy, inexpensive, fast, ethically safe. Can study several outcomes. Helpful to health planner.	Establishes only association, not causality or event sequence; susceptible to selection and information bias; cannot provide true risk or relative risk.	Prevalence and/or incidence bias; potential survivor bias.

(continued)

TABLE 1.1 *(continued)*

Type of Study/Descripton	Measure of Effect	Advantages	Disadvantages	Principle Problem/ Source of Bias
Case-control: Subjects are selected for study based on whether or not they have disease or condition; their history is then reviewed for presence of possible causal exposure. *Controls* persons who do not have disease but have had same opportunity for exposure as cases.	Odds ratio or risk ratio. Can estimate relative risk when prevalence of disease is low.	Useful for rare disorders. Relatively inexpensive. Short duration. Can study many exposures. Odds ratio approximates relative risk in rare diseases. Easy to manipulate statistically.	Does not yield prevalence, incidence, or relative risk. Time sequence can be only inferred. Selection of appropriate control groups is difficult. Susceptible to confounding, as well as to selection and information bias. Can study only one outcome variable.	Sampling bias; recall bias; measurement bias; Berkson bias; exposure suspicion bias.
Prospective cohort: Subjects selected according to whether or not they have a given exposure. At start of the study, no subject has disease. Subjects followed to see who develops disease.	Relative risk, excess risk (RR-I), and odds ratio often used due to ease of statistical analysis.	Establishes true time sequence. Yields incidence and relative risk rates. Less susceptible to information and selection bias. Blinding easily done. Good for rare exposures, many outcomes.	Costly. Loss to follow-up. Can study only one exposure variable, except in nested case-control studies. Not good for rare outcomes. Often need large sample sizes.	Loss to follow-up; diagnostic suspicion bias.
Nested case-control: Case-control study with cases and controls drawn from cohorts in a prospective cohort study.	Odds ratio.	Effects from confounding may be reduced.	Must be nested within larger cohort. Requires bank of samples stored until outcome occurs. Not generalizable if involvement in cohort has effect on sample population.	Loss to follow-up. Cases may be controls for other cases, and controls may become cases.
Retrospective cohort: Subjects selected according to whether or not they have a given exposure. At start of study, some subjects in each exposure group already have disease. Used most often for occupational cohorts.	Relative risk; population attributable risk (PAR) because unexposed cohort often not available; odds ratio.	Similar to prospective cohort, but less expensive and faster. Good for occupational cohorts. Can study very rare exposures.	Similar to prospective cohort. No control over selection of subjects and outcome measurements; measurements used are often no longer relevant. Loss to follow-up	Healthy worker effect; loss to follow-up; diagnostic suspicion bias.
Randomized clinical trial (RCT): Experimental trial in which participants are assigned either to receive intervention being tested or else an alternative treatment or placebo.	Relative risk; excess risk; odds ratio.	Establishes true time sequence and relative risk. Least susceptible to information and selection bias. Double or triple blinding easy to do. Can study many outcomes.	Most costly. Loss to follow-up. Ethical considerations limit studies conducted. Often need large sample sizes. Favorite choice of well-funded drug companies so negative results less likely to be reported.	Non-response/ volunteer bias; loss to follow-up.
Cross-over design: Method of comparing two or more treatments in which subjects, on completion of one treatment, are switched to another.	Relative risk; odds ratio.	As with randomized clinical trial.	Effects of first treatment may carry over into period when the second treatment is given.	Loss to follow-up; generalizability.
Metaanalysis: Method using statistics to combine results of different studies. Often used to pool data from small number of randomized clinical trials, none of which demonstrates significance alone but in aggregate can achieve significance.	Odds ratio.	Can calculate summary risk measure for an outcome and exposures.	Many potential analytical and methodological problems; outcome and exposures may be measured differently. Studies may show very different results making a summary odds ratio less accurate, with greater variance about the estimate.	Problems with completeness of data and consistency of collection.

Source: Adapted from Mausner, 1985; Hennekens and Buring, 1987; Hulley and Cummings, 1988, Lillienfeld and Stolley, 1994; CU, 1997; and Rothmar, 1998.

Bias

- Bias is any systematic error in design, conduct, or analysis of a study that results in a mistaken estimate of exposure's effect on risk of disease (see Table 1.2) (Schlesselman, 1982). Bias must be distinguished from random error (commonly referred to as "noise"), which always yields a distortion of results toward the null.

TABLE 1.2 TYPES OF BIAS

Type of Class	Definition	Solution
Selection bias	Systematic error in choosing a study population	Random sampling methods
Berkson bias	Selection bias in which hospital cases and controls are different from each other, with higher rate of disease in cases	Nonhospitalized cases
Sampling bias	Error arising from not sampling from entire universe in which all have chance of selection	Probability sampling methods
Misclassification bias	Error in the assignment of cases or controls	Stricter case and control definitions
Surveillance bias	Error in which cases are more likely to be identified when under medical surveillance	Masking; stratification by medical care facility
Observer bias	Difference between a true value and that detected due to observer variation	Masking; blinding
Information bias	Flaw in measuring an exposure or outcome which results in differential quality (accuracy) of information between compared groups	Well constructed definitions for cases and controls
Recall bias	Error due to differences in accuracy or completeness of memory recall of prior events or experiences by study participants	Prospective or nested-case control studies
Nonresponse bias/ withdrawal bias	Difference between the true value and that actually observed in a study due to the characteristics of participants who withdrew	Intention-to-treat analysis

Source: Last et al., 2001.

Confounding (Jhu, 1992; Cu, 1997; Rothman and Greenland, 1998)

- Confounding is not bias. Confounders are noncausal associations between exposure and outcome of interest. For a third factor to be a true confounder, the following criteria must be met:
  1. The third factor must be an independent risk factor for the disease.
  2. The third factor must be associated with (but not cause) the exposure of interest.
  3. The third factor must not be an intermediate step in the pathway from exposure to disease.
- Confounders are addressed either in the design or the analysis phase of a study (JHU, 1991). Methods of handling confounders in the design phase include:
  1. Randomization to evenly distribute confounders among cases and controls.
  2. Restriction so that all subjects in the study do not have the confounder.
  3. Matching so that comparison pairs both either have or do not have the confounder.
- Methods of controlling for confounders in the analysis phase include:
  1. Stratification by the Mantel-Haenzsel chi-square.
  2. Direct or indirect adjustment.
  3. Multivariate regression analysis to control at once for multiple confounders mathematically.

Interaction or Effect Modification (Mausner and Kramer, 1985; Rothman and Greenland, 1998)

- An interacting variable modifies the effect of a causal factor. For example, the relationship between an exposure and disease may vary depending upon the level of a third variable. If an interaction exists, the data must be presented in a stratified analysis. The data must not be presented as a crude or summary measure of effect, as interaction cannot be controlled. Effect modifiers are a reason to measure many exposures in a study, even if they are not part of the original study hypotheses.

Measures of Association (Table 1.3) (Kahn and Sempos, 1989; Selvin, 1991; Rothman and Greenland, 1998)

TABLE 1.3 MEASURES OF ASSOCIATION*

	Disease +	Disease −	
Exposure +	A	B	**A + B**
Exposure −	C	D	**C + D**
	A + C	**B + D**	**A + B + C + D**

* Relative risk: A/(A + B) ÷ C/(C + D); prospective studies odds ratio (OR): A/B ÷ C/D → OR = AD/BC; case-control OR: A/C ÷ B/D → OR = AD/BC; matched case-control OR: ratio of discordant pair = B/C.

- **Incidence:** The number of new cases of disease during a period of time divided by the total population at risk for the disease.
- **Prevalence:** The number of disease cases at a specific point in time divided by the total population at risk for the disease. (Note: Prevalence equals incidence times disease duration. If disease incidence is low but duration long, then disease prevalence is high; if disease incidence is high but duration short, then disease prevalence is low).
- **Correlation coefficient:** A measure of how well two values vary with one another. The correlation coefficient varies from −1 to 0 (inversely correlated) and 0 to 1 (positively correlated). Correlation >0.70 is highly positively correlated.
- **Relative risk (RR):** The proportion of diseased people among those exposed to a relevant risk factor (incidence in exposed) divided by the proportion of diseased people among those not exposed to the risk factor (incidence in nonexposed). This is the likelihood of developing disease in the exposed group relative to that in the nonexposed group. An RR of 1.0 indicates no association between the variables; an RR of 0 to 1 indicates a protective effect; and an RR of 1 to infinity indicates a risk factor.
- **Odds ratio (OR):** A comparison of the presence of a risk factor for disease in a sample of diseased subjects and nondiseased controls. In prospective cohort studies, the OR is the ratio of the odds of exposed people developing the disease to the odds of nonexposed people developing the disease; in case-control studies, the OR is the ratio of the odds of exposure among the people with disease to the odds of exposure among the controls. An OR of 1.0 indicates no relationship between the variables; an OR of 0 to 1 indicates a protective effect; and an OR of 1 to infinity indicates a risk factor. In addition, the OR can estimate the RR when:
  1. The cases are representative of all people with the disease in the population.
  2. The controls are representative of all people without the disease.
  3. The disease is rare.
- **Confidence interval (CI):** A range of values intended to contain the parameter of interest with a certain degree of assurance. The 95% CI has a 95% chance of including the true size of the effect (which can never be known exactly). When the 95% CI includes 1.0, then the estimate of risk is not statistically significant (*Clinical Evidence 2000*, 2000).
- **Attributable risk:** The proportion of disease incidence (risk) that can be attributed to a specific exposure (for an entire population or for exposed persons only). Attributable risk varies from 0 to 1.
- **Intention-to-treat analysis:** An analysis of the data from all participants initially enrolled into the study as if they had remained in the group into which they were randomized, regardless of whether they remained until the end or withdrew from the trial early. Intention-to-treat analysis is the opposite of *completer analysis*, which is the analysis of data from only those participants who remained at the end of the study (*Clinical Evidence 2000*, 2000).

Statistical Significance (Kahn and Sempos, 1989; Selvin, 1991;*Clinical Evidence 2000*, 2000)

- Look at p-value (α) or CIs to assess if study outcome can be explained by chance alone.
- Significance is commonly cited at 5% level (p-value <0.05), which indicates that the observed result would occur by chance alone in 1 of 20 similar studies (i.e., there is a 5% chance that the null hypothesis has been rejected when it is in fact true, a phenomenon called *type I error*).

- CIs should not include 1.0 (the null value). CIs are often set at 95%, which is equivalent to a p-value of 0.05.

Power

- Power $(1 - \beta)$ is the statistical ability to detect a postulated difference between two treatment groups, if one truly exists. The following are guidelines to determine if a study's power is sufficient.
  1. The larger the sample size, the better the power.
  2. The larger the proposed difference between the two groups (OR or RR), the more power a study has to detect it, regardless of sample size.
  3. The higher the level of statistical significance claimed by a study $(1 - \alpha)$, the higher the level of power needed to detect an association of any given size.
- In general, an acceptable level of power is 0.80 or 80%.
- For reference, it is useful to remember that for 80% power, with a type I error of 5% (two-sided) in a case-control study with a postulated OR of 2.0, there should be approximately 200 cases and 200 controls. If the postulated OR is 1.2, there should be approximately 4000 in each group; and if it is 3.0, there should be approximately 60 in each group.

Generalizability

- Are study results significant? Determine by looking at magnitude of p-value and/or size of CIs.
- Are study results important? Assess quality of study's subject and hypothesis.
- Are study results generalizable? Determine if study subjects are representative of the population to which results will be applied (e.g., studies using subjects of one race, ethnicity, or gender have limited generalizability).

EVALUATION OF DIAGNOSTIC AND SCREENING TESTS (TABLE 1.4) (JAESCHKE ET AL., 1994)

TABLE 1.4 VALIDITY, SENSITIVITY, AND SPECIFICITY

	Disease +	Disease −
Test +	True positive (TP)	False positive (FP)
Test −	False negative (FN)	True negative (TN)

- When evaluating whether to perform tests, consider what will be done with the results. Is there good treatment? Will knowledge of future illness alter the patient's quality of life? Are treatments noxious?
- **Validity:** The accuracy of a test, or the degree to which the test measures what it purports to measure (Last, 2001).
- **Sensitivity** = TP/(TP + FN) (see Table 1.4): The proportion of truly diseased persons identified as diseased.
- **Specificity** = TN/(TN + FP) (see Table 1.4): The proportion of truly nondiseased persons correctly identified as disease-free.
- **Positive predictive value (PPV)** = TP/(TP + FP) (see Table 1.4): The proportion of persons identified as diseased who are truly diseased. PPV is dependent upon the prevalence of disease and the specificity of the test (increased specificity increases PPV).
- **Negative predictive value (NPV)** = TN/TN + FN (see Table 1.4): The proportion of persons identified as disease-free who are truly disease-free. NPV is dependent upon the prevalence of disease and the sensitivity of the test (increased sensitivity increases NPV).
- **Reliability:** The precision or repeatability of a test, or the degree of stability exhibited when a measurement is repeated under identical conditions. There can be intrasubject, intraobserver, and interobserver variation. The latter two can be evaluated by the percent agreement and by the kappa statistic, which measures the percent observed agreement as a factor of the percent agreement expected by chance alone (JHU, 1991).

SELECTED REFERENCES

1. *Clinical evidence 2000.* London: BMJ Publishing Group, 2000.
2. Dans AL, Dans LF, Guyatt GH, et al. Users' guides to the medical literature. XIV. How to decide on the applicability of clinical trial results to your patient. The Evidence-based Medicine Working Group. *JAMA* 1998; 279:545–549.
3. Guyatt GH, Sackett DL, Cook DJ. Users' guides to the medical literature. II. How to use an article about therapy or prevention. The Evidence-based Medicine Working Group. *JAMA* 1994;271:59–63.
4. Hennekens C, Buring J. *Epidemiology in medicine.* Boston: Little, Brown & Company, 1987.
5. Hulley SB, Cummings SR, ed. *Designing clinical research.* Baltimore: Williams & Wilkins, 1988.
6. Jaeschke R, Guyatt GH, Sackett DL. Users' guides to the medical literature. III. How to use an article about a diagnostic test. The Evidence-based Medicine Working Group. *JAMA* 1994;271:703–707.
7. Johns Hopkins University School of Hygiene and Public Health. Epidemiology 2 (course syllabus). Baltimore: Johns Hopkins University School of Hygiene and Public Health, 1992.
8. Johns Hopkins University School of Hygiene and Public Health. Principles of epidemiology (course syllabus). Baltimore: Johns Hopkins University School of Hygiene and Public Health, 1991.
9. Joseph Mailman School of Public Health at Columbia University. Principles of epidemiology (course syllabus). New York: Joseph Mailman School of Public Health at Columbia University, 1997.
10. Kahn HA, Sempos CT. *Statistical methods in epidemiology.* New York: Oxford University Press, 1989.
11. Last JM, Spasoff R., Harris S. *A dictionary of epidemiology,* 4th Edition. New York: Oxford University Press, 2001.
12. Lillienfeld D, Stolley P. *Foundations of epidemiology.* New York: Oxford University Press, 1994.
13. Mausner J, Kramer S. *Epidemiology, an introductory text.* Philadelphia: W. B. Saunders, 1985.
14. Oxman AD, Sackett DL, Guyatt GH. Users' guides to the medical literature. I. How to get started. The Evidence-based Medicine Working Group. *JAMA* 1993;270:2093–2095.
15. Richardson WS, Wilson MC, Guyatt GH, et al. Users' guides to the medical literature. XV. How to use an article about disease probability for differential diagnosis. The Evidence-based Medicine Working Group. *JAMA* 1999;281:1214–1219.
16. Rothman K, Greenland S. *Modern epidemiology,* 2nd ed. New York: Lippincott, Williams & Wilkins, 1998.
17. Sackett DL, Rosenberg WM, Gray JA, et al. Evidence based medicine: what it is and what it isn't. *BMJ* 1996; 312(7023):71–72.
18. Schlesselman JJ. *Case-control studies, design, conduct, analysis.* New York: Oxford University Press, 1982.
19. Selvin S. *Statistical analysis of epidemiological data.* New York: Oxford University Press, 1991.

2

HEALTH MAINTENANCE AND SCREENING

INTRODUCTION

- The concept of a "healthy visit" for adults came about early this century and has come under scrutiny over the last 20 years (see Tables 2.1 to 2.3).
- This chapter outlines evidence-based recommendations for general internists seeing healthy patients, based on United States Preventive Services Task Force (USPSTF) recommendations and other published guidelines.
- Suggested minimum visit frequency for healthy adults:
  ⇒ Age 18 to 39: once every 2 years.
  ⇒ Age 40 and over: once a year.

TABLE 2.1 HEALTHY EXAM GUIDELINESS APPLICABLE TO ALL AGE GROUPS

History (hx)	Physical Examination	Screening	Counseling	Interventions
Past medical history	**Blood pressure**	**Depression**	**EtOH/substance**	**Tetanus/diptheria (Td)***
Medications	Q 2 years if	**Alcohol (EtOH)**	abuse	Q 10 years or once at
Prescription drugs	normal	CAGE questionaire	**Tobacco cessation***	age 50
Herbs	Q year if	**Domestic Violence**	**Diet/nutrition**	**Hepatitis A vaccine**
Over-the-counter	130–139/85–89	Women or homosexual men	Reduce fat intake*	Traveling/working in
drugs	**Height**	**Glucose (fasting)**	Increase fiber	endemic area;
Vitamins/supplements	Q 10 years	Consider if family hx, gestational diabetes	**Obesity**	homosexual men;
Family hx	**Weight**	hx, marked obesity, high density	**Physical activity**	illegal drugs (IV or
Social hx	Q year	lipoprotein (HDL) <35, triglycerides	Exercise for	not); chronic liver
Sexual hx	Calculate body	>250, hypertension, some ethnic groups	cardiovascular	disease (including
Safety	mass index	(Native Americans, Latinos, African	fitness (30	chronic hepatitis B or
Seat belts	(BMI)	Americans)	minutes/day, 3	C)
Guns	**Oral cavity**	**Cholesterol/HDI**	times/week)*	**Hepatitis B vaccine***
Helmets	If alcohol or	Q 5 years if ratio <4.5, q 1–2 years if	**Infectious**	Health care worker;
Smoke detectors	tabacco use	mildly increased and fewer than 2	diseases/STDs	IVDU; STDs; HD;
Habits	**Thyroid**	cardiac risk factors (CRF)	Sexual abstinence or	clotting factor tx;
Alcohol	Consider if	Full panel if CAD or multiple CRF	monogomy*	homosexual;
Tobacco	received	**HIV* (Human immunodeficiency virus)**	Regular condom	multiple sexual
Drugs	childhood	Consider if homosexual; history of sexually	use*	partners; partner of
Functional	radiation	transmitted disease (STD), intravenous	Avoidance of	positive patient;
assessment	therapy	drug use (IVDU), sex for drugs or	contaminated	traveler to endemic
consider advance	**Cardiac**	money; HIV+ sexual partners; blood	needles*	area
directives	Consider at initial	transfusion between 1978 and 1985	**Injury Prevention**	**Varicella zoster virus**
Review of systems	visit	**RPR***	Bike helmets*	**(VZV) vaccine**
			Fire arms	

(continued)

TABLE 2.1 *(continued)*

History (hx)	Physical Examination	Screening	Counseling	Interventions
	Skin exam	Consider if HIV+; close contact with tuberculosis (TB); chest x-ray (CXR) consistent with TB; prednisone >15mg/day or equivalent; immigrant; IVDU; resident or employee of high risk setting; cancer; diabetes mellitus (DM); end-stage renal disease (ESRD); weight loss >10%; gastrectomy; jejuno-ileal bypass **Hepatitis A and B** Consider prevaccination testing in high-risk patients **Hepatitis C** Consider if blood transfusion before 1982; IVDU; needle stick exposure; long-term hemodialysis (HD); history of STD, HIV, hepatitis B, multiple sexual partners; homosexual male; tattoos; shared cocaine straws	**Motor vehicle injury prevention** Seat belt use Air bag use* Avoiding drinking and driving* **Depression/suicide** Be aware of major symptoms of depression and evaluate risk factors **Skin protection** Sun avoidance, protective clothing Sunscreen with sun protection factor (SPF) ≥15 **Self breast exam for women and self testicular exam for men**	Consider if no history of chicken pox, especially if teachers, day-care, or health-care workers **Lyme diseae vaccine** Residents of high-risk areas; exposure to ticks **Calcium (Ca)/Vitamin D (Women only)** Premenopause: 1000 mg Ca and 400–800 IU vitamin D/day Postmenopause: 1500 mg Ca and 400–800 IU vitamin D/day

Q, every; EtOH, alcohol; CAD, coronary artery diseae; RPR, rapid plasma reagin; PPD, purified protein derivative.
* United States Preventive Services Task Force (USPTSF) recommendation "A," consistent with good evidence to support recommendation for inclusion of service in periodic health exam.

TABLE 2.2 HEALTHY EXAM GUIDELINES SPECIFIC TO CERTAIN AGE GROUPS

Age	Physical Examination	Screening	Counseling	Interventions
19–39	**(F) Breast exam Q 3 yrs (M) Testicular exam**	**(F) Chlamydia/STD screening** Under 25: annually Over 25: annually if unsafe sex, new/multiple partners, history of STD, cervical ectopy **(F) Pap smear*** Start at 18 or sexually active Q 1–3 yrs per risk factors **(F) TSH** If post partum	**(M) Testicular self exam** If cryptorchidism, orchiopexy consider for all patients **(F) Preconception counseling** Teratogens of early pregnancy, including alcohol Daily folate **(F) Osteoporosis prevention** Weight bearing exercise Smoking cessation Calcium/vitamin D	**Flu shot** If chronic disease, health care worker, essential personnel, or if patient requests it **Pneumovax** If chronic disease, HIV+, asplenia, immunocompromised Consider revaccination 5 yrs after first dose in highest risk patients **Measles/mumps** If born before 1956 and not reimmunized Consider second measles-mumps-rubella (MMR) if work/school overcrowded, healthcare worker, international travel, contacts of cases **Meningococcal vaccine** Consider for college freshmen living in dorms; asplenia; complement deficiency **(F) Rubella** Check titer and vaccinate if not pregnant **(F) Folate** 0.4 mg for women of childbearing age

(continued)

TABLE 2.2 *(continued)*

Age	Physical Examination	Screening	Counseling	Interventions
40–49	**(F) Breast exam** Annually	**Fasting plasma glucose** Consider q 3 yrs (over age 45) **Chlamydia/STD screening** Annually if unsafe sex, new/multiple partners, history of STD, cervical ectopy **Colon cancer screening** If history in first degree relative, irritable bowel disease, hereditary syndrome, high risk polyps **(M) Prostate specific antigen (PSA)** Only if family history of disease or African American **(F) Pap smear*** Q 1–3 yrs per risk factors **(F) BMD** Consider if would change treatment in menopausal women with personal or family history of adult fx, cigarette use, weight under 127 lbs, or premenopausal amenorrhea greater than 1 yr **(F) Mammography** Discuss risks and benefits	**(F) Preconception counseling** Teratogens of early pregnancy, including alcohol Daily folate **(F) Menopause and HRT discussion** **(F) Osteoporosis prevention** Weight-bearing exercise Smoking cessation Calcium/vitamin D	**Flu shot** If chronic disease, health care worker, essential personnel, or if patient requests it **Pneumovax** If chronic disease, HIV+, asplenia, immunocompromised Consider revaccination 5 yrs after first dose in highest risk patients **Measles/mumps*** If born before 1956 and not reimmunized; consider second MMR if high risk (see above) **Glaucoma screening** Annually if African American, family history of disease, severe myopia **ASA** Consider if CAD risk factors present **(F) Rubella** Check titer and vaccinate if not pregnant **(F) Folate** 0.4 mg for women of childbearing age
50–64	**(F) Breast exam** Annually **Snellen eye exam** Q 3 yrs **Hearing** If symptomatic	**Fasting plasma glucose** Consider q 3 yrs **Chlamydia/STD testing** Annually if unsafe sex, new/multiple partners, history of STD, cervical ectopy **Colon cancer screening** Annual FOBT and/or sig q 5 yrs or colonoscopy q 10 ys or double contrast BE q 10 yrs **Cognitive function/ADLs screen** **(M) PSA/digital rectal exam (DRE)** Discuss and proceed per doctor/patient discretion **(F) Pap smear*** Q 1–3 yrs per risk factors **(F) BMD** Consider if would change treatment in menopausal women with risk factors **(F) Mammogram*** Annually **Electrocardiogram (ECG) or ETT** Consider if would change treatment in patients with multiple cardiac risk factors	**(F) Menopause and HRT discussion** **(F) Osteoporosis prevention** Weight-bearing exercise Smoking cessation Calcium/vitamin D	**Flu Shot** Annually (note change from previous guidelines of patients over age 65) **Pneumovax** If chronic disease, HIV+, asplenia, immunocompromised Consider revaccination 5 yrs after first dose in highest risk patients **Glaucoma screening** Annually if African American, family history of disease, severe myopia **ASA** Consider if CAD risk factors present
65+	**(F) Breast exam** Annually **Snellen eye exam** Q 3 yrs **Hearing** If symptopmatic	**Fasting plasma glucose** Consider q 3 yrs **Chlamydia/STD testing** Annually if unsafe sex, new/multiple partners, history of STD, cervical ectopy **Colon cancer screening** Annual FOBT and/or sigmoidoscopy q 5 yrs or colonoscopy q 10 yrs or double contrast barrium enema q 10 yrs **Cognitive function/ADL screen** **Elder abuse screen** **(M) PSA/DRE** Discuss and proceed per doctor/patient discretion consider risks, benefits, and life expectancy	**Fall prevention** **Choking prevention** **Fire/burn prevention** **(F) Menopause and HRT discussion** **(F) Osteoporosis prevention** Weight-bearing exercise Smoking cessation Calcium/vitamin D	**Flu Shot** Annually **Pneumovax** Once and then consider revaccination 5 yrs after dose if under age 65 at time of initial vaccination **Glaucoma screening** Q 1–2 yrs **ASA** Consider if CAD risk factors

(continued)

TABLE 2.2 *(continued)*

Age	Physical Examination	Screening	Counseling	Interventions
		(F) Pap smear* Q 1–3 yrs per doctor discretion Consider stopping if consistently normal **(F) BMD** Consider in all women if would change treatment **(F) Mammography** Annually to age 69 Over age 69 at discretion of doctor/patient ECG or ETT Consider if would change treatment in patients with multiple cardiac risk factors		

TSH, thyroid stimulatory hormone; BMD, bone mineral density; fx, family history; HRT, hormone replacement therapy; ASA, aspirin; CAD, coronary artery disease; FOBT, fecal occult blood test; ADL, activities of daily life; ETT, exercise tolerance test.

* USPTSF recommendation "A": good evidence to support recommendation for inclusion of service in periodic health exam. (Although the effectiveness of counseling to relieve a health care aim is not always "A" recommendation.

TABLE 2.3 CANCER SCREENING RECOMMENDATIONS

Type of Cancer	USPSTF	American Cancer Society	American College of Physicians	MGH/PCOI
Breast	Mammography every 1–2 yrs age 50–69 CBE may added yearly, ages 50–69 Other ages, use clinical judgment Self breast exam (SBE): limited data	Mammography every yr starting at age 40 CBE every 3 yrs; ages 20–39 and yearly starting at age 40 SBE monthly starting at age 20	Mammography every 1–2 yrs, ages 50–74: annually in high-risk women starting at age 40 CBE annually starting at age 40	Mammography every 1–2 yrs, ages 50–74: discuss with patients ages 40–49 or over age 74 CBE annually ages 40–74; discuss if over age 74 SBE instruction may be prudent
Cervical	Pap smear at least every 3 yrs if sexually active or age 18 or over Consider stopping at age 65 if consistently normal No need to screen after hysterectomy for benign disease	Pap smear annually starting when sexually active or age 18; may decrease frequency if 3 normal consecutive tests Regular Pap smear postmenopause Discuss posthysterectomy for benign disease	Ages 20–65: Pap smear every 3 yrs or every 2 yrs if high risk Ages 66–75: Pap smear every 3 yrs if not screened in the 10 yrs before age 66 Initial Pap smears may be done annually for the first 2 or 3 examinations	Ages 18–65: Pap smear every 1–3 yrs, starting when sexually active or at age 18. Annually present if risk factors At age 65 stop Pap smears if consistently normal No need to screen after hysterectomy for benign disease
Colorectal	Annual FOBT and/or flexible sigmoidoscopy starting at age 50; earlier if affected first degree relative. Colonoscopy if very high risk. Discuss strategy with patients Insufficient evidence regarding routine digital rectal examination (DRE), Barium enema (BE), colonoscopy	Starting at age 50, annual FOBT or every 5 yrs or both (preferred); or double-contrast BE every 5 yrs or colonoscopy every 10 yrs. Starting at age 50 DRE at same time as sig, colonoscopy, BE	FOBT annually and flexible sigmoidoscopy every 3–5 years, starting at age 50 High-risk individuals: BE every 3–5 years or colonoscopy	If over age 50 discuss screening strategy Annual FOBT or flexible sigmoidosscopy every 5 yrs or both starting at age 50: earlier if affected relative. Colonoscopy if very high risk DRE stool guaiac discouraged
Ovarian	Routine screening not recommended	No specific recommendations	Routine screening not recommended. Refer women with family history of hereditary syndrome	Routine screening not recommended, counsel women at high risk

(continued)

TABLE 2.3 *(continued)*

Type of Cancer	USPSTF	American Cancer Society	American College of Physicians	MGH/PCOI
Prostate	Routine screening not recommended. Informed decision-making by patient	Offer annual PSA and DRE starting at age 50; starting at age 45 in African Americans or if first degree family history. Informed decision-making	Routine screening not recommended. Informed decision-making by patient	Routine screening not recommended. Discuss PSA with patients ages 50–74; benign prostate hyperplasia (BPH) screen those who ask. Informed decision-making by patient
Skin	Insufficient evidence regarding physician exams, sunscreen. Counseling about sun exposure if high risk. Dermatology referral if precursor lesions present	Physician exam every 3 yrs ages 20–39; annually over age 40		Insufficient evidence regarding physician exams. Counsel about sun exposure. Dermatology referral if precursor lesions present
Testicular	Insufficient evidence for screening by physician exam or self-exam. Discuss screening in men at higher risk	Self-exams monthly. Sunscreen use encouraged. Physician exam as part of cancer checkup every 3 yrs, ages 20–39. Individual decision regarding self-exam		Obtain history and examine for atrophy. Men at higher risk or all men under age 40: self-exam, physician exam at visits, although insufficient evidence
Lung	No screening recommendations from any group listed			

USPSTF, United States Preventive Services Task Force; MGH/PCOI, Massachusetts General Hospital/Primary Care Operations Improvement.

SELECTED REFERENCES

1. American Cancer Society. *Cancer facts and figures 2001*. Atlanta: American Cancer Society, 2001.
2. American Thoracic Society and Centers for Disease Control. Targeted tuberculin testing and treatment of latent tuberculosis infection. *Am J Respir Crit Care Med* 2000;161:S221–227.
3. Boland BJ, Wollan PC, Silverstein MD. Yield of laboratory tests for case-finding in the ambulatory general medical examination. *Am J Med* 1996;101:142–152.
4. Czeizel AE, Dudas I. Prevention of the first occurrence of neural tube defects by periconceptional vitamin supplementation. *N Engl J Med* 1992;327:1832–5.
5. Eddy DM, ed. *Common screening tests*. Philadelphia: American College of Physicians, 1991.
6. Executive Committee for the Asymptomatic Carotid Atherosclerosis Study. Endarterectomy for asymptomatic carotid artery stenosis. *JAMA* 1995;273:1421–1428.
7. Gianrossi R, Detrano R, Mulvihill D, et al. Exercise-induced ST depression in the diagnosis of coronary artery disease: a meta-analysis. *Circulation* 1989;80:87–98.
8. *Guide to clinical preventive services. Report of the US preventive services task force.* 2nd ed. Baltimore: Williams & Wilkins, 1995.
9. Henschke CI, McCauley DI, Yankelevitz DF, et. al. Early lung cancer action project: overall design and findings from baseline screening. *Lancet* 1999;354:99–105.
10. The HOPE Investigators. Vitamin E supplementation and cardiovascular events in high-risk patients. *N Engl J Med* 2000;342:154–160.
11. Lee TH, Cook EF, Weisberg MC, et al. Impact of the availability of a prior electrocardiogram on the triage of a patient with acute chest pain. *J Gen Intern Med* 1990;5:381–388.
12. Liberman UA, Weiss SR, Broll J, et al. Effect of oral alendronate on bone mineral density and the incidence of fractures in post-menopausal osteoporosis. *N Engl J Med* 1995;333:1437–1443.
13. Marcus PM, Bergstralh EJ, Fagerstrom RM, et al. Lung cancer mortality in the Mayo lung project: Impact of extended follow-up. *J Natl Cancer Inst* 2000;92(16):1308–1316.
14. MGH Primary Care Operations Improvement web site (www.mgh.pcoi.org). Contributors: Michael Barry, MD, Nancy Rigotti, MD, Steve Atlas, MD, Blair Fosburgh, MD, James Meigs, MD, Mary Morgan, Liz Mort, MD, Brit Nicholson, MD, Will Schmitt, MD, Sue Clifford.
15. Murphy SL. Deaths: final data from 1998. *Natl Vital Stat Rep* 2000;48(11):1–106.
16. Nichol KL, Wuorenma J, von Sternberg T. Benefits of influenza vaccination for low-, intermediate-, and high-risk senior citizens. *Arch Intern Med* 1998;158:1769–1776.
17. Rosen HN, Basow DS. Screening for osteoporosis. UpToDate, 2000 (www.uptodate.com).
18. Scholes D, Stergachis A, Heidrich FE. Prevention of pelvic inflammatory disease by screening for cervical chlamydial infection. *N Engl J Med* 1996;334:1362–1366.

19. Shapiro ED, Berg AT, Austrian R et al. The protective efficacy of polyvalent pneumococcal polysaccharide vaccine. *N Engl J Med* 1991;325:1453–1460.
20. Siscovic DS, Ekelund LJ, Johnson JL, et al. Sensitivity of exercise electrocardiography for acute cardiac events during moderate and strenuous physical activity: the lipid research clinics coronary primary prevention trial. *Arch Intern Med* 1991;151:325–330.
21. Steering Committee of the Physicians' Health Study Research Group. Final report on the aspirin component of the ongoing Physicians' Health Study. *N Engl J Med* 1989;321:129–135.
23. Thun MJ, Peto R, Lopez AD, et. al. Alcohol consumption and mortality among middle aged and elderly U.S. adults. *N Engl J Med* 1997;337:1705–1714.

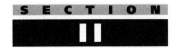

CARDIOVASCULAR

3

HYPERTENSION

INTRODUCTION

- Hypertension has a 24% incidence in adult U.S. population (Burt et al., 1995).
- Hypertension is a risk factor for coronary artery disease, congestive heart failure, stroke, retinopathy, and renal failure.
- After 10 years, 30% of people with untreated mild hypertension develop atherosclerosis, and 50% experience end-organ damage (Williams, 1997).
- Only 53% of hypertensives are treated, and only half of those being treated have adequate blood pressure control (Burt et al., 1995).

PATHOPHYSIOLOGY

- 2 to 5% of hypertension has clear etiology (often renal/adrenal disease); the remaining 95% is designated *essential hypertension.*
- Underlying pathophysiology of essential hypertension remains unclear (probably heterogeneous).
- Although rare, secondary hypertension should always be considered because it may be treatable (see Table 3.1).

TABLE 3.1 SELECTED CAUSES OF SECONDARY HYPERTENSION

Disease*(Incidence)	Symptoms	Initial Workup
Renal parenchymal disease (2–3%)	Elevated creatinine, abnormal urinalysis	Depends on abnormality
Renovascular disease (1–2%): • Atherosclerotic • Fibromuscular dysplasia (FMD)	History of arterial vascular disease, sudden onset in older or younger patient, renal failure induced by ACEIs, abdominal bruits	Captopril renal scan, renal MRI/MRA, renal angiogram
Primary hyperaldosteronism (0.3%)	Unprovoked hypokalemia	Renin and aldosterone levels; 24-hour urine aldosterone

ACEIs, angiotensin-converting enzyme inhibitors; MRI, magnetic resonance imaging; MRA, magnetic resonance arteriography.
*Also consider: Cushing's disease/syndrome, pheochromocytoma, coarctation of aorta, thyroid disease, hyperparathyroidism.
Source: Adapted from Williams GH. Chapter 246: Hyptertensive vascular disease. In: Fanci A, Braunwald E, Isselbacher K, et al., eds. *Harrison's principles of internal medicine*, 14th ed. New York: McGraw-Hill, 1998:1380–1394.

EVALUATION

Overall Goals

- Identify potential secondary cause.
- Estimate total cardiovascular risk.

Diagnosis/definition

- Current use of antihypertensive medication; or
- Systolic blood pressure (SBP) >140 or diastolic blood pressure (DBP) >90, using the average of two readings, taken two minutes apart, at each of two or more visits.

History

- Identify comorbid conditions, including cardiovascular disease, cerebrovascular accidents, renal disease, diabetes mellitus, and hyperlipidemia. Identify symptoms of target organ damage (TOD), including angina, dyspnea, transient weakness or blindness, claudication, and loss of visual acuity.
- Obtain medication history, especially the use of estrogens, androgens, corticosteroids, sympathomimetics, over-the-counter medications (such as decongestants), and herbs and supplements.
- Identify relevant behaviors, including the use of tobacco, alcohol, and illicit drugs, weight gain, exercise, and diet.

Risk Stratification (Table 3.2)

- The Framingham Heart Study (D'Agostino et al., 2000) illustrates that the presence of other cardiovascular risk factors (CRFs) synergistically increases risk of developing coronary disease.
- CRFs: smoking, dyslipidemia, diabetes mellitus, age greater than 60, men or postmenopausal women, family history of cardiovascular disease in men under age 55 and/or women under age 65.
- The Sixth Report of the Joint National Committee on Detection, Evaluation, and Treatment of High Blood Pressure (JNC-VI) recommends risk stratification, (a) to identify patients at greatest risk as determined by degree of hypertension, comorbid risk factors, and TOD, and (b) to identify groups that will benefit most from aggressive treatment.
- Target organ damage (TOD): heart disease (left ventricular hypertrophy, angina, prior myocardial infarction, prior coronary revascularization, heart failure), stroke or transient ischemic attack, nephropathy, peripheral arterial disease, retinopathy.

TABLE 3.2 RISK STRATIFICATION AND TREATMENT OF HYPERTENSION IN ADULTS

Blood pressure stage (mm Hg)	Risk group A No CRF or TOD	Risk group B One or more CRF (not DM) and no TOD	Risk group C TOD and/or DM
High to normal (130–139/85–89)	Lifestyle modification	Lifestyle modification	Lifestyle modification and drug therapy if heart failure, DM, or renal insufficiency are present
Stage I (140–159/90–99)	Lifestyle modification (up to 12 months) Drug therapy and lifestyle modification	Lifestyle modification (up to 6 months) and drug therapy if more than one risk factor present	Drug therapy and lifestyle modification
Stages 2 and 3 (>160/100)		Drug therapy and lifestyle modification	Drug therapy and lifestyle modification

CRF, Cardiovascular risk factor; TOD, target organ damage; DM, diabetes mellitus.
Adapted from the Joint National Committee on Prevention, Detection, Evaluation, and Treatment of High Blood Pressure. The Sixth Report of the Joint National Committee on Prevention, Detection, Evaluation, and Treatment of High Blood Pressure. *Arch Intern Med* 1997; 157: 2413–2446.

Physical Exam

- Accurate blood pressure measurement depends on proper patient positioning (patient should sit with arm at heart level). Patients should not smoke, ingest caffeine or other stimulants, or

exercise within 30 minutes of measurement. Cuff size must be appropriate (bladder of cuff must surround more than 80% of patient's arm). Bilateral measurement should be considered.
- Include heart rate and funduscopic, vascular, and neurologic exams.

Data

- Include blood chemistries, hematocrit, urinalysis, lipid profile, and electrocardiogram.
- Consider 24-hour creatinine clearance, urine microalbumin, calcium, uric acid, hemoglobin A1C, thyroid stimulating hormone, and echocardiogram.

TREATMENT

Goals

- Reduce long-term complications of hypertension.
- Balance cardiovascular benefits with side effects.
- Target values: SBP <140 and DBP <90.
- Modified goals in select situations:
  ⇒ Diabetes: blood pressure <130/85.
  ⇒ Renal failure with proteinuria (>1g/24h): blood pressure <125/75.
  ⇒ Elderly patients with severe isolated systolic hypertension: SBP <160.

Lifestyle Modification (Table 3.3)

- Should be the foundation of all therapy. Can control mild hypertension without medication.
- Enhances effectiveness of antihypertensives; reduces overall cardiovascular risk.

TABLE 3.3 LIFESTYLE MODIFICATIONS TO REDUCE BLOOD PRESSURE

Lifestyle Modification	Efficacy In Clinical Trials
Sodium restriction: No added salt (4 g/day) or low sodium diet (2 g/day). Can control mild hypertension and enhances effectiveness of antihypertensive medications.	Meta-analysis of randomized controlled trials of low-salt diets shows reduction of systolic/diastolic blood pressure by 3–5/2–3 mm Hg (Midgley et al., 1996).
Diet: All patients should eat a diet low in fat/sodium, rich in fruits and vegetables, include only low-fat dairy products.	DASH study demonstrated reduction in blood pressure by 11.4 mm Hg SBP and 5.5 mm Hg DBP (Sacks et al., 2001).
Weight reduction: Patients more than 15% above ideal body weight (body mass index >27) should lose weight.	TAIM study showed 4.5 kg weight loss as effective in lowering DBP as low-dose medication (Wassertheil-Smoller et al., 1992).
Limit alcohol consumption: Limit alcohol intake to less than 1 oz per day (less than 0.5 oz per day in women and thin people).	Consumption of more than 2 oz alcohol per day is associated with increased rate of hypertension (Stamler et al., 1997)
General: Exercise 30–45 min 3 days/wk, stop smoking.	Improve overall cardiovascular health, but never shown to affect blood pressure in a large clinical trial.

DASH, Dietary Approaches to Stop Hypertension; TAIM, Trial of Antihypertensive Interventions and Management; SBP, systolic blood pressure; DBP, diastolic blood pressure.

Medications (Tables 3.4 and 3.5)

- Four major classes of first-line antihypertensives: thiazide diuretics, beta-blockers, angiotensin-converting enzyme inhibitors (ACEIs), calcium channel blockers. Each has similar efficacy reducing blood pressure in head-to-head trials (Materson et al., 1993). A large, ongoing prospective trial (with more than 200,000 patients) is comparing all four antihypertensives (ALLHAT Collaborative Research Group, 2000).
  ⇒ Thiazides reduce mortality and incidence of stroke and myocardial infarction (Psaty et al., 1997). Should be used only in low doses given safety concerns (and because additional efficacy is not gained at higher doses).

⇒ Beta-blockers reduce cardiovascular morbidity and mortality in hypertensives (Psaty et al., 1997). Provide cadioprotection following myocardial infarction (Freemantle et al., 1999). Not as good as diuretics for uncomplicated essential hypertension in the elderly (Messerli, 1998).

⇒ ACEIs are first-line agent in all diabetics with proteinuria and nondiabetics with glomerular disease to reduce progression of renal disease (GISEN Group, 1997; Giatras et al., 1997; Maschio et al., 1996; Weidmann et al., 1995). Shown in white men to reduce stroke by 33%, myocardial infarction by 22%, and mortality by 24% (HOPE Study Investigators, 2000). Shown to reduce mortality in patients with congestive heart failure or systolic dysfunction following myocardial infarction (Flather et al., 2000; Latini et al., 2000).

⇒ Calcium channel blockers: Short-acting dihydropyridines no longer routinely used because of demonstrated dangers immediately following acute myocardial infarction (Furberg et al., 1995). No increased risk of coronary artery disease mortality with long-acting forms (D'Agostino et al., 2000). Protection from myocardial infarction, stroke, and cardiovascular death equivalent to that of conventional therapy.

TABLE 3.4 ADVERSE EFFECTS OF FIRST LINE ANTIHYPERTENSIVE MEDICATIONS

Class Examples	Potential Adverse Effects
Thiazide diuretics Hydrocholorothiazide, chlorthalidone	Hypokalemia, increased insulin resistance, allergic response, erectile dysfunction
Beta-blockers Atenolol, metoprolol, propanolol, carvedilol	Bronchospsam, derpression, fatigue, impotence, increased total cholesterol, increased insulin resistance
Angiotensin-converting enzyme inhibitors Captropril, enalapril, ramipril	Dry cough (10%), hyperkalemia, renal failure
Calcium channel blockers Verapamil, diltiazem, nifedipine, amlodipine	Verapamil (negative inotrope): conduction defects Dihydropyridines (vasodilators): reflex tachycardia, edema

TABLE 3.5 SECOND-LINE ANTIHYPERTENSIVE MEDICATIONS

Agent/Mechanism of Action	Clinical Effects/Efficacy
Angiotension receptor blockers (ARBs): Block binding of angiotensin II to type-1 receptors. **Alpha-blockers:** Inhibit post-synaptic α-1-receptors thereby preventing catecholamine-mediated arterial/venous vasoconstriction.	Safe and effective at lowering blood pressure (Willenheimer, 1999). Decrease mortality with congestive heart failure (CHF) (Pitt et al., 2000). Doxazosin vs. chlorthalidone had two-fold increase in CHF and significantly higher rate of stroke (ALLHAT Collaborative Research Group, 2000).
Loop diuretics: Antihypertensive effects similar to thiazide diuretics.	Short duration of action and potent diuretic effect make these less attractive than thiazides.
Potassium-sparing diuretics: Commonly coupled with thiazides to ameliorate potassium loss.	Severe hyperkalemia is potential side effect. Decreased mortality in patients with congestive heart failure (Pitt et al., 1999).

● Choosing a first-line agent:

⇒ Monotherapy is sufficient in 60% to 80% of patients.

⇒ Individualize therapy based on comorbid conditions (see Table 3.6).

TABLE 3.6 CONSIDERATIONS FOR INDIVIDUALIZING ANTIHYPERTENSIVE THERAPY

Indication	Antihypertensive Drug
Compelling Indications (unless contraindicated)	
Diabetes mellitus with microalbuminuria	ACEIs
Nondiabetic chronic renal failure with proteinuria	ACEIs (questionable value once plasma creatinine >3 mg/dL)
Congestive heart failure	ACEIs, beta-blockers, diuretics
Myocardial infarction	Beta-blockers (without ISA), ACEIs (with systolic dysfunction or anterior infarct)
Isolated systolic HTN in the elderly	Diuretics (preferred), calcium blockers (long-acting DHP)
Possible effects on comorbid conditions	
Angina pectoris	Beta-blockers, calcium channel blockers
Atrial tachycardia and fibrillation	Beta-blockers diltiazem, verapamil
Congestive heart failure	Spironolactone, losartan
Osteoporosis	Thiazide diuretics
Preoperative hypertension	Beta-blockers
Benign prostatic hypertrophy	Alpha-blockers
Contraindicated	
Bronchospastic disease	Beta-blockers
Pregnancy	ACEIs angiotensin II receptor antagonists
Second- or third-degree heart block	Beta-blockers, diltiazem, verapamil
Possible adverse effect on comorbid conditions	
Depression	Beta-blockers, methyldopa
Diabetes mellitus (types I and II)	Beta-blockers, high-dose diuretics
Gout	Diuretics
Renovascular disease	ACEIs, angiotensin II receptor antagonists

ACEI, angiotensin-converting enzyme inhibitor; ISA, intrinsic sympathomimetic activity; HTN, hypertension; DHP, dihydropyridines.

Follow-up

- See patient within 1 to 2 months of initiating therapy and every 3 to 6 months once patient stabilizes.
- If drug is well tolerated, but blood pressure response is inadequate, a second drug from another class should be added. If the first drug was not a diuretic, one should be considered now as the second agent, as low-dose diuretics often enhance effects of other drugs. Consider possible reasons for lack of response, including:
  ⇒ Pseudoresistance: "white-coat hypertension," undersized cuff, pseudohypertension of the elderly related to decreased arterial compliance
  ⇒ Nonadherence to therapy
  ⇒ Volume overload (caused by salt intake or renal disease)
  ⇒ Drug-related causes: inadequate dosage; rapid inactivation; possible drug interactions with sympathomimetics (decongestants, appetite suppressants), cocaine, oral contraceptives, steroids, caffeine or other stimulants, licorice, erythropoietin, nonsteroidal antiinflammatory drugs (NSAIDs), cyclosporine, and antidepressants
  ⇒ Associated conditions: smoking, increasing obesity, obstructive sleep apnea, alcohol use or abuse, anxiety, chronic pain
- After 1 year, consider decreasing dosage and/or number of agents in well-controlled patients who have succeeded in making lifestyle modifications.

SELECTED REFERENCES

1. ALLHAT Collaborative Research Group. Major cardiovascular events in hypertensive patients randomized to doxazosin vs. chlorthalidone: the Antihypertensive and Lipid-Lowering Treatment to Prevent Heart Attack Trial (ALLHAT). *JAMA* 2000;283:1967–1975.
2. Andersen S, Tarnow L, Rossing P, et al. Renoprotective effects of angiotensin II receptor blockade in type 1 diabetic patients with diabetic nephropathy. *Kidney Int* 2000;57:601–606.
3. Australia/New Zealand Heart Failure Research Collaborative Group. Randomised, placebo-controlled trial of carvedilol in patients with congestive heart failure due to ischaemic heart disease. *Lancet* 1997;349:375–380.

4. Bristow MR, Gilbert EM, Abraham WT, et al., for the MOCHA Investigators. Carvedilol produces dose-related improvements in left ventricular function and survival in subjects with chronic heart failure. *Circulation* 1996;94:2807–2816.

5. Brown MJ, Palmer CR, Castaigne A, et al. Morbidity and mortality in patients randomised to double-blind treatment with a long-acting calcium-channel blocker or diuretic in the International Nifedipine GITS study: Intervention as a Goal in Hypertension Treatment (INSIGHT). *Lancet* 2000;356:366–372.

6. Burt VL, Whelton P, Roccella EJ, et al. Prevalence of hypertension in the US adult population. Results from the Third National Health and Nutrition Examination Survey, 1988-1991. *Hypertension* 1995;25:305–313.

7. CIBIS-II Investigators and Committees. The Cardiac Insufficiency Bisoprolol Study II (CIBIS-II): a randomised trial. *Lancet* 1999;353:9–13.

8. Cohn JN, Tognoni G, Glazer R, et al. Baseline demographics of the Valsartan Heart Failure Trial. Val-HeFT Investigators. *Eur J Heart Fail* 2000;2(4):439–446.

9. D'Agostino RB, Russell MW, Huse DM, et al. Primary and subsequent coronary risk appraisal: new results from the Framingham study. *Am Heart J* 2000;139:272–281.

10. Davis BR, Cutler JA, Gordon DJ, et al. Rationale and design for the Antihypertensive and Lipid-Lowering Treatment to Prevent Heart Attack Trial (ALLHAT). *Am J Hypertens* 1996;9:342–360.

11. Flather MD, Yusuf S, Kober L, et al. Long-term ACE-inhibitor therapy in patients with heart failure or left-ventricular dysfunction: a systematic overview of data from individual patients. *Lancet* 2000;355:1575.

12. Freemantle N, Cleland J, Young P. B-Blockade after myocardial infarction: systematic review and meta regression analysis. *BMJ* 1999;318(7200):1730–1737.

13. Furberg CD, Psaty BM, Meyer JV. Nifedipine: dose-related increase in mortality in patients with coronary heart disease. *Circulation* 1995;92:1326–1331.

14. Giatras I, Lau J, Levey AS. Effect of angiotensin-converting enzyme inhibitors on the progression of nondiabetic renal disease: a meta-analysis of randomized trials. Angiotensin-Converting-Enzyme Inhibition and Progressive Renal Disease Study Group. *Ann Intern Med* 1997;127:337.

15. The GISEN Group. Randomised placebo-controlled trial of effect of ramipril on decline in glomerular filtration rate and risk of terminal renal failure in proteinuric, non-diabetic nephropathy. *Lancet* 1997;349:1857.

16. Hansson L, Hedner T, Lund-Johansen P, et al. Randomised trial of effects of calcium antagonists compared with diuretics and [beta]-blockers on cardiovascular morbidity and mortality in hypertension: the Nordic Diltiazem (NORDIL) study. *Lancet* 2000;356:359–365.

17. Hansson L, Lindholm L, Ekbom T, et al., for the STOP Hypertension-2 Study Group. Randomized trial of old and new antihypertensive drugs in elderly patients: cardiovascular mortality and morbidity, the Swedish Trial in Old Patients with Hypertension-2 study. *Lancet* 1999;354:1751–1756.

18. Heart Outcomes Prevention Evaluation (HOPE) Study Investigators. Effects of ramipril on cardiovascular and microvascular outcomes in people with diabetes mellitus: Results of the HOPE study and MICRO-HOPE substudy. *Lancet* 2000;355:253.

19. Joint National Committee on Detection, Evaluation, and Treatment of High Blood Pressure. The Sixth Report of the Joint National Committee on Prevention, Detection, Evaluation, and Treatment of High Blood Pressure. *Arch Intern Med* 1997:157:2413–2446.

20. Latini R, Tognoni G, Maggioni AP, et al. Clinical effects of early angiotensin-converting enzyme inhibitor treatment for acute myocardial infarction are similar in the presence and absence of aspirin: systematic overview of individual data from 96,712 randomized patients. Angiotensin-converting Enzyme Inhibitor Myocardial Infarction Collaborative Group. *J Am Coll Cardiol* 2000; 35:1801–1807.

21. Maschio G, Alberti D, Janin G, et al. Effect of the angiotensin-converting-enzyme inhibitor benazepril on the progression of chronic renal insufficiency. *N Engl J Med* 1996; 334:939.

22. Materson BJ, Reda DJ, Cushman WC, et al. Single-drug therapy for hypertension in men: a comparison of six antihypertensive agents with placebo. *N Engl J Med* 1993;328:914–921.

23. Messerli FH, Grossman E, Goldbourt U. Are beta-blockers efficacious as first-line therapy for hypertension in the elderly?: A systematic review. *JAMA* 1998:279(23):1903–1907.

24. Midgley JP, Matthew AG, Greenwood CMT, et al. Effect of reduced dietary sodium on blood pressure: a meta-analysis of randomized controlled trials. *JAMA* 1996;275:1590–1597.

25. Packer M, Colucci WS, Sackner-Bernstein JD, et al., for the PRECISE Study Group. Double-blind, placebo-controlled study of the effects of carvedilol in patients with moderate to severe heart failure: the PRECISE trial. *Circulation* 1996;94:2793–2799.

26. Pitt B, Poole-Wilson PA, Segal R, et al. Effect of losartan compared with captopril on mortality in patients with symptomatic heart failure: randomized trial-the Losartan Heart Failure Survival Study ELITE II. *Lancet* 2000;355:1582–1587.

27. Pitt B, Zannad F, Remme WJ, et al. The effect of spironolactone on morbidity and mortality in patients with severe heart failure. *N Engl J Med* 1999;341:709–717.

28. Psaty BM, Smith NL, Siscovick DS, et al. Health outcomes associated with antihypertensive therapies used as first-line agents: a systematic review and meta-analysis. *JAMA* 1997;277:739–745.

29. Sacks FM, Svetkey LP, Vollmer WM, et al. Effects on blood pressure of reduced dietary sodium and the Dietary Approaches to Stop Hypertension (DASH) diet. *N Engl J Med* 2001;344(1):3–10.

30. SHEP Cooperative Research Group. Prevention of stroke by antihypertensive drug treatment in older persons with isolated systolic hypertension: final results of the Systolic Hypertension in the Elderly Program (SHEP). *JAMA* 1991;265:3255–3302.

31. Stamler J, Caggiula AW, Grandits GA. Chapter 12: relation of body mass and alcohol, nutrient, fiber, and caffeine intakes to blood pressure in the special intervention and usual care groups in the Multiple Risk Factor Intervention Trial. *Am J Clin Nutr* 1997;65(suppl):338S–365S.

32. Wassertheil-Smoller S. Oberman A. Blaufox MD, et al. The Trial of Antihypertensive Interventions and Management (TAIM) Study. Final results with regard to blood pressure, cardiovascular risk, and quality of life. *Am J Hypertens* 1992;5(1):37–44.

33. Weidmann P, Schneider M, Böhlen L. Therapeutic efficacy of different antihypertensive drugs in human diabetic nephropathy: an updated meta-analysis. *Nephrol Dial Transplant* 1995;10(Suppl 9):39–45.

34. Williams GH. Disorders of the cardiovascular system (Part 8). In: Braunwald E, Hauser S, Fauci A, et al., eds. *Harrison's principles of internal medicine*, 15th ed., New York: McGraw-Hill, 2001.

35. Williams GH. Part 8: Disorders of the cardiovascular system, Section 4: Vascular disease, Chapter 246: Hypertensive vascular disease. In: Fauci A, Braunwald E, Isselbacher K, et al., eds. *Harrison's Priciples of Internal Medicine*, 14th ed. New York: McGraw-Hill, 1998:1380–1394.

36. Willenheimer R, Dahlof B, Rydberg E, et al. AT1-receptor blockers in hypertension and heart failure: clinical experience and future directions. *Eur Heart J* 1999;20(14):997–1008.

4

HYPERLIPIDEMIA

INTRODUCTION

- Hyperlipidemia is a major risk factor for coronary artery disease (CAD), cerebrovascular disease, and peripheral vascular disease (Kannel et al., 1979).
- More than 100 million people in United States have total cholesterol exceeding the desirable limit (200 mg/dL) (American Heart Association, 2000).
- 10% decrease in cholesterol may result in 30% reduction of CAD (Cohen, 1997).
- Pharmacologic lipid lowering has been shown safe and effective for primary/secondary CAD prevention.

PATHOPHYSIOLOGY

- Etiologies: diet, obesity, diabetes mellitus, hypothyroidism, alcohol use, renal disease, cholestatic liver disease, use of drugs (oral contraceptive pills, steroids); minority of cases attributable to inherent defect in lipid transport/metabolism.
- Clinical management requires basic understanding of lipid metabolism.
  - ⇒ Ingested fats are emulsified in small intestine by bile salts and converted to triglycerides (TG) for transport into the blood/lymphatics, where they reassemble into lipoproteins.
  - ⇒ Lipoproteins are macromolecular aggregates that consist of a hydrophobic lipid core surrounded by TG and cholesteryl esters along with phospholipid and specialized proteins known as apolipoproteins. The five major families of lipoproteins are chylomicrons, very-low-density lipoproteins (VLDL), low-density lipoproteins (LDL), intermediate-density lipoproteins (IDL), and high-density lipoproteins (HDL).
  - ⇒ Lipoproteins are carried through the bloodstream and targeted by interactions between apolipoproteins and lipoprotein receptors. The liver is the primary site of lipoprotein metabolism, although extrahepatic tissues are also involved.
  - ⇒ Enzymes such as lipoprotein lipase and hepatic lipase contribute to metabolic processing of lipoproteins. Other enzymes such as hydroxymethylglutaryl CoA (HMG-CoA) reductase more specifically control the metabolism of cholesterol.
- Medications targeting lipoprotein metabolism such as fibric acid derivatives (fibrates) and HMG-CoA reductase inhibitors (the "statins") can alter systemic lipid levels by altering enzyme function.

EVALUATION

History/Screening

- Screen for symptoms of cardiovascular disease; ask about potential causes of secondary hyperlipidemia (diabetes, hypothyroidism, alcohol use, renal disease, cholestatic liver disease, medications).
- Assess for presence of known cardiac risk factors (CRFs): target lipid levels are determined by the established presence or likelihood of CAD (see Table 4.1). Emerging CRFs not yet widely accepted include TG, lipoprotein (a), homocysteine, apolipoprotein B, small, dense LDL, prothrombotic markers (such as fibrinogen), proinflammatory markers (such as C-reactive protein), and ECG abnormalities (such as left ventricular hypertrophy [LVH]) (Grundy et al., 1999).

TABLE 4.1 CARDIAC RISK FACTORS IN ADDITION TO ELEVATED LDL

Family history	First-degree relative with CAD (first-degree relative: men under age 55, women under age 65)
Age	Men over age 45, women over age 55
Tobacco	Prior use within 15 years
Hypertension	Even if controlled with medications
Diabetes	Considered equivalent to CAD in NCEP guidelines
HDL	<40 mg/dL (HDL >60 mg/dL, will allow you to subtract one of the other risk factors)
Obesity	BMI >25 (not included in calculations for risk in NCEP guidelines)

LDL, low-density lipoproteins; CAD, coronary artery disease; NCEP, National Cholesterol Education Program; HDL, high-density lipoproteins; BMI, body mass index.

- LDL level correlates with accelerated coronary heart disease and is used to guide therapy (see Table 4.2).
- Recommendations from the National Cholesterol Education Program Adult Treatment Panel III (NCEP ATPIII) (Expert Panel on Detection, 2001):
  ⇒ Obtain fasting lipid profile including total cholesterol, LDL, HDL, and TG for all adults over age 20, at least every 5 years (must fast 9 to 12 hours prior to testing).

TABLE 4.2 NCEP ATPIII CLASSIFICATION: CHOLESTEROL, LDL, HDL, TRIGLYCERIDES

Total Cholesterol		LDL Cholesterol*	
<200 mg/dL	Desirable	<100 mg/dL	Optimal
200–239 mg/dL	Borderline high	100–129 mg/dL	Near optimal
≥240 mg/dL	High	130–150 mg/dL	Borderline high
		160–189 mg/dL	High
Triglycerides		≥190 mg/dL	Very high
<150 mg/dL	Normal		
150–199 mg/dL	Borderline high	**HDL cholesterol**	
200–499 mg/dL	High	<40	Low
>500 mg/dL	Very high	≥60	High

* LDL is difficult to measure directly, but may be indirectly calculated from measured lipids using the Friedewald formula: LDL = total cholesterol − HDL − TG/5 (Friedewald et al., 1972)

  ⇒ In patients with moderate to severe hypertriglyceridemia (TG >400 mg/dL), LDL calculations become inaccurate, and it may be necessary to use a direct LDL assay such as reflex LDL (RLDL).
- NCEP ATPIII has identified a subset of patients having the "metabolic syndrome" (see Table 4.3), typified by metabolic derangements that predispose the patient to insulin resistance and carry a high risk for coronary artery disease (CAD). These patients should be identified and treated earlier and more aggressively.

TABLE 4.3 METABOLIC SYNDROME*

Risk Factor	Defining Level
Abdominal Obesity	Waist circumference
Men	>102 cm (>40 in)
Women	>88 cm (>35 in)
Triglycerides	>150 mg/dL
HDL cholesterol	
Men	<40 mg/dL
Women	<50 mg/dL
Blood pressure	>130/85 mm Hg
Fasting glucose	>110 mg/dL

HDL, high-density lipoprotein.
* Defined as having any three risk factors.

Physical exam

- Check for signs of hyperlipidemia: corneal arcus, lipemia retinalis, xanthelasma, palmar tendon xanthomas (may indicate primary hereditary hyperlipidemia).
- Examine patients with known hyperlipidemia for evidence of cardiac, cerebrovascular, and peripheral vascular disease.

TREATMENT

Diet

- Dietary modification, weight management, and exercise (together known as "therapeutic lifestyle change") are recommended in all patients with hyperlipidemia before and along with appropriate drug therapy.
- Collaborate with clinical nutritionist to develop appropriate dietary strategy.
- American Heart Association (AHA) 2000 guidelines emphasize a healthy, balanced diet for all, minimizing calories while increasing physical activity (Krauss et al., 2000).
  ⇒ Limit fat intake to 30% of calories, with up to 10% of calories from saturated fat, and limit cholesterol to less than 300 mg per day. This translates to less than 60 grams of fat per day per woman and less than 80 grams of fat per day per man. Avoid butter, margarine, oils (except olive oil), fried foods, all red meats, whole milk, and fatty prepared foods (e.g., muffins). Substitute whole grains and unsaturated fatty acids from vegetables, fish, legumes, and nuts for high-calorie, high-fat foods.
  ⇒ In patients with known CHD or diabetes, saturated fat should be less than 7% of caloric intake and cholesterol should be kept under 200 mg per day.
  ⇒ Increase dietary fiber.
- In contrast, NCEP ATPIII guidelines suggest the following for all: saturated fat should comprise less than 7% of caloric intake; cholesterol should be kept under 200 mg per day; soluble fiber intake should be between 10 and 25 g per day; and intake of plant stanols of 2 g per day.

Exercise and Weight Loss

- Advocate exercise and weight management for all patients with hyperlipidemia (obesity is a cause of secondary hyperlipidemia).
- Set reasonable goals: Begin by getting patients into a routine. Gradually work individuals up to 85% of maximum heart rate 3 times a week for 30 minutes.
- Sedentary patients with multiple risk factors: Consider exercise tolerance testing before initiating exercise program.
- Patients identified as having the "metabolic syndrome" (see Table 4.3) should be particularly encouraged to reduce weight and increase physical activity.

Drug therapy

- Medical therapy should be tailored toward individuals' fasting lipid profiles in stepwise fashion.
- Initiation and management of therapy are guided by LDL and risk category, as determined by number of cardiac risk factors (see Table 4.4).

TABLE 4.4 NCEP ATPIII LDL CHOLESTEROL LEVELS AT WHICH TO INITIATE THERAPY

Risk Category	LDL Goal	LDL at Which to Initiate Therapeutic Lifestyle Changes	LDL at Which to Begin Drug Therapy
High: CAD or CAD risk equivalents (10-year risk >20%)	<100 mg/dL	≥100 mg/dL	≥130 mg/dL (100–129 mg/dL, optional)
Moderate: 2 or more risk factors (10-year risk ≤20%)	<130 mg/dL	≥130 mg/dL	≥130 mg/dL (10-year risk 10–20%) ≥160 mg/dL (10-year risk <10%)
Low: 0–1 Risk Factor	<160 mg/dL	≥160 mg/dL	≥190 mg/dL (160-189 mg/dL, optional)

LDL, low-density lipoprotein; CAD, coronary artery disease.

● Four major classes of drugs used to treat hyperlipidemia are nicotinic acid (niacin), bile acid sequestrants, HMG-CoA reductase inhibitors (the statins), and fibric acid derivatives (fibrates) (see Table 4.5).

TABLE 4.5 AGENTS USED FOR HYPERLIPIDEMIA AND DOSING CONSIDERATIONS

Drug Class	LDL	HDL	TG	Side Effects	Contraindications	Agents and Considerations
Nicotinic Acid	↓↓	↑↑↑↑	↓↓	• Flushing • Pruritis • Hyperuricemia • GI upset • Hyperglycemia • Hepatotoxicity	**Absolute:** • Severe gout • Chronic liver disease • Risk of pregnancy **Relative:** • Diabetes • Hyperuricemia • Active PUD	• Initial dose of immediate release (crystalline) niacin 100 mg tid with meals and with ASA qam for first 2 wks to prevent prostaglandin-mediated flushing; gradually increase to 500 mg po tid with max 1000 mg po tid. • Extended release niacin 1–2 g po qd • Sustained release niacin 1–2 g po qd • Check LFT's every 3 mo
Bile acid sequestrants	↓↓	↑	↑	• GI distress • Constipation • Decreased absorption of other medications	**Absolute:** • TG > 400 mg/dL • Dysbeta-lipoproteinemia **Relative:** • TG > 250 mg/dL	• Cholestyramine: 4 g po qd to 12 g po bid • Colestipol: 5 g po qd to 30 g po qd • Colesevelam: 2.6 to 3.8 g po qd • Mix in water, applesauce, gelatin or popsicles • No other meds 2 hrs before or 4 hrs after cholestyramine
Statins	↓↓↓↓	↑↑	↓	• Mild GI upset • Liver toxicity • Myositis (rare)	**Absolute:** • Chance of pregnancy • Active or chronic liver disease **Relative:** • Medications: cyclosporine, antifungal, CyP45O inhibitors, fibrates, niacin	• Atorvastatin 10–80 mg qhs • Fluvastatin 20 mg qhs to 20 mg bid • Lovastatin 20 mg qd to 40 mg bid with meals • Pravastatin 20-40 mg qhs • Simvastatin 10 mg qhs to 40 mg bid • Check LFTs at baseline, then after 1 and 6 mo (Maron, 2000)
Fibrates	↓	↑↑	↓↓↓	• Mild GI upset • Dyspepsia • Gallstones • Myopathy	**Absolute:** • Severe renal disease • Severe liver disease • Risk of pregnancy	• Germfibrozil 600 mg bid • Fenofibrate 201 mg po qd with breakfast* • Check LFTs ev 6 week (Staels, 1998)

LDL, low-density lipoproteins; HDL, high-density lipoproteins; TG, triglycerides; GI, gastrointestinal; PUD, peptic ulcer disease; tid, three times a day; ASA, aspirin; qam, every morning; po, by mouth; qd, every day; LFTs, liver function tests; bid, twice a day; qhs, every night.
* Fenofibrate is an alternative to gemfibrozil in familial hypertriglyceridemias, which decreases TG synthesis and enhances clearance. It may cause GI upset and has significant risk of cholelithiasis, coumadin potentiation, myositis, hepatitis, and agranulocytosis (requiring monthly bloodwork) (Dais, 2001).

● **Elevated LDL:** Statins are drugs of choice as initial agents.
⇒ Start at moderate dose, check liver function tests (LFTs) and creatine phosphokinase (CPK) at baseline. Repeat fasting lipids and LFTs 8 to 12 weeks after initiation. If target LDL not achieved, consider increasing dose or adding a bile acid sequestrant or niacin. If LDL goals cannot be attained after 12 weeks, consider consultation with lipid specialist. Once target LDL is achieved, follow patients every 4 to 6 months.
⇒ Patients with LDL above 190 mg/dL often have inherited form of hyperlipidemia; may require combination drug therapy. Consider screening patient's relatives.
⇒ Controversy exists whether all statin drugs are equivalent. Some experts believe there is a class effect; others argue that only agents specifically studied should be recommended.
⇒ Most large trials have shown pravastatin (LIPID, 1998; Pfeffer et al., 1995; Sacks et al., 1996; Shepherd et al., 1995), simvastatin (Scandinavian Simvastatin Survival Study Group, 1994), and lovastatin (Downs et al., 1998), and to a lesser degree, atorvastatin (Pitt et al., 1999; Schwartz et al., 2001) to be effective for both primary and secondary prevention. Fluvastatin effective in limited clinical trial data (Ballantyne et al., 1999; Herd et al., 1997).

- **Elevated TG:** Fibrates such as gemfibrozil are drugs of choice.
  - ⇒ Growing body of data implicate TG as independent cardiac risk factor (Cullen, 2000).
  - ⇒ TG can be elevated by conditions such as the metabolic syndrome (see Table 4.3), obesity/overweight, physical inactivity, cigarette smoking, alcohol use, diabetes, chronic renal insufficiency, nephritic syndrome and use of certain medications (e.g., steroids, estrogens, and high-dose beta-blockers).
  - ⇒ NCEP ATPIII identifies the contribution of TG to cardiac risk as a function of "non-HDL cholesterol" (the difference between total cholesterol and HDL, biologically comprised of LDL and VLDL). When treating patients with elevated TG, a secondary goal should be adjusting the non-HDL level (see Table 4.6).

TABLE 4.6 LDL AND NONHDL GOALS FOR PATIENTS WITH ELEVATED TG

Risk Category	LDL Goal	NonHDL Goal*
High: CHD OR CHD risk equivalents (10-year risk >20%)	<100 mg/dL	<130 mg/dL
Moderate: 2+ Risk factors (10-year risk ≤20%	<130 mg/dL	<160 mg/dL
Low: 0–1 risk factor	<160 mg/dL	<190 mg/dL

LDL, low-density lipoproteins; HDL, high-density lipoproteins.
* NonHDL is defined as total cholesterol minus HDL.

- **Elevated LDL and TG:** Focus first on achieving both LDL and non-HDL goals with either (a) an LDL lowering agent (e.g., a statin), (b) a fibrate either with or without niacin, or (c) both (watch for side effects). NCEP ATPIII recommends initial emphasis on treating TG greater than 500 mg/dL to avoid pancreatitis, and then turning attention to reaching the target LDL.
  - ⇒ Add niacin if necessary (generally underused as an inexpensive and highly effective agent). Use is limited by side effects, in particular flushing, which improve over time and with nighttime dosing. Extended-release formulations of niacin such as Niaspan are associated with a lower incidence of adverse side effects, but may have increased risk of hepatotoxicity (Goldberg, 1998; Morgan et al., 1998).
- **Decreased HDL:** Numerous options exist. Selection should be based on remainder of lipid profile. NCEP ATPIII does not identify a goal HDL for patients with decreased HDL, although early trials suggest that raising HDL decreases risk of adverse cardiovascular events (Ballantyne et al., 1999; Robins et al., 2001). All four classes of agents may be effective (Table 4.5). Exercise and achievement of LDL and non-HDL cholesterol goals should remain the focus of treatment until further data emerge (Gotto, 2001).

RESOURCES

- American College of Cardiology: www.acc.org
- American Diabetes Association: www.diabetes.org
- American Heart Association: www.americanheart.org
- National Cholesterol Education Program: www.nhlbi.nih.gov/about/ncep/index.htm
- National Heart, Lung, and Blood Institute: www.nhlbi.nih.gov

SELECTED REFERENCES

1. American Heart Association. *2001 Heart and Stroke Statistical Update.* Dallas: American Heart Association, 2000.
2. Ballantyne CM, Herd JA, Ferlic LL, et al. Influence of low HDL on progression of coronary artery disease and response to fluvastatin therapy. *Circulation* 1999;99:736–743.

3. Cohen JD. A population-based approach to cholesterol control. *Am J Med* 1997;102:23–25.
4. Cullen P. Evidence that triglycerides are an independent coronary heart disease risk factor. *Am J Cardiol* 2000; 86:943–949.
5. Diabetes Atherosclerosis Intervention Study (DAIS). Effects of fenofibrate on progression of coronary-artery disease in type 2 diabetes: the Diabetes Atherosclerosis Intervention Study, a randomised study. *Lancet* 2001; 357:905–910.
6. Downs JR, Clearfield M, Weis S, et al. Primary prevention of acute coronary events with lovastatin in men and women with average cholesterol levels: results of AFCAPS/TexCAPS. Air Force/Texas Coronary Atherosclerosis Prevention Study. JAMA 1998;279:1615–1622.
7. Expert Panel on Detection, Evaluation, and Treatment of High Blood Cholesterol in Adults. Executive Summary of the Third Report of the National Cholesterol Education Program (NCEP) Expert Panel on Detection, Evaluation and Treatment of High Blood Cholesterol in Adults (Adult Treatment Panel III). *JAMA* 2001;285:2486–2497.
8. Friedewald WT, Levy RI, Fredrickson DS. Estimation of the concentration of low-density lipoprotein cholesterol in plasma, without use of the preparative ultracentrifuge. *Clin Chem* 1972;18:499–502.
9. Goldberg AC. Clinical trial experience with extended-release niacin (Niaspan): dose- escalation study. *Am J Cardiol* 1998;82:35U–38U(discussion 39U–41U).
10. Goldberg RB, Mellies MJ, Sacks FM, et al. Cardiovascular events and their reduction with pravastatin in diabetic and glucose-intolerant myocardial infarction survivors with average cholesterol levels: subgroup analyses in the cholesterol and recurrent events (CARE) trial. The Care Investigators. *Circulation* 1998;98:2513–2519.
11. Gotto AM. Low high-density lipoprotein cholesterol as a risk factor in coronary heart disease: a working group report. *Circulation* 2001;103:2213–2220.
12. Grundy SM, Pasternak R, Greenland P, et al. Assessment of cardiovascular risk by use of multiple-risk-factor assessment equations: a statement for healthcare professionals from the American Heart Association and the American College of Cardiology. *Circulation* 1999;100:1481–1492.
13. Herd JA, Ballantyne CM, Farmer JA, et al. Effects of fluvastatin on coronary atherosclerosis in patients with mild to moderate cholesterol elevations [Lipoprotein and Coronary Atherosclerosis Study (LCAS)]. *Am J Cardiol* 1997;80:278–286.
14. Kannel WB, Castelli WP, Gordon T. Cholesterol in the prediction of atherosclerotic disease. New perspectives based on the Framingham study. *Ann Intern Med* 1979;90:85–91.
15. Krauss RM, Eckel RH, Howard B, et al. AHA Dietary Guidelines: revision 2000: a statement for healthcare professionals from the Nutrition Committee of the American Heart Association. *Circulation* 2000;102:2284–2299.
16. The Long-Term Intervention with Pravastatin in Ischaemic Disease (LIPID) Study Group. Prevention of cardiovascular events and death with pravastatin in patients with coronary heart disease and a broad range of initial cholesterol levels. *N Engl J Med* 1998;339:1349–1357.
17. Maron DJ, Fazio S, Linton MF. Current perspectives on statins. *Circulation* 2000;101:207–213.
18. Morgan JM, Capuzzi DM, Guyton JR. A new extended-release niacin (Niaspan): efficacy, tolerability, and safety in hypercholesterolemic patients. *Am J Cardiol* 1998;82:29U–34U(discussion 39U–41U).
19. Pfeffer MA, Sacks FM, Moye LA, et al. Cholesterol and recurrent events: a secondary prevention trial for normolipidemic patients. CARE Investigators. *Am J Cardiol* 1995;76:98C–106C.
20. Pitt B, Waters D, Brown WV, et al. Aggressive lipid-lowering therapy compared with angioplasty in stable coronary artery disease. Atorvastatin versus Revascularization Treatment Investigators. *N Engl J Med* 1999; 341:70–76.
21. Robins SJ, Collins D, Wittes JT, et al. Relation of gemfibrozil treatment and lipid levels with major coronary events. VA-HIT: a randomized controlled trial. *JAMA* 2001;285:1585–1591.
22. Sacks FM, Pfeffer MA, Moye LA, et al. The effect of pravastatin on coronary events after myocardial infarction in patients with average cholesterol levels. Cholesterol and Recurrent Events Trial investigators. *N Engl J Med* 1996;335:1001–1009.
23. Scandinavian Simvastatin Survival Study Group. Randomised trial of cholesterol lowering in 4444 patients with coronary heart disease: the Scandinavian Simvastatin Survival Study (4S). *Lancet* 1994;344:1383–1389.
24. Schwartz GG, Olsson AG, Ezekowitz MD, et al. Effects of atorvastatin on early recurrent ischemic events in acute coronary syndromes. The MIRACL study: a randomized controlled trial. *JAMA* 2001;285:1711–1718.
25. Shepherd J, Cobbe SM, Ford I, et al. Prevention of coronary heart disease with pravastatin in men with hypercholesterolemia. West of Scotland Coronary Prevention Study Group. *N Engl J Med* 1995;333:1301–1307.
26. Staels B, Dallongeville J, Auwerx J, et al. Mechanism of action of fibrates on lipid and lipoprotein metabolism. *Circulation* 1998;98:2088–2093.

CORONARY ARTERY DISEASE AND ANGINA

INTRODUCTION

- Coronary artery disease (CAD) is the leading cause of death and disability in industrialized nations, with increasing prevalence worldwide.
- Mortality of myocardial infarction (MI): 30% acutely, 5% to 10% over first year.
- Mortality in patients with chronic stable angina: 2% to 12% per year.

PATHOPHYSIOLOGY

- Atherosclerosis causes CAD. Atheromatous plaques develop over years in arterial intima, particularly at sites of high turbulence. Plaques have central core of cholesterol, lipid-laden macrophages, and necrotic debris, all covered by a subendothelial fibrous cap.
- Disruption of plaque surface can lead to intracoronary thrombosis and obstruction of distal blood flow. Depending on degree and/or duration of myocardial ischemia and concomitant myocardial oxygen demand, intracoronary thrombosis may result in tissue injury or infarction.
- Manifestations of CAD:
  ⇒ Ischemia: chronic stable angina (fixed coronary stenoses), silent (asymptomatic), unstable angina (unstable plaques at risk for fissuring and/or precipitating intracoronary thrombosis)
  ⇒ Myocardial cell death: non-Q–wave MI (NQWMI), ST elevation MI (STEMI)
  ⇒ Arrhythmias: ventricular tachycardia, ventricular fibrillation, possibly leading to sudden death
  ⇒ Left ventricular dysfunction/ischemic cardiomyopathy: symptoms of congestive heart failure (CHF)

DIFFERENTIAL DIAGNOSIS (CHEST PAIN)

- Musculoskeletal pain: tends to occur with movement or slight changes in position; usually reproducible by palpation
- Gastrointestinal discomfort: reflux disease, gastritis, esophagitis, cholecystitis, esophageal spasm, esophageal stricture, peptic ulcer disease
- Pleuritic pain: sharp and knifelike, brought on by respiratory movements or coughs; potentially secondary to pneumonia or pulmonary embolism
- Aortic dissection: tearing chest pain, often radiating to the back
- Panic disorder
- Pain that can be localized with one finger, radiates to lower extremities, is present for a few seconds or less, or has been constant for days is usually not indicative of angina

EVALUATION

History

- **Assess cardiac risk factors** (defined by the Framingham Heart Study): age (men over age 55, women over age 65); dyslipidemia [elevated total cholesterol and/or low high-density lipoproteins (HDL)]; peripheral vascular disease; diabetes; hypertension; cigarette smoking; postmenopausal women; family history of premature CAD (males under age 55, females under age 65).
- **Evaluation of chest pain/angina:**
  - ⇒ Quality of chest pain is least reliable part of history.
  - ⇒ Exertional symptoms relieved with rest are more reliable indicators of CAD. Progressive decline in activity level may also be a sign of ischemia.
  - ⇒ Associated symptoms include shortness of breath, diaphoresis, nausea, palpitations, syncope, and near-syncope.
  - ⇒ Determine whether angina is stable (symptoms occur with consistent level of exertion/are relieved by consistent level of rest or by nitroglycerin) or unstable (symptoms increasing in frequency/intensity, occurring while at rest, requiring increasing nitroglycerin to relieve, or new onset under 60 days).

Physical Exam

- Signs of heart disease/CAD risk factors: xanthelasmas, xanthomata, premature arcus, hypertension (blood pressure, retinal vasculopathy), elevated jugular venous pressure (JVP), lower extremity edema, hepatojugular reflux, right ventricular (RV) and/or left ventricular (LV) S3 or S4 gallops, ventricular lifts, cardiac murmurs, pulmonary rales, palpable abdominal aortic aneurysm, abdominal/peripheral/carotid bruits, decreased carotid/peripheral pulses.

Diagnostic Studies

- **Pretest probability:** For diagnostic tests with fixed sensitivity and specificity, the posttest likelihood of disease (CAD) depends on the pretest probability of disease. Data gathered from history and physical exam can be used to estimate likelihood (pretest probability) that patient has CAD. Important factors include age, gender, reversible cardiac risk factors, association between symptoms and exertion, and responsiveness to nitrates (Wilson, 1998).
- **Resting electrocardiogram (ECG):** Usually nondiagnostic in the absence of symptoms; may help select appropriate type of stress test; can reveal evidence of old MI (suggesting existing CAD) or LV hypertrophy (risk factor for increased mortality).
- **Exercise tolerance test (ETT)/pharmacologic stress test** (see Tables 5.1 and 5.2): Increases myocardial oxygen demand and looks for evidence of ischemia (by ECG, echo wall motion abnormalities, or radionucleotide imaging); pharmacologic tests look for differences in regional myocardial blood flow after infusion of coronary vasodilators (persantine, adenosine).
  - ⇒ **Primary diagnosis:** Evaluate chest pain of unknown etiology. Screen patients over age 40 with multiple risk factors, sedentary patients over age 40 prior to initiating exercise program, or patients in whom a cardiac event would endanger the public (e.g., pilots, bus drivers).
  - ⇒ **Secondary evaluation:** Evaluate patients preoperatively (especially higher risk patients or before higher risk operations); evaluate patients post-MI (low-level ETT 4 to 7 days post-MI, full level test 4 to 6 weeks post-MI); evaluate adequacy of antiischemic regimen.
  - ⇒ **Contraindications to stress testing:** Current acute MI or unstable angina; critical aortic stenosis or severe dynamic outflow obstruction (if suspected on physical, obtain echocardiogram prior to ETT); hypotension, uncontrolled hypertension, decompensated CHF; advanced atrioventricular block (Wenckebach with symptoms, Mobitz II, or complete heart block); patients who are not candidates for revascularization [relative contraindication, as the main purpose of ETT is to identify patients who would benefit from or are able to undergo percutaneous transluminal coronary angioplasty (PTCA) or coronary artery bypass grafting (CABG)].

⇒ **Post-test probability after ETT:** Treat (or not) patients with extremely high (or low) pretest probabilities of CAD on the basis of their pretest likelihood of CAD alone. ETT testing in these patients has an increased chance of generating false negative (or positive) values; most helpful in patients with an intermediate pretest probability of CAD (Diamond and Forrester, 1979).

TABLE 5.1 TYPES OF EXERCISE TOELRANCE TESTS (ETTS)

Type of ETT	Technique	Evaluation
Standard ETT	Exercise leads to an increase in heart rate (HR), systolic blood pressure (SBP), O_2 consumption. Maximally predictive test requires: a) > 5–6 METS (metabolic equivalents); measures workload. b) Peak double product (PDP) >20,000: peak HR × SBP; correlates linearly to cardiac workload. c) Predicted maximum HR (PMHR) ≥85%: 220 – patient's age; necessary to achieve adequate sensitivity.	Myocardial ischemia assessed by electrocardiogram (ECG). Positive: ≥1 mm horizontal or downward-sloping ST depression in ≥2 contiguous leads. Sensitivity 65% –70%; specificity 80%–85%. Good screen in males with normal baseline ECG; poor sensitivity in women, patients with baseline ECG abnormalities (LVH, LBBB), patients on digoxin, and patients with mitral valve prolapse/Wolff-Parkinson-White syndrome.
ETT with thallium sestamibi	Radionucleotide uptake in viable myocardium examined along with ECG. Patterns of uptake/redistribution distinguish well-perfused, ischemic, and infarcted myocardium. Sestamibi better than thallium for obese patients or women with large breasts (gives better signal).	Better indication of anatomy and degree of ischemia than standard ETT. Extent of ischemic territory correlates with prognosis (Brown et al., 1983). Sensitivity approx. 85%, specificity approx 95%.
Persantine/adenosine stress with thallium sestamibi	For patients unable to exercise to adequate HR. Persantine and adenosine act as coronary vasodilators; healthy arteries have increased blood flow relative to arteries with fixed stenoses. Areas of relative ischemia detected with imaging tracers (thallium or sestamibi).	Less sensitive/specific for diagnosis of ambulatory chest pain than ETT/thallium, but equally useful for post MI or preop evaluation. Use adenosine cautiously with bronchospasm, increased PR interval, or heart block.
Dobutamine with thallium sestamibi	Provides a pharmacologic HR increase in patients unable to exercise.	Sensitivity and specificity similar to regular ETT/thallium studies.
Dobutamine stress echocardiogram	Additional data about ejection fraction and valvular function. Useful in patients who cannot exercise or receive adenosine.	Sensitivity and specificity in a technically proficient lab and in "optimal patients" (thin, without COPD) comparable to ETT/thallium studies.

LVH, left venticular hypertrophy; LBBB, left bundle branch block; MI, myocardial infarction; COPD, chronic obstructive pulmonary disease.

TABLE 5.2 POOR PROGNOSTIC FACTORS IN EXERCISE TOLERANCE TESTING

Duration <6 METS
Sustained decrease in SBP ≥10 mm Hg
ST depressions ≥2 mm at low workload
ST depresions ≥5 leads lasting ≥5 minutes
ST elevation
Sustained or symptomatic ventricular ectopic activity
Increased pulmonary uptake
Reversible left ventricular dilation
Multiple territories with defects

METS, metabolic equivalents; SBP, systolic blood pressure.

- **Cardiac catheterization:** Gold standard for diagnosis, but relatively contraindicated in many (including patients with contrast allergy or renal failure). Indications for outpatient catheterization: evidence of large amount of cardiac territory at risk; symptoms of CAD with known LV dysfunction; CAD in combination with severe valvular disease; strong patient preference to undergo catheterization to reach definitive diagnosis.

- **Prognosis:** Related to left ventricular function (ejection fraction); extent of CAD (number and location of stenoses); severity of myocardial ischemia; occurrence of acute ischemia in the previous 6 months; arrhythmia (ventricular tachycardia or premature ventricular contractions); LV hypertrophy; uncorrected risk factors.

TREATMENT

- **Risk factor reduction:** Smoking cessation (50% reduction in recurrent cardiovascular events); blood pressure control; cholesterol reduction; control of diabetes (efficacy unproven, but likely important); weight reduction/graded exercise program.
- **Cardiac rehabilitation:** Good trial data indicate reduction of events.
- **Aspirin (ASA):** 325 mg every day unless bleeding contraindication. Physicians' Health Study showed 44% reduction in risk of acute MI using ASA 325 mg every other day (with subgroup analysis suggesting benefit only in patients under age 50). For secondary prevention, meta-analysis showed reduction of vascular mortality by 13% and nonfatal MI by 31% (Antiplatelet Trialists Collaboration, 1988).
- **Beta-blockers:** 26% decrease in mortality after MI (American Beta-Blocker Heart Attack Trial, 1982). Beta-1 selective agents may cause less bronchospasm (atenolol, metoprolol), while water-soluble agents may cause fewer central nervous system CNS side effects (atenolol, nadolol). Greater benefit in patients with low ejection fraction (EF) (Norwegian Multicenter Study Group, 1981).
- **Nitrates:** All patients with CAD should carry sublingual nitroglycerin (SL TNG) (0.3 mg or 0.4 mg tablets); prescription should be renewed every 6 months (older tablets lose efficacy). Isosorbide dinitrate may help reduce anginal symptoms, but does not reduce mortality or major ischemic events. The antiimpotence drug sildenafil (Viagra) is contraindicated in patients taking nitrates.
- **Angiotensin-converting enzyme inhibitors (ACEIs):** Reduce mortality in post-MI patients, especially with anterior infarctions, EF under 40%, and patients with symptomatic CHF (Pfeffer, 1992). The HOPE trial (Weinsaft et al., 2000) found significant benefit to ramipril in patients at high risk for CAD (diabetes and one other risk factor or peripheral vascular disease) in reducing both cardiac events and mortality.
- **Calcium channel blockers:** Second line to beta-blockers; not shown to decrease mortality and some may increase mortality in patients with low EF.
- **PTCA with or without stent:** May decrease anginal symptoms, but no proven impact on mortality.
- **CABG:** Shown to improve mortality in patients with: left main disease; 3-vessel disease with EF under 50%; 2-vessel disease with LV dysfunction or severe proximal left main disease; possibly superior when compared to PTCA in diabetics (Detre et al., 2000).

FUTURE DIRECTIONS

- Future research which will likely impact management:
  ⇒ Genetic polymorphisms that further define risk for CAD
  ⇒ Advantages of percutaneous coronary interventions in the coronary stent era
  ⇒ Noninvasive modalities (CT, MRI) to diagnose coronary disease and to risk-stratify patients
  ⇒ Prevention of sudden death with implantable defibrillators in high-risk patients (Buxton, et al., 1999).
  ⇒ Potential links between CAD and chronic infection/inflammation.
  ⇒ Markers of inflammation as prognostic factors, such as C-reactive protein.
  ⇒ Disparities in the treatment of CAD in women and minorities.

SELECTED REFERENCES

1. American Beta-Blocker Heart Attack Trial. *JAMA* 1982;247:1707–1714.
2. Antiplatelet Trialists Collaboration. Secondary prevention of vascular disease by prolonged antiplatelet treatment. *BMJ* 1988;295:320.

3. Brown KA, Boucher CA, Okada RD, et al. Prognostic value of exercise thallium-201 imaging in patients presenting for evaluation of chest pain. *J Am Coll Cardiol* 1983;1:994–1001.

4. Buxton AE, Lee KL, Fisher JD, et al., for the MUST trial. A randomized study of the prevention of sudden death in patients with coronary artery disease. *N Engl J Med* 1999; 341:1882–1890.

5. Detre KM, Lombardero MS, Brooks MM, et al. The effect of previous coronary-artery bypass surgery on the prognosis of patients with diabetes who have acute myocardial infarction. *N Engl J Med* 2000;342:989–997.

6. Diamond GA, Forrester JS. Analysis of probability as an aid in the clinical diagnosis of coronary artery disease. *N Engl J Med* 1979;300:1350–1358.

7. Norwegian Multicenter Study Group. Timolol-induced reduction in mortality and reinfarction in patients surviving acute myocardial infarction. *N Engl J Med* 1981;304:80.

8. Nurses' Health Study. *N Engl J Med* 1991;325:756.

9. Passamani E, Davis K, Gillespie M, et al. A randomized study of coronary artery bypass surgery: survival of patients with low ejection fraction. *N Engl J Med* 1985; 312:1665–1671.

10. Pfeffer M, Braunwald E, Moye E, et al. Effect of captopril on mortality and morbidity in patients with left ventricular dysfunction after myocardial infarction: results of the survival and ventricular enlargement trial. *N Engl J Med* 1992;327:669–677.

11. Physicians Health Study. *N Engl J Med* 1989;321:129–135.

12. The Bypass Angioplasty Revascularization Investigation (BARI) Investigators. Comparison of coronary bypass surgery with angioplasty in patients with multivessel disease. *N Engl J Med* 1996;335:217–225.

13. Weinsaft JW, O'Rourke MF, Nichols WW, et al. Effects of an angiotensin-converting-enzyme inhibitor, ramipril, on cardiovascular events in high risk patients. The Heart Outcomes Prevention Evaluation Study Investigators. *N Engl J Med* 2000;342;145–153.

14. Wilson PWF. Prediction of coronary artery disease using risk factor categories. *Circulation* 1998;97:1837–1847.

CONGESTIVE HEART FAILURE

SYSTOLIC HEART FAILURE

Introduction

- Failure of heart to pump blood at rate commensurate with metabolic requirements (or doing so only at expense of causing elevated filling pressure).
- Affects 4.8 million Americans; accounts for more than 3 million annual office visits; leading cause of hospital admissions for patients over age 65; annual expenditure $20 billion (Massie, 1997).
- Despite advances in therapy, prognosis remains poor: 1-year survival, 76%; 5-year survival, 35%.

Pathophysiology

- Involves neurohormonal activation and ventricular remodeling (see Fig. 6.1).

Differential Diagnosis

- Coronary artery disease (CAD); hypertension; valvular heart disease
- Cardiomyopathy: idiopathic dilated; infectious (viral, bacterial, fungal, protozoal); infiltrative (amyloid, hemochromatosis, sarcoid); toxic (cocaine, alcohol, adriamycin, cyclophosphamide); endocrine/metabolic diseases (diabetes, thyroid disease)

Evaluation

Classification of Evidence

- Elements of patient evaluation have varying degrees of consensus/evidence, classified by American College of Cardiology (ACC)/American Heart Association (AHA) (Hunt, 2001) (see Table 6.1).

TABLE 6.1 EVIDENCE CLASSIFICATIONS

Class of Evidence	Level of Evidence
Class I: evidence and/or general agreement that procedure or treatment is useful	Level A: data derived from multiple randomized clinical trials
Class II: conflicting evidence and/or divergence of opinion about usefulness or efficacy	Level B: data derived from single randomized trial or nonrandomized studies
Class III: evidence and/or general agreement that procedure is not useful or effective	Level C: data derived from consensus and/or opinion of experts

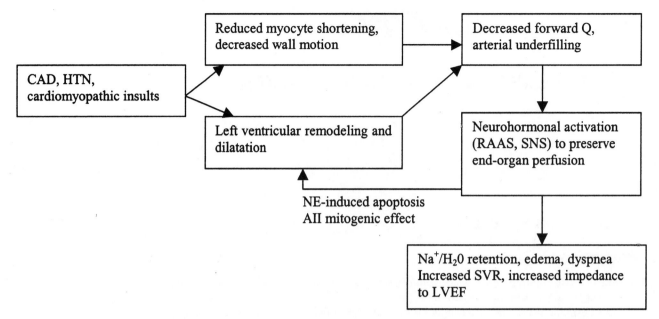

FIGURE 6.1. Pathophysiology of systolic heart failure. CAD, coronary artery disease; HTN, hypertension; Q, cardiac output; RAAS, renin-angiotensin-aldosterone system; SNS, sympathetic nervous system; NE, nore-pinephrine; AII, angiotensin II.

History (Class I, Evidence C)

- Patient history is best discriminator of acuity, etiology, rate of progression.
    ⇒ Risk factors: coronary risk factors (establish probability of ischemic cardiomyopathy); rheumatic fever, alcohol/cocaine use, hypertension, HIV risk factors, thyroid dysfunction
    ⇒ Family history: sudden cardiac death, premature CAD, heart failure
    ⇒ Acute/subacute congestive heart failure (CHF): Usually characterized by dyspnea, orthopnea, paroxysmal nocturnal dyspnea (PND), occasionally right upper quadrant (RUQ) pain. Common precipitants include diet and medication noncompliance, ischemia, arrhythmia, infection
    ⇒ Chronic CHF: fatigue, anorexia, edema (may be more pronounced than dyspnea because pulmonary venous capacitance adapts to chronic volume overload)

Physical Exam (Class 1, Evidence C)

- Assess volume status, ventricle size, peripheral perfusion:
    ⇒ Weight, blood pressure, pulse, "pulsus alternans" (evenly spaced alternating strong and weak pulses; virtually pathognomonic for severe left ventricular dysfunction)
    ⇒ Volume overload: jugular venous distension (JVD), rales, peripheral edema, ascites, hepatosplenomegaly, hepato-jugular reflux
    ⇒ Left ventricular (LV) size: apical impulse displaced beyond midclavicular line typifies enlarged LV
    ⇒ Secondary pulmonary hypertension: right ventricular (RV) heave, palpable pulmonic tap (felt in second intercostal space), accentuated P2

Laboratory Evaluation

- Class I, evidence C: complete blood count (CBC), urinalysis, electrolytes, blood urea nitrogen (BUN), creatinine, liver function tests, glucose, phosphorus, magnesium, calcium, albumin, thyroid-stimulating hormone (TSH)
- Class II, evidence C: On basis of clinical suspicion, consider serum iron, ferritin/transferrin

saturation, antinuclear antibody (ANA), rheumatoid factor (RF), urinary vanillylmandelic acid (VMA)/metanephrines, serum protein electrophoresis (SPEP), urine protein electrophoresis (UPEP), HIV screening, urine toxicology screen for cocaine, myocarditis labs [creatine kinase (CK)/troponin, erythrocyte sedimentation rate (ESR)].

Diagnostic Studies

- Class I:
  ⇒ Chest radiograph: cardiomegaly (cardiac-to-thoracic width ratio greater than 50%), cephalization of pulmonary vessels, Kerley B-lines, pleural effusions. Rule out confounding pulmonary disease (evidence C).
  ⇒ Electrocardiogram (ECG): evidence of ischemic heart disease: QS-waves, poor R-wave progression, left ventricular hypertrophy, conduction system disease such as left bundle branch block (LBBB) (evidence C)
  ⇒ Echocardiography: valvular/pericardial disease, chamber size, sphericity, wall motion abnormalities, left ventricular ejection fraction (LVEF), right ventricular ejection fraction (RVEF) (evidence C)
  ⇒ Cardiac catheterization/coronary arteriography: patients with angina who are candidates for revascularization (evidence B); noncoronary cardiac lesions in need of correction (e.g., aortic stenosis) along with risk factors for CAD (evidence C); large areas of ischemic or hibernating myocardium evident on stress testing (evidence B); patients with history of myocardial infarction (e.g., QS-waves on ECG) (evidence C)
- Class II:
  ⇒ Cardiac catheterization/coronary arteriography: heart failure (HF) of unknown etiology (evidence C)
  ⇒ Noninvasive stress imaging: to detect ischemia in patients with known coronary artery disease (CAD) (evidence C)
  ⇒ Endomyocardial biopsy: Consider for systemic disease present with possible cardiac involvement (hemochromatosis, sarcoid, amyloid, endomyocardial fibroelastosis); to differentiate giant cell from other causes of myocarditis with better prognoses; to differentiate primary restrictive from amyloid cardiomyopathy if initial workup is inconclusive (evidence C).
- Class III, evidence C:
  ⇒ Routine endomyocardial biopsy, holter monitoring, and signal-averaged ECG are not recommended.
  ⇒ Multiple echocardiographic or radionuclide studies for routine follow-up of HF are not indicated.

Prognosis

- Strong independent predictors of mortality include older age, higher New York Heart Association (NYHA) functional class, reduced LVEF, and being male.
- Risk among patients with severe left ventricular dysfunction can be further stratified on basis of RVEF and oxygen consumption during peak exercise.
- Presence of arrhythmias, such as atrial fibrillation or nonsustained ventricular tachycardia (NSVT), increases the risk of death.

Management

Goals

- Ameliorate symptoms; maximize functional capacity; limit hospitalizations; minimize ventricular remodeling; reduce risk of sudden cardiac death
- Identify reversible etiologies; manage three major predisposing conditions: diabetes, hypertension, CAD
- Pharmacotherapy (see Table 6.2)

TABLE 6.2 PHARMACOTHERAPY FOR HEART FAILURE (HF)

Agent	Indications	Dosing (Initial Dose/Target Dose)	Comment
Angiotensin-converting enzyme inhibitors (ACEI)	ACC/AHA and Heart Failure Society of America (HFSA) recommend ACEIs as drug of choice for inhibiting RAAS in heart failure (Class I, evidence A). Mortality benefit, in all classes of HF. **NYHA Class I:** Reduces HF incidence and hospitalizations in asymptomatic EF <35%, beneficial within 24 hrs of acute MI. **NYHA Class II:** Shown superior to hydralazine/isordil.	Captopril (6.25 mg tid/50 mg tid) Enalapril (2.5 mg bid/10 mg bid) Ramipril (1.25–2.5 mg qd/5 mg bid) Lisinopril (2.5–5 mg qd/20–40 mg qd) (Note: improved morbidity/mortality with lisinoporil 22.5 mg/d vs. 3.2 mg/d (Packer, 1999)	15%–20% of patients do not tolerate (most commonly to cough). Less common adverse effects: hypotension (2%), renal insufficiency (2%), hyperkalemia, angioneurotic edema.
Angiotensin II receptor blockers (ARB)	May be used in ACEI intolerant patients (evidence C). Similar mechanism to ACEI; superior tolerability but unproven equivalence. Losartan superior to captopril in small trial but inferior in larger trial. Unclear benefit of concomitant use with ACEI.	Losartan 50 mg qd–100 mg qd/50 mg qd) Valsartan (80 mg qd/160 mg bid)	
Beta-blockers	Effective for all classes of compensated HF (Class I, evidence A/B). Believed to blunt sympathetic overdrive of HF. Mortality benefit for carvedilol, long-acting metoprolol, bisoprolol.	Metoprolol XL (12.5–25 mg qd/200 mg qd) Bisoprolol (1.25 mg qd/10 mg qd) Carvedilol (3.125–6.25 mg bid/25–50 mg bid) (Note: Carvedilol offers advantage of lower-dose pills than metoprolol, but is more expensive.)	Can acutely worsen HF signs and symptoms, so should only be initiated after clinical stability and fluid overload corrected. Clinical evaluation should precede each up-titration to assess for fatigue, fluid retention, and decreased exercise capacity. Avoid rapid withdrawal.
Digoxin	Improves symptoms, quality of life, and exercise tolerance in patients with NYHA II–III HF (Class I, evidence A). Neutral effect on mortality. Although clinical trial data is lacking for patients with severe NYHA IV HF, digoxin is thought to work across spectrum of left verticular (LV) systolic dysfunction (Class I, evidence C). Inhibition of Na-K ATPase increases intramyocyte calcium which results in increased contractility. Extracardiac Na-K ATPase inhibition results in sympathoinhibition, and reduction in renal tubular Na reabsorption.	No evidence for escalating dose. For normal renal function: 0.25 mg qd. For CrCl: <50 mL/min: age >60, small stature: 0.125 mg qd	Dose adjustments typically based on digoxin levels 2–3 wks following drug initiation or if toxicity suspected.
Anticoagulation	Treatment with warfarin (INR 2–3) is standard of care for patients with HF (class II-IV) plus atrial fibrillation or history of thromboembolic disease (Class I, evidence A); no RCTs address role of warfarin in HF in absence of these conditions.	See Chapter 43, Anticoagulation in Primary Care	NA
Antiplatelet agents	Concern exists about aspirin's potential role in attenuating ACEI induced augmentation of prostaglandin synthesis and thus reducing the efficacy of ACEI (Nguyen, 1997). Insufficient data at present. 1999 HFSA guidelines recommend consideration of both agents on the basis of their individual merits, especially since a large proportion of HF patients have a history of ischemic heart disease for which aspirin has proven efficacy (Class IIb, evidence B).	See Chapter 5, Coronary Artery Disease and Angina	NA
Antiarrhythmic therapy	The common occurrence of ventricular arrhythmias in HF has prompted trials with class Ia and Ic agents and dofetilde and D-sotalol, none of which have offered mortality benefit (Class III, evidence A). Amiodarone trials have yielded conflicting results.	NA	Due to toxicity profile, not recommended for primary prevention of death in HF (Class IIb, evidence B).
Aldosterone antagonists	30% reduction in death and 35% reduction in hospitalizations in Class III-IV HF patients already on ACEI, diuretics, +/– digoxin.	Maintain on 12.5–25 mg qd	Frequent monitoring of K+ and renal function; forewarn of potential gynecomnastia (10% vs. 1% with placebo).

ACC/AHA, American College of Cardiology/American Heart Association; RAAS, renin-angiotensin-aldosterone system; MI, myocardial infarction; NYHA, New York Heart Association; EF, ejection fraction; tid, three times a day; bid, twice a day; qd, every day; INR, international normalized ratio; RCT, randomized controlled trial; NA, not applicable.

Device Therapy

- Implantable cardiac defibrillators (ICD) improve mortality in ventricular fibrillation survivors and in postinfarction patients with low ejection fraction (EF), non-sustained ventricular tachycardia (NSVT), or inducible ventricular tachycardia (VT). At present there is insufficient evidence that routine ICD placement prolongs survival in all patients with HF (Class III, evidence C).

DIASTOLIC HEART FAILURE

Introduction

- Risk factors: age, hypertension, diabetes, left ventricular hypertrophy, CAD.
- Women and African Americans affected disproportionately for unclear reasons (Vasan, 1995).
- Annual mortality: 9% to 28% [thought to be 50% of that for systolic HF, but 4 times that of general population (Vasan et al., 1999)].
- Despite prevalence of diastolic dysfunction (30% to 50% of HF cases), there is little evidence to guide therapy.

Pathophysiology

- Increased resistance to filling in one or both ventricles raises diastolic pressure-volume curve during terminal phase of cardiac cycle, raising atrial pressures and resulting in pulmonary or systemic congestion.

Evaluation

- Difficult to make definitive diagnosis: based on signs/symptoms of HF; documentation of preserved LVEF and absence of valvular disease; direct evidence of impaired left ventricular relaxation and filling indices (historically based on cardiac catheterization) (Vasan and Levy, 2000).
- Since widespread catheterization is not feasible, noninvasive methods using Doppler echocardiography have been developed; limited by wide variation in cardiac filling patterns with frequent changes in cardiac loading conditions.

Treatment

- Few randomized trials given difficulties inherent in verifying diagnosis, heterogeneity of underlying causes, and occurrence in elderly patients with multiple comorbidities.
- Current treatment recommendations stem from physiologic principles:
  ⇒ Strict blood pressure control according to published guidelines (see Chapter 3: Hypertension) (Class I, evidence A)
  ⇒ Avoiding excess sodium intake
  ⇒ Cautious use of diuretics to relieve pulmonary congestion (without excessive reduction of preload) (Class I, evidence C)
  ⇒ Rate control of atrial fibrillation (see Chapter 7: Atrial Fibrillation) (Class I, evidence C); restoration of sinus rhythm in atrial arrhythmias (Class IIb, evidence C)
  ⇒ Consider atrial pacing (elderly patients with sick-sinus syndrome requiring pacemakers have been shown to have less severe HF when atrially paced instead of ventricularly paced). Preservation of atrial contribution to diastolic function may account for this benefit (Class IIa, evidence C).
  ⇒ Correct precipitating factors, including ischemia; consider revascularization (Class IIa, evidence C).
- Consider drug therapy: addition of angiotensin-converting enzyme inhibitor (ACEI), beta-blocker, angiotensin II receptor blocker (ARB), or calcium antagonist may improve symptoms of HF (Class IIb, evidence C).
  ⇒ Trials of ACEI, beta-blockers, ARBs for all classes of diastolic HF ongoing. No proven mortality benefit, but potential utility for controlling blood pressure/heart rate.
  ⇒ Digoxin and diuretics may provide symptomatic relief in class II-IV diastolic HF, but no proven mortality benefit.

SELECTED REFERENCES

1. Baker DW. Management of heart failure. III. The role of revascularization in the treatment of patients with moderate or severe left ventricular systolic dysfunction. *JAMA* 1994;272:1528–1534.
2. The Digitalis Investigation Group. The effect of digoxin on mortality and morbidity in patients with heart failure. *N Engl J Med* 1997;336:525–533.
3. European Heart Failure Training Group. Experience from controlled trials of physical training in chronic heart failure. *Eur Heart J* 1998;19:466–475.
4. Hunt SA, Baker DW, Chin MH, et al. ACC/AHA guidelines for the evaluation and management of chronic heart failure in the adult: executive summary. A report of the American College of Cardiology/American Heart Association Task Force on Practice Guidelines (Committee to Revise the 1995 Guidelines for the Evaluation and Management of Heart Failure) developed in collaboration with the International Society for Heart and Lung Transplantation endorsed by the Heart Failure Society of America. *J Am Coll Cardiol* 2001;38(7): 2101–2113.
5. Massie BM, Shah MB. Evolving trends in the epidemiologic factors of heart failure: rationale for preventative strategies and comprehensive disease management. *Am Heart J* 1997;133:703–712.
6. Nguyen KN. Interaction between enalapril and aspirin on mortality after acute myocardial infarction: subgroup analysis of the Cooperative New Scandinavian Enalapril Survival Study II (CONSENSUS II). *Am J Cardiol* 1997;79:115–119.
7. Packer M. Comparative effects of low and high doses of the angiotensin-converting enzyme inhibitor, lisinopril, on morbidity and mortality in chronic heart failure. ATLAS Study Group. *Circulation* 1999;100(23): 2312–2318.
8. Packer M. Withdrawal of digoxin from patients with chronic heart failure treated with angiotensin-converting-enzyme inhibitors. RADIANCE Study. *N Engl J Med* 1993;329:1–7.
9. Pitt B, Poole-Wilson PA, Segal R, et al. Effect of losartan compared with captopril on mortality in patients with symptomatic heart failure: randomized trial—the Losartan Heart Failure Survival Study ELITE II. *Lancet* 2000;355(9215):1582–1587.
10. Scanlon PJ. ACC/AHA guidelines for coronary angiography. A report of the American College of Cardiology/American Heart Association Task Force on practice guidelines (Committee on Coronary Angiography). Developed in collaboration with the Society for Cardiac Angiography and Interventions. *J Am Coll Cardiol* 1999;33(6):1756–1824.
11. SOLVD Investigators. Effect of enalapril on survival in patients with reduced left ventricular ejection fractions and congestive heart failure. *N Engl J Med* 1991;325:293–302.
12. SOLVD Investigators. Effect on mortality and the development of heart failure in asymptomatic patients with reduced left ventricular ejection fractions. *N Engl J Med* 1992;327:685–691.
13. Vasan RS. Prevalence, clinical features and prognosis of diastolic heart failure: an epidemiologic perspective. *J Am Coll Cardiol* 1995;26:1565–1574.
14. Vasan RS, Larson MG, Benjamin EJ, et al. Congestive heart failure in subjects with normal versus reduced left ventricular ejection fraction: prevalence and mortality in a population-based cohort. *J Am Coll Cardiol* 1999; 33:1948–1955.
15. Vasan RS, Levy D. Defining diastolic heart failure: a call for standardized diagnostic criteria. *Circulation* 2000; 101:2118–2121.
16. Williams JF. Guidelines for the Evaluation and Management of Heart Failure Report of the American College of Cardiology/ American Heart Association Task Force on Practice Guidelines (Committee on Evaluation and Management of Heart Failure). *Circulation* 1995;92:2764–2784.

7

ATRIAL FIBRILLATION

INTRODUCTION

- Atrial fibrillation (AF) is the most common cause of systemic embolism; increases stroke rate fivefold (Wolf et al. 1978; Flegel et al., 1987).
- Incidence of AF doubles with each decade of life; overall prevalence is 0.95%; affects 4% of people over age 60 and 9% over age 80 (Go, 2001; Narayan, 1997).
- Most common arrhythmia leading to hospital admission.

PATHOPHYSIOLOGY

- AF likely depends on presence of multiple small circuits in the atria. Ectopic beats from pulmonary vein foci are often the source (Haissaguerre, 1998). Sustained AF is promoted by fibrosis/inflammation (decrease conduction velocity), thyrotoxicosis (decrease refractoriness), ischemia/autonomic tone (decrease both) (Narayan, 1997).
- AF is frequently associated clinically with hypertension (50%) and coronary artery disease (CAD) (20%).
- *AF begets AF*: Chronic AF causes remodeling (atrial enlargement, atrial fibrosis) and shortened atrial refractoriness (Wijffels et al., 1995).

EVALUATION

- Initial workup includes 12-lead electrocardiogram (ECG), thyroid stimulating hormone (TSH), and transthoracic echocardiogram (TTE).
- Hospitalization is not required, but may be considered for hemodynamic compromise, highly symptomatic palpitations, high risk of embolism, and/or candidacy for early cardioversion (Falk, 2001).
- In the absence of evidence of ischemia, ruling out myocardial infarction is not necessary (acute coronary syndromes rarely present as AF).

TREATMENT
Goals

- Stroke prevention
- Ventricular rate control
- Restoration and maintenance of normal sinus rhythm

Stroke prevention/anticoagulation

- See Chapter 43: Anticoagulation in Primary Care.

Ventricular Rate Control

- Rate control is important for: control of symptomatic palpitations; prevention of hemodynamic compromise [congestive heart failure (CHF) due to tachycardia and decreased ventricular filling in decompensated states]; and prevention of tachycardia-mediated cardiomyopathy (occurs after 3 to 5 weeks of experimental rapid pacing) (Shinbane et al., 1997).
- Calcium channel blockers and beta-blockers have rapid onset of action (Salerno et al., 1989).
- Digoxin generally has slow onset of action, although it may significantly slow heart rate within 2 hours of administration [The Digitalis in Acute Atrial Fibrillation (DAAF) Trial Group Investigators, 1997]. Not as effective in situations where catecholamines are released (e.g., exercise or stress), because mode of action is via enhancement of parasympathetic system.

Restoration of Normal Sinus Rhythm

- Restoration of sinus rhythm has potential advantages over rate control alone: resolution of symptoms, possible elimination of need for anticoagulation, physiological rate control, atrial contribution to cardiac output. No data yet comparing restoration of sinus rhythm vs. rate control and anticoagulation (AFFIRM study will address) (Waldo, 1999).
- Spontaneous conversion to sinus rhythm occurs within 24 hours in up to two-thirds of patients (Danias et al., 1998).
- Consider:
  ⇒ The longer the duration of AF, the more likely patient will remain in AF. After being in AF for over 1 year, only 20% of patients are cardioverted successfully.
  ⇒ Larger atria (greater than 50 to 60 mm) are more likely to remain in AF.
  ⇒ Balance the need for antiarrhythmic therapy with risk of proarrhythmia (especially if pre-existing structural heart disease).

Anticoagulation and Cardioversion

- If AF has lasted less than 48 hours, immediate cardioversion may be attempted.
- If AF has lasted more than 48 hours or duration unknown, two options (no significant differences after eight weeks) (Klein et al., 2001):
  1. Anticoagulation for 3 to 4 weeks prior to cardioversion.
  2. Screen for atrial thrombus with transesophageal echocardiography (TEE), then consider cardioversion if negative.
- Risk of embolic event with cardioversion after AF lasting more than 48 hours (without anticoagulation) is 1% to 5%; reduced to 1% with anticoagulation for 3 to 4 weeks before and after cardioversion [international normalized ratio (INR) goal: 2.0 to 3.0] (Prystowsky et al., 1996).
- After cardioversion for AF lasting more than 48 hours, anticoagulation must be continued for 3 to 4 weeks secondary to atrial stunning, regardless of mode of cardioversion (chemical or electric).

Methods of Cardioversion

- When cardioversion is considered, refer patient to a cardiologist. Methods include electrical or chemical.
  ⇒ **External electrical cardioversion:** Success rate between 67% and 94% (Naccarelli et al., 2000); failures may benefit from oral amiodarone or intravenous ibutilide prior to re-cardioversion (Cappuci et al., 2000; Oral et al., 2000).
  ⇒ **Intravenous pharmacological agents:** Include ibutilide, procainamide, and amiodarone; often work quickly with benefit of avoiding anesthesia and/or electrical shock; risks include proarrhythmia (especially in cases of structural heart disease).
  ⇒ **Oral pharmacological agents:** Include flecainide, propafenone, and dofetilide. Digoxin does not significantly increase conversion to sinus rhythm when compared to placebo (The Digitalis in Acute Atrial Fibrillation [DAAF] Trial Group Investigators, 1997).

Maintenance of Sinus Rhythm

- Antiarrhythmic therapy is often needed for maintenance of sinus rhythm after cardioversion.
- Most drugs have similar efficacy, although the recent Canadian Trial of Atrial Fibrillation study showed amiodarone superior to sotalol/propafenone at 12-month follow-up (Roy et al., 2000).
- Following recommendations are based on theory and side effect profiles due to lack of clear-cut comparative studies (Reiffel, 2000):
  ⇒ Patients with lone AF: Class IC agents (flecainide, propafenone) are agents of choice; sotalol, amiodarone, dofetilide, disopyramide are second choices.
  ⇒ Patients with hypertension: Propafenone is first line, sotalol and amiodarone are second line (association of increased torsades with left ventricular hypertrophy in experimental models).
  ⇒ Patients with ischemic heart disease: Class I agents are contraindicated; racemic sotalol, dofetilide and beta-blocker, and amiodarone are first line (offer beta-blocking activity).
  ⇒ Patients with poorly decompensated CHF: Amiodarone is preferred because of established safety in this setting; dofetilide is an alternative.

Nonpharmacological Options

- Radiofrequency ablation may be curative (atrial flutter ablation, pulmonary vein ablative isolation, atrioventricular nodal ablation).
- Atrial pacing may have role in paroxysmal AF with increased vagal tone (e.g., AF during sleep) or intraatrial conduction delay (Cannom, 2000).
- Maze surgical procedure is controversial (atrial appendages are excised and mazelike pathways created to prevent formation of large reentrant loops that propagate AF).
- Implantable atrial defibrillators: role is not yet determined.

SELECTED REFERENCES

1. Cannom DS. Atrial fibrillation: nonpharmacological approaches. *Am J Cardiol* 2000;85:25D–35D.
2. Cappuci A, Villani GQ, Aschieri D, et al. Oral amiodarone increases the efficacy of direct-current cardioversion in restoration of sinus rhythm in patients with chronic atrial fibrillation. *Eur Heart J* 2000;21:66–73.
3. Danias PG, Caulfield TA, Weigner MJ, et al. Likelihood of spontaneous conversion of atrial fibrillation to sinus rhythm. *J Am Coll Cardiol* 1998;31:588–92.
4. Falk RH. Atrial fibrillation. *N Engl J Med* 2001;344:1067–1078.
5. Flegel KM, Shipley MJ, Rose G. Risk of stroke in nonrheumatic atrial fibrillation. *Lancet* 1987;1:526–529.
6. Go AS, Hylek EM, Philips KA, et al. Prevalence of diagnosed atrial fibrillation in adults. National implications for rhythm management and stroke prevention: the AnTicoagulation and Risk Factors in Atrial Fibrillation (ATRIA) Study. *JAMA* 2001;285:2370–2375.
7. Haissaguerre M, Jais P, Shah DC, et al. Spontaneous initiation of atrial fibrillation by ectopic beats originating in the pulmonary veins. *N Engl J Med* 1998;339:659–66.
8. Klein AL, Grimm RA, Murray RD, et al. Use of transesophageal echocardiography to guide cardioversion in patients with atrial fibrillation. *N Engl J Med* 2001;344:1411–1420.
9. Naccarelli GV, Dell'Orfano JT, Wolbrette DL, et al. Cost-effective management of acute atrial fibrillation: role of rate control, spontaneous conversion, medical and direct current cardioversion, transesophageal echocardiography and antiembolic therapy. *Am J Cardiol* 2000;85:36D–45D.
10. Narayan SM, Cain ME, Smith JM.. Atrial fibrillation. *Lancet* 1997;350:943–950.
11. Oral H, Souza JJ, Michaud GF, et al. Facilitating transthoracic cardioversion of atrial fibrillation with ibutilide pretreatment. *N Engl J Med* 1999;340:1849–1854.
12. Ozcan C, Jahangir A, Friedman PA, et al. Long-term survival after ablation of the atrioventricular node and implantation of a permanent pacemaker in patients with atrial fibrillation. *N Engl J Med* 2001;344:1043–1051.
13. Prystowsky EN, Benson DW Jr, Fuster V, et al. Management of patients with atrial fibrillation: a statement for healthcare professionals. From the Subcommittee on Electrocardiography and Electrophysiology, American Heart Association. *Circulation* 1996;93:1262–1277.
14. Rieffel JA. Drug choices in the treatment of atrial fibrillation. *Am J Cardiol* 2000;85:12D–19D.
15. Roy D, Talajic M, Dorian P, et al. Amiodarone to prevent recurrence of atrial fibrillation. Canadian Trial of Atrial Fibrillation Investigators. *N Engl J Med* 2000;342:913–920.
16. Salerno DM, Dias VC, Kleiger RE, et al. Efficacy and safety of intravenous diltiazem for treatment of atrial fibrillation and atrial flutter. The Diltiazem-Atrial Fibrillation/Flutter Study Group. *Am J Cardiology* 1989;63:1048–1051.

17. Shinbane JS, Wood MA, Jensen DN, et al. Tachycardia-induced cardiomyopathy: a review of animal models and clinical studies. *J Am Coll Cardiol* 1997;29:709–715.
18. The Digitalis in Acute Atrial Fibrillation (DAAF) Trial Group Investigators. Intravenous digoxin in acute atrial fibrillation: results of a randomized, placebo-controlled multicentre trial in 239 patients. *Eur Heart J* 1997;18:649–654.
19. Waldo AL for the AFFIRM investigators. Management of atrial fibrillation: the need for AFFIRMative action. *Am J Card* 1999;84:698–700.
20. Wijffels MC, Kirchhof CJ, Dorland R, et al. Atrial fibrillation begets atrial fibrillation: a study in awake chronically instrumented goats. *Circulation* 1995;92:1954–1968.
21. Wolf PA, Dawber TR, Thomas HE Jr, et al. Epidemiologic assessment of chronic atrial fibrillation and risk of stroke: the Framingham study. *Neurology* 1978;28:973–977.

LOWER EXTREMITY EDEMA

INTRODUCTION

- Edema is an increase in the interstitial component of extracellular fluid volume.
- May occur in isolation or as sign of underlying pathology.
- Etiology can often be determined without diagnostic testing.
- Low-dose diuretics often given, but benefit not well-supported in the literature.

PATHOPHYSIOLOGY

- Edema results from alterations in Starling forces that promote increased filtration from plasma space to interstitium. Can be produced by elevated capillary hydraulic pressure, increased capillary permeability, increased interstitial oncotic pressure, or decreased plasma oncotic pressure.
- Underlying mechanism may be produced at systemic level (e.g., congestive heart failure, nephrotic syndrome, pregnancy, cirrhosis) or local level (e.g., lymphatic obstruction, venous insufficiency).
- To maintain tissue perfusion, overall extracellular volume becomes overexpanded through renal sodium and water retention prior to the clinical appearance of edema (Martin and Schrier, 1995). Clinical appearance usually does not occur until interstitial volume has increased by at least 2.5 to 3 liters (except with localized edema such as occurs with an allergic reaction).

DIFFERENTIAL DIAGNOSIS

- Unilateral acute edema:
  ⇒ Deep venous thrombosis (DVT): Virchow's triad (hypercoagulability, stasis, endothelial injury). Many clinical signs (warmth, superficial venous dilatation, Homans' sign) are suggestive but not specific.
  ⇒ Popliteal (Baker's) cyst rupture.
  ⇒ Rupture of gastrocnemius medial head (follows injuries involving acute dorsiflexion of ankle while knee is extended or foot is planted; assess for asymmetry in muscle contours).
  ⇒ Cellulitis: Elicit history of cellulitis, diabetes, trauma, and coexisting lymphedema. Examine for marginated border of erythema, swelling, and/or tenderness. May have an identifiable portal of entry (e.g., puncture wound, insect bite, interdigital skin breaks from tinea).
  ⇒ Compartment syndrome: Assess for history of recent trauma, overuse injury, or surgery to an extremity. Exam that reveals acute loss of pulses distal to area of painful swelling may represent a surgical emergency.
- Unilateral chronic edema:
  ⇒ Venous insufficiency: Heavy, fatigued, or "aching" feeling in the leg(s) that worsens as the day progresses, but may improve with elevation. Look for varicosities, hemosiderin deposition in skin (so-called "brawny edema"), or stasis dermatitis with ulcer formation over medial malleolus. Difficult to distinguish from cellulitis if stasis dermatitis is present (history may help). May be bilateral.

⇒ Lymphedema: Firm swelling, rarely tender, often nonpitting and involving the digits. May be family history of this condition. Evaluate for inguinal lymphadenopathy or lymphatic obstruction from pelvic pathology.

⇒ Reflex sympathetic dystrophy: History of burning pain, hyperesthesia, or hyperhidrosis. Generally occurs several weeks after trauma. Trophic changes in skin and/or bone with pain out of proportion to exam.

⇒ Malignancy: Consider venous compression by pelvic masses or Kaposi's sarcoma (Merli and Spandorfer, 1995).

- Bilateral acute edema:
  ⇒ Usually implies catastrophic change in venous system, such as inferior vena cava (IVC) thrombosis/compression, or altered permeability (as in acute angioedema). May be subacute, over days, in salt-retaining states.
- Bilateral chronic edema:
  ⇒ History and physical exam can often differentiate between systemic and local etiologies (can stratify by primary alteration in Starling forces) (Table 8.1).

TABLE 8.1 CAUSES OF BILATERAL CHRONIC LOWER EXTREMITY EDEMA

Mechanism	Systemic Etiologies	Local Etiologies
Elevated capillary hydraulic pressure	• Congestive heart failure: orthopnea, paroxysmal nocturnal dyspnea • Constrictive pericarditis: history of pericardiotomy or acute pericarditis, right heart failure symptoms, hepatic congestion, ascites, jugular venous distention • IVC compression/thrombosis: underlying malignancy or hypercoagulable state • Medication affecting salt handling: NSAIDs, glucocorticoids, estrogen, anabolic steroids (Christy and Shaver, 1974)	• Bilateral DVT • Pregnancy: late or multiple gestation, due to venous compression by gravid uterus • Lymphatic obstruction: malignancy, history of local XRT or lymph node dissection, filariasis
Increased capillary permeability	• Vasculitis: history of Bartonella infection, sarcoid, cryglobulinemia; erythema nodosum changes may be present on skin of affected extremities. • Medication effect on vascular permeability: calcium channel blockers, minoxidil, diazoxide, hydralazine	• Hypothyroid myxedema: proposed mechanism of increased capillary permeability to plasma protein with leak into interstitium and slowed lymphatic egress (Parving et al., 1979).
Decreased plasma oncotic pressure	• Enhanced albumin loss: large surface-area burns, nephrotic syndrome, protein-losing enteropathy • Reduced albumin production: starvation, protein malnutrition, cirrhosis	• NA
Other	• Lipedema: foot-sparing, nonpitting, not prone to cellulites (differentiates it from lymphedema and most venous abnormalities). Begins in teens to twenties, almost exclusively in women. Swelling is soft, consistent with fat tissue (Rudkin and Miller 1994).	• NA

IVC, inferior vena cava; NSAIDs, nonsteroidal antiinflammatory drugs; DVT, deep venous thrombosis; XRT, radiation therapy; NA, not applicable.

EVALUATION

History

- Symptoms: lower extremity swelling, pain, difficulty walking, infection, altered habitus due to swelling
- Distribution: isolated to lower extremities or systemic (periorbital, anasarca, dyspnea/orthopnea, abdominal enlargement); unilateral or bilateral
- Medications
- History of underlying disease: cardiac, renal, hepatic, hypothyroidism (weight gain, cold intolerance, fatigue), infection, malignancy, hypercoagulable state (DVT, thrombophlebitis), local trauma
- Variation: diurnal, menstrual, positional
- History of interventions to pelvis/groin

- Family history of clotting or lymphedema
- Travel to areas with high prevalence of filariasis (*Wuchereria bancrofti, Brugia malayi*)

Physical Exam

- Assess for nutritional status, evidence for recent weight loss, periorbital edema, jugular venous pressure, pulmonary congestion, ascites, lymphadenopathy (local or systemic), stigmata of chronic liver dysfunction (spider angiomata, palmar rubor, gynecomastia), stigmata of hypothyroidism (skin or hair changes, delayed deep tendon reflex recovery), pelvic masses (male/female genitourinary malignancies). Measure leg sizes (reproducibility with consistent method important for follow-up, such as a calf diameter of 10 cm below tibial tubercle).

Laboratory Data

- Used to limit differential diagnosis established by history/physical exam. May include:
  ⇒ Hematologic evaluation for suspected underlying malignancy or hypercoagulable state
  ⇒ Evaluation of cardiac, renal, hepatic function by imaging, chemical analysis, or estimation of function
  ⇒ Noninvasive vascular imaging
  ⇒ Abdominal/pelvic imaging
  ⇒ Culture data
  ⇒ Rheumatologic serologies

TREATMENT

Underlying Causes

- Treatment should be directed at identified underlying etiology (thrombosis, malignancy, infection, rheumatologic disease, trauma, nephrotic syndrome, heart failure, cirrhosis, etc.).
- Discontinue suspected culprit medications.

Symptomatic Treatment

- Difficult if permanent damage to venous and/or lymphatic systems has occurred from prolonged obstruction or inherent insufficiency.
- Aimed at reducing movement of fluid from plasma to interstitium. Available therapies, in ascending order of hydrostatic support, are:
  ⇒ Support pantyhose: widely available, self-selected by size
  ⇒ TED stockings: available in knee-high and thigh-high lengths (thigh-high length is more effective)
  ⇒ Jobst stockings (over the counter): size determined by height and weight charts
  ⇒ Fitted support stockings (Jobst and other brands): require prescription and measurement of patient. Many medical suppliers custom make them and can tailor amount/location of support.
- Lifestyle modification and leg elevation may offer some improvement.
- Low-dose diuretics often given, but benefit not well supported in the literature.
- Surgery for varicosities or to remove excess tissue (as in lipedema) is occasionally effective, but has not been shown useful for lymphedema or chronic venous insufficiency.

SELECTED REFERENCES

1. Alguire PC, Mathes BM. Chronic venous insufficiency and venous ulceration. *J Gen Intern Med* 1997;6:374–383.
2. Christy NP, Shaver JC. Estrogens and the kidney. *Kidney Int* 1974;6:366.
3. Ciocon JO, Fernandez BB, Ciocon DG. Leg edema: clinical clues to the differential diagnosis. *Geriatrics* 1993; 48:34–45.
4. Martin PY, Schrier RW. Renal sodium excretion and edematous disorders. *Endocrinol Metab Clin North Am* 1995;3:459–479.

5. Merli GJ, Spandorfer J. The outpatient with unilateral leg swelling. *Med Clin North Am* 1995;2:435–447.
6. Parving HH, Hansen JM, Nielsen SL, et al. Mechanisms of edema formation in myxedema: increased protein extravasation and relatively slow lymphatic drainage. *N Engl J Med* 1979;301:460.
7. Powell AA, Armstrong MA. Peripheral edema. *Am Fam Physician* 1997;5:1721–1726.
8. Rudkin GH, Miller TA. Lipedema: a clinical entity distinct from lymphedema. *Plast Reconstr Surg* 1994;94: 841–847.
9. Russell RP. Side effects of calcium channel blockers. *Hypertension* 1988;11(Suppl II):42–44.

9

SURGICAL CONSULTATION

INTRODUCTION

- Goal of the medical consultant: assess preoperative risk; manage medical problems in the peri-operative period.

GENERAL RISKS OF SURGERY AND ANESTHESIA

- 0.3% of all operations result in death; 55% of deaths occur within 48 hours
- Age over 70: 4- to 8-fold increased risk
- Emergency surgery: 2-fold increased risk
- High-risk procedures in terms of overall perioperative mortality: craniotomy, cardiac surgery, exploratory laparotomy, large bowel surgery
- Patient and surgery-related factors are more important than types of anesthesia

ROUTINE PREOPERATIVE LABS (TABLE 9.1)

- Little role for preoperative "routine" bloodwork (Kaplan et al., 1985). Laboratory work done in previous 3 to 4 months need not be repeated, with the exception of β-HCG (Macpherson et al., 1990).

TABLE 9.1 PREOPERATIVE TESTING GUIDELINES FOR PATIENTS WITH MEDICAL PROBLEMS RECEIVING GENERAL ANESTHESIA

Test	Indications	Test	Indications
CBC	Procedure with potentially significant blood loss Women age 50 and over, Men over age 65 Infants under 6 months Cardiovascular disease Anemia Abnormal bleeding history Smoking over 40 pack-years Renal disease Malignancy, malnutrition Radiation therapy Intracranial disease Anticoagulant use	Electrocardiogram (ECG)	Women over age 50 Men over age 40 Cardiovascular disease Pulmonary disease Diabetes Intracranial disease Radiation therapy Morbid obesity Sleep apnea Digoxin
Type and screen	Procedure with potential for significant blood loss	Urinalysis	Suspected urinary tract infection Procedure involving catheter
PT/PTT	Known bleeding disorder Hepatic disease Leukemia Malnutrition Anticoagulant use	Chest x-ray	Cardiovascular disease Pulmonary disease Malignancy Radiation therapy Goiter Rheumatoid arthritis
b-HCG	Possible pregnancy	Pulmonary function tests	(See Pulmonary Risk Assessment and Management section) Known liver disease
CHEM-7	Diabetes Renal disease Diuretics, digoxin, steroids Intracranial disease Over age 65	Liver function tests	Exposure to hepatitis virus Alcohol abuse Bleeding disorder

CARDIAC RISK ASSESSMENT AND MANAGEMENT

- History, physical exam, and electrocardiographic (ECG) assessment should focus on identification of cardiac risk factors (such as hypertension, diabetes, age, and hyperlipidemia), evidence of coronary artery disease, angina, prior myocardial infarction (MI), congestive heart failure, and arrhythmias.
- Identify disease severity, stability, prior treatment, comorbid conditions, type of surgery, and patient's baseline premorbid functional status.
- American Heart Association/American College of Cardiology: algorithm for cardiac assessment and preoperative testing based on patient's clinical characteristics, type of surgery, and functional capacity (see Figs. 9.1 and 9.2 and Table 9.3).
- Cardiac stress testing or intervention [percutaneous transluminal coronary angioplasty (PTCA) or coronary artery bypass graft (CABG)] usually not necessary unless already indicated before the question of surgery. Test only if it might affect treatment.

Perioperative Beta-Blockade

- Reduces tachycardia/hemodynamic instability during intubation and surgical manipulation; fewer episodes of myocardial ischemia and arrhythmias in the presence of beta-blockers.
- Significant mortality benefit in high-risk patients undergoing noncardiac surgery; 3% mortality in patients treated with bisoprolol vs. 34% mortality in the placebo group (90% relative risk reduction) (Poldermans et al., 1999; Mangano et al., 1996).
- Consider eligibility for beta-blockers in all patients undergoing surgery, particularly those with known coronary disease or cardiac risk factors.

CARDIAC RISK ASSESSMENT AND MANAGEMENT IN NONCARDIAC SURGERY (ACC/AHA TASK FORCE, 1996) (TABLE 9.2 AND FIGURES 9.1 AND 9.2)

Intraoperative and Postoperative ST-segment Monitoring

- Most postoperative MIs occur in the first three days following surgery; the majority (61%) of these events occur without anginal pain.
- Patients at high risk for cardiovascular complications should have postoperative ECG analysis through day 3, with checking of cardiac markers only if there is a suggestion of ischemia.
- Intraoperative ST-segment changes predict perioperative MI; such patients are at higher risk for cardiac death or future MI, and need evaluation for revascularization.

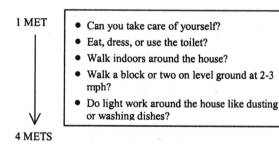

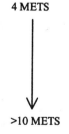

FIGURE 9.1. Estimated energy requirements for various activities. (Adapted from Hlatkyma, et al. Duke activity status index. *Am J Cardiol* 1989;64:651–654.)

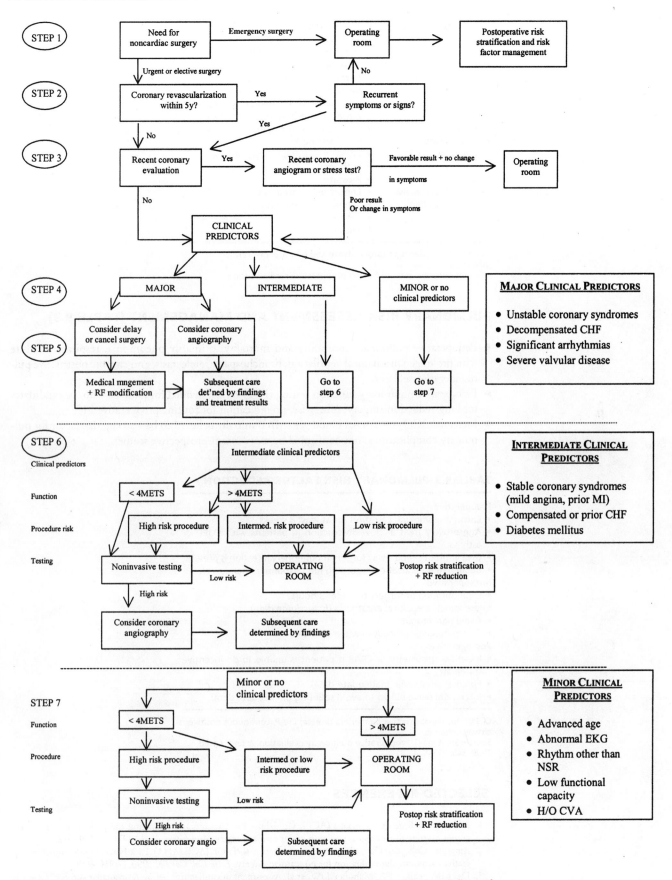

FIGURE 9.2. Stepwise approach to preoperative cardiac assessment. [Adapted from American College of Cardiology/American Heart Association (ACC/AHA) Task Force. Guidelines of perioperative cardiovascular evaluation for noncardiac surgery. *J Am Coll Cardiol* 1996;27:910–948.]

TABLE 9.2 CARDIAC RISK[a] STRATIFICATION FOR NONCARDIAC SURGICAL PROCEDURES

High (Reported cardiac risk often >5%)	• Emergent major operations, particularly in the elderly • Vascular • Anticipated prolonged procedures with large fluid shifts and/or blood loss
Intermediate (Reported cardiac risk generally <5%)	• Carotid endarterectomy • Head and neck • Intrathoracic and intraperitoneal • Orthopedic
Low[b] (Reported cardiac risk generally <1%)	• Prostate • Endoscopic procedures • Superficial procedures • Cataract • Breast

[a] Combined incidence of cardiac death and nonfatal myocardial infarction.
[b] Do not generally require further preoperative cardiac testing.

PULMONARY RISK ASSESSMENT AND MANAGEMENT (TABLE 9.3)

- Perioperative pulmonary morbidity and mortality: primarily pneumonia, respiratory failure with prolonged mechanical ventilation, bronchospasm, atelectasis, and chronic obstructive pulmonary disease flares.
- Preoperative pulmonary function testing (PFT) recommended for patients who are candidates for lung-reduction surgery; otherwise, no indication for routine preoperative PFT.
- Increased PCO_2 on arterial blood gas (ABG) initially believed to be a strong risk factor for pulmonary complications; not confirmed by more recent prospective studies.

TABLE 9.3 PULMONARY RISK FACTOR REDUCTION

Preoperative
- Encourage smoking cessation for at least 8 weeks.
- Aggressively treat airflow obstruction in patients with COPD or asthma.
- Give antibiotics and delay surgery if pulmonary infection is present.
- Begin patient education regarding lung-expansion maneuvers.

Intraoperative
- Limit duration of surgery to under 3 hours.
- Use spinal or epidural anesthesia (inadequate data).
- Avoid pancuronium.
- Do laparoscopic procedure when possible.

Postoperative
- Incentive spirometry or CPAP if patient is unable to do incentive spirometry
- Epidural anesthesia (inadequate data)
- Intercostal nerve blocks to avoid splinting (inadequate data)

COPD, chronic obstructive pulmonary disease; CPAP, continuous positive airway pressure.
Source: Smetana G. Preoperative pulmonary evaluation. *N Engl J Med* 1999; 340: 937–944.

SELECTED REFERENCES

1. American College of Physicians (ACP). Guidelines for assessing and managing the perioperative risk from coronary artery disease associated with major cardiac surgery. *Ann Intern Med* 1997;127:309–312.
2. American College of Cardiology/American Heart Association (ACC/AHA) Task Force. Guidelines of perioperative cardiovascular evaluation for noncardiac surgery. *J Am Coll Cardiol* 1996;27:910–948.
3. Das MK, Pellikka PA, Mahoney DW, et al. Assessment of cardiac risk before nonvascular surgery. *J Am Coll Cardiol* 2000;35:1647–1653.

4. Eagle KA, Coley CM, Newell JB, et al. Combining clinical and thallium data optimizes preoperative assessment of cardiac risk before major vascular surgery. *Ann Intern Med* 1989;110:859–66.
5. Goldman L, Lee T, Rudd P. Ten commandments for effective consultations. *Arch Intern Med* 1983;143: 1753–1755.
6. Hollenberg SM. Preoperative cardiac risk assessment. *Chest* 1999;115:51S–57S.
7. Kaplan EB, Sheiner LB, Boeckmann AJ, et al. The usefulness of preoperative laboratory screening. *JAMA* 1985;253:3576–3581.
8. Lee TH, Marcantonio ER, Mangione CM, et al. Derivation and prospective validation of a simple index for prediction of cardiac risk of major noncardiac surgery. *Circulation* 1999;100:1043–1049.
9. Macpherson DS. Preoperative laboratory testing: should any tests be "routine" before surgery? *Med Clin North Am* 1993;77:289–308.
10. Macpherson DS, Snow R, Lofgren RP. Preoperative screening: value of previous tests. *Ann Intern Med* 1990; 113:969–973.
11. Mangano DT, Goldman L. Preoperative assessment of patients with known or suspected coronary disease. *N Engl J Med* 1995;333:1750–1756.
12. Mangano DT, Layug EL, Wallace A, et al. Effect of atenolol on mortality and cardiovascular morbidity after noncardiac surgery. *N Engl J Med* 1996;335:1713–1720.
13. Palda VA, Detsky AS. Perioperative assessment and management of risk from coronary artery disease. *Ann Intern Med* 1997;127:313–328.
14. Poldermans D, Boersma E, Bax JJ, et al. The effect of bisoprolol on perioperative mortality and myocardial infarction in high risk patients undergoing vascular surgery. *N Engl J Med* 1999;341:1789–1794.
15. Schein OD, Katz J, Bass EB, et al. The value of routine preoperative medical testing before cataract surgery. *N Engl J Med* 2000;342:168–175.
16. Smetana G. Preoperative pulmonary evaluation. *N Engl J Med* 1999;340:937–944.

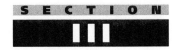

PULMONARY

CHRONIC COUGH

INTRODUCTION

- Chronic cough is defined as persistent and/or recurrent cough lasting more than 3 weeks.
- Chronic cough is found in 14% to 23% of nonsmoking adults.
- Fifth most common symptom in outpatients, accounting for 30 million visits annually.
- $600 million per year is spent on prescription and over-the-counter antitussives.

PATHOPHYSIOLOGY

- Coughing removes inhaled/aspirated foreign material from respiratory tract to protect lung from injury and is under both voluntary and involuntary control.
- Full coughing function requires intact diaphragm, glottis, and muscles of expiration (both intercostal and abdominal).
- Receptors for cough stimuli are found in airways and lung parenchyma, as well as in the tympanic membranes, esophagus, and pericardium.

DIFFERENTIAL DIAGNOSIS

- Three most common causes account for majority of cases: postnasal drip (34%), bronchial asthma (28%), gastroesophageal reflux disease (18%) [assumes normal chest x-ray (CXR), not on angiotensin-converting enzyme inhibitors (ACEIs), and not post-infectious] (see Table 10.1). The remaining differential is wide, and etiology is often suggested by history or CXR findings (Table 10.2).
- Chronic cough can result simultaneously from more than one condition in 18% to 93% of cases (Irwin and Madison, 2000).

TABLE 10.1 COMMON CAUSES OF COUGH

Etiology	Definition/Diagnosis	Treatment
Post-upper respiratory tract infection	Persistence up to 2 months after a viral upper respiratory infection (URI) is normal.	Cough suppression: +/− bronchodilators +/− inhaled steroids
Postnasal drip	Causes: allergic or nonallergic, vasomotor rhinitis, nasopharyngitis, sinusitis Symptoms: dripping sensation in back of throat, cough, clearing of secretions, or asymptomatic Signs: cobblestoning of oropharyngeal mucosa, no reliable radiographic findings	Acute onset: oral antihistamine/decongestant Chronic: nasal inhaled corticosteroids Refractory: sinus films/CT +/− 6-week course of antibiotics
Cough-variant asthma	Symptoms: dry, constant cough made worse by URI, seasonal allergies, exercise, or cold Diagnosis: spirometry/PFTs, methacholine inhalation challenge, improvement of symptoms with 1 week of bronchodilators	Bronchodilators Inhaled steroids Systemic steroids

continued

TABLE 10.1 *(continued)*

Etiology	Definition/Diagnosis	Treatment
Gastroesophageal reflux disease (GERD)	75% with GERD-induced cough have no symptoms of heartburn. Symptoms: cough worse with meals or at night, with or without dyspepsia or waterbrash Diagnosis: empiric antacid trial first, esophageal pH monitoring (gold standard), endoscopy	Bed elevation Regular meals H$_2$ blockers Proton-pump inhibitors Metoclopramide Inhaled anticholinergics
Angiotensin-couverting enzyme inhibitors (ACEIs)	Causes: Bradykinins and prostaglandins Switching ACEIs generally does not help. Symptoms may start after beginning medication. Signs: Dry cough without secretions or airflow obstruction. Affects men more often than women.	Resolves days to weeks after discontinuation of ACEIs. Consider angiotensin II receptor antagonist.
Bordetella pertussis	As many as 17% of patients with chronic cough have evidence of recent *Bordetella pertussis* by serology (Birkebaek et al., 1999).	Macrolides do not reduce duration of cough but have effects on transmission.
Chronic bronchitis	Persistent cough for more than 3 months for 2 consecutive years. Occurs in smokers and is productive of a whitish sputum.	Stopping smoking, 4-week trial bronchodilators No role for steroids

PFTs, pulmonary function tests.

TABLE 10.2: ADDITIONAL CAUSES OF CHRONIC COUGH

If CXR abnormal, consider:
Allergic alveolitis
Bronchogenic cancer
Lung abscess
Sarcoidosis
Tuberculosis
Medication-induced:
ACEIs
Amiodarone
Aspirin
Beta-blockers (including ophthalmic)
Cholinesterase inhibitors
Nitrofurantoin
NSAIDs
Tryptophan
Other common causes:
Bordetella pertussis infection
Bronchiectasis
Chronic bronchitis (smokers)
Eosinophilic bronchitis
Interstitial lung disease
Left ventricular dysfunction
Postinfectious cough
Sinusitis

CXR, chest x-ray; ACEIs, angiotensin-converting enzyme inhibitors; NSAIDs, nonsteroidal antiinflammatory drugs.

EVALUATION

History

- In assessment of chronic cough in a nonsmoker without hemoptysis, normal or no CXR, and not immunocompromised, evaluate for history of recent upper respiratory infection (URI), postnasal drip, known sinusitis, cough-variant asthma, gastroesophageal reflux disease (GERD), use of ACEIs, cardiac condition(s), occupational exposures, and/or tobacco exposure.

Physical Exam

- Ear, nose, throat: oropharyngeal abnormalities, auditory canal foreign body/cerumen, nasal polyps, or "cobblestone" appearance of nasal mucosa.

- Lung: wheezes, prolonged expiratory phase
- Cardiac: evidence of cardiac disease, congestive heart failure

Laboratory Studies

- Consider pulmonary function tests (PFTs)/spirometry/methacholine challenge, complete blood count (CBC), sinus films, CXR (CXR useful in only 7% of cases; must consider pretest probability of tuberculosis, cancer).
- Bronchoscopy useful only if CXR is abnormal, wheezing is localized on exam, or patient is over age 40 and has strong smoking history (or if all other workup negative).

Response to Empiric Therapy

- Often used to diagnose etiology.

Assess for Complications of Cough

- Asymptomatic elevation of creatine phosphokinase (CPK), rectus abdominus muscle rupture, rib fractures
- Pneumomediastinum, pneumothorax, pneumatosis intestinalis, laryngeal trauma, exacerbation of asthma, subcutaneous emphysema, bronchospasm
- Bradycardia due to elevated vagal tone, hypotension, rupture of subconjunctival/nasal/anal veins, dislodgment of intravascular catheters
- Cough syncope from valsalva [commonly found in middle-aged men with chronic obstructive pulmonary disease (COPD)]
- Stress incontinence, abdominal hernias, wound dehiscence
- Disturbed sleep, daytime somnolence, lack of concentration, social isolation, fear of cancer. Psychosocial burden may outweigh physiologic burden for many patients (French et al., 1998).

TREATMENT

Approach

- Strategies (outlined in table 10.1) attacking the three most common causes (postnasal drip, bronchial asthma, gastroesophageal reflux disease) yield higher than 90% response rates with specific therapy.

Nonspecific Therapy

- Recommended if cough serves no useful purpose (nonproductive) or has accompanying complications, particularly sleep interference.
  - ⇒ Cough suppressants [e.g., Tessalon (benzonatate)] act centrally on cough center in medulla. Opiates (e.g., codeine) are most effective; nonopiates (e.g., dextromethorphan) are widely available over the counter.
  - ⇒ Cough drops useful for symptomatic sore throat. Any sucking candy can be as effective as "cough" drops.
  - ⇒ Expectorants (e.g., guaifenesin) increase volume of secretions.
  - ⇒ Mucolytics (e.g. N-acetyl-cysteine) decrease/alter mucus production.
  - ⇒ Local anesthetics (e.g., levodropropizine) can be used.
  - ⇒ Anticholinergics (e.g., ipratropium bromide) can be used.

Over-the-Counter Medications

- Cough syrup "DM" contains guaifenesin plus dextromethorphan
- Combination antihistamine and decongestant, most commonly containing diphenhydramine and pseudoephedrine. (Brand names Sudafed, Contac, Sinutab, Actifed, Tavist-D, Drixoral: often in combination with acetaminophen.)
- Generic formulations of above compounds often 33% to 50% less expensive than brand names.

RESOURCES

- American College of Chest Physicians: 1-800-343-2227 or http://www.chestnet.org/
- Useful online patient handout: http://familydoctor.org/handouts/237.html

SELECTED REFERENCES

1. Birkebaek NH, Kristiansen M, Seefeldt T, et al. Bordetella pertussis and chronic cough in adults. *Clin Infect Dis* 1999;29:1239–1242.
2. French CL, Irwin RS, Curley FJ, et al. Impact of chronic cough on quality of life. *Arch Intern Med* 1998;158: 1657–1661.
3. Irwin RS, Curley FJ, French CL. Chronic cough. The spectrum and frequency of causes, key components of the diagnostic evaluation, and outcome of specific therapy. *Am Rev Respir Dis* 1990;141:640–647.
4. Irwin RS, Madison JM. The diagnosis and treatment of cough. *N Engl J Med* 2000;343:1715–1721.
5. Lawler WR. An office approach to the diagnosis of chronic cough. *Am Fam Physician* 1998;58:2015–2022.
6. Mello CJ, Irwin RS, Curley FJ. Predictive values of the character, timing, and complications of chronic cough in diagnosing its cause. *Arch Intern Med* 1996;156:997–1003.
7. Ours TM, Kavuru MS, Schilz RJ, et al. A prospective evaluation of esophageal testing and a double-blind, randomized study of omeprazole in a diagnostic and therapeutic algorithm for chronic cough. *Am J Gastroenterol* 1999;94:3131–3138.
8. Pratter MR, Bartter T, Akers S, et al. An algorithmic approach to chronic cough. *Ann Intern Med* 1993;119: 977–983.

ALLERGIC RHINITIS

INTRODUCTION

- Allergic rhinitis is defined as episodic sneezing, itching, rhinorrhea, and nasal obstruction.
- It afflicts 8% to 16% of Americans and accounts for $1.2 billion in direct costs (medications, health care visits), plus more in indirect costs such as missed work (Weiss and Sullivan, 2001).

PATHOPHYSIOLOGY

- Two types: seasonal and perennial (chronic symptoms caused by dust mites and molds).
- Characterized by type 1 Gell/Coombs hypersensitivity reaction (Kay, 2001).
- Initial allergen exposure → presentation to antigen processing cell (macrophage, dendritic cells) → activation of specific helper Th2 lymphocytes → Th2 cells release cytokines (i.e., IL-4, IL-5) → formation of memory-resident T helper cells and plasma cells that produce specific immunoglobulins, particularly exaggerated levels of IgE.
- Subsequent allergen exposure → IgE bound to mast cells/basophils on respiratory mucosa forms cross links → mast cell degranulation results in release of histamine, tryptase, kinase, and eosinophil chemotactic factors.
- *Early phase* is characterized by sneezing, itching, watery rhinorrhea, and nasal congestion.
- *Late phase* begins 2 to 4 hours after allergen exposure, peaks at 6 to 9 hours, and is characterized by cellular inflammatory response and nasal congestion.

DIFFERENTIAL DIAGNOSIS

- Allergic
- Infectious (viral, bacterial)
- Idiopathic (hyperresponsiveness to strong smells)
- Hormonal (pregnancy, puberty, acromegaly, hypothyroidism)
- Drug induced [angiotensin-converting enzyme inhibitors (ACEIs), beta-blockers, nonsteroidal antiinflammatory drugs (NSAIDs), aspirin (ASA)]
- Gustatory (hot spicy foods, food allergies)
- Rhinitis medicamentosa (overuse of nasal decongestants)
- Nasal obstruction (deviated nasal septum, polyps, turbinate hypertrophy, tumors, foreign bodies)
- Emotional (stress, sexual arousal)
- Nonallergic with or without eosinophilia

EVALUATION

- Based on history and physical exam. Further workup is not cost-effective and should be reserved for refractory cases.

History

- Sneezing, nasal pruritus, postnasal drip, nasal congestion, eye watering/tearing/itching, nasal and pharyngeal itching
- Patient may have history of chronic mouth breathing, postnasal discharge, cough, headaches.
- Reaction may correspond with specific exacerbating factors, time of onset, or inciting agents (pets, carpeting, moldy basement).
- Family history: A child with one parent with known allergic rhinitis has a 30% probability of developing inhalant allergy symptoms (60% if both parents are affected).

Physical Exam

- Allergic "shiners" (infraorbital edema and cyanosis due to obstructed vascular drainage), allergic "salute" (wiping nose leads to nasal crease across nasal bridge), nasal polyps, enlarged erythematous to bluish nasal turbinates with watery mucus

Nasal Cytology

- Nasal secretions show predominance of eosinophils (allergic rhinitis) vs. neutrophils (infectious rhinitis); little supportive evidence for clinical utility.

Diagnostic Tests

- Reserve for severe and/or refractory cases.
- Immediate hypersensitivity skin testing is gold standard; identifies allergen and patient's relative sensitivity to allergen.
  - ⇒ Common modalities include skin-prick testing (application of small amount of concentrated allergen to skin and then pricking skin through solution into epidermal layer) and intradermal testing (introduction of measurable amount of allergen into intradermal layer). The latter is more sensitive and reproducible.
- RAST (radioallergosorbent test) immunoassay test reliably detects allergen-specific IgE antibodies in serum and quantitates serum concentrations of antibodies; slightly less sensitive than skin testing.

TREATMENT

- Treatment is three-tiered: (1) avoidance of allergens; (2) antiallergic drug therapy; and (3) immunotherapy (see Fig. 11.1).
- Inadequate treatment can result in chronic state of nasal inflammation, which has been linked to asthma, sinusitis, and otitis media (Skoner, 2000).

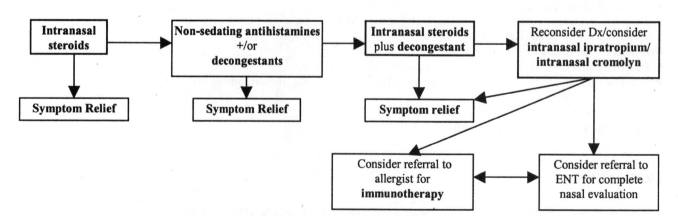

FIGURE 11.1. Drug treatment algorithm for allergic rhinitis.

Avoidance of Allergens

- Most effective and simple approach is avoidance of allergens (often impossible to attain) (see Table 11.1).

TABLE 11.1 AVOIDANCE SUGGESTIONS FOR VARIOUS ALLERGENS

Pollen	Wear sunglasses to decrease exposure to allergen.
	Keep windows in cars and buildings shut.
	Remain indoors in the morning when pollen counts are highest.
	Stay inside on sunny or windy days and avoid open grassy places when outdoors.
	Avoid airborne chemical irritants (tobacco smoke, insect sprays, air pollution, fresh tar or paint), which exacerbate pollen allergic response.
Mold	Have nonallergic person mow lawn and rake leaves often.
	Correct all plumbing, drainage, and construction defects.
Dust mites	Fit vacuum cleaner with HEPA (high-efficiency particulate air) filter.
	Dust-proof bedroom (no wall-to-wall carpets, Venetian blinds, full closets, or down comforters or pillows; bedding must be covered in zippered plastic cover).
Pet dander	Brush animal daily and bathe it weekly.
	Keep pets out of bedroom.
	Use mask while cleaning pets.
	Fit vacuum with HEPA filter.

Antiallergic Drug Therapy

- Medications become necessary when avoidance of allergens is not possible or is inadequate; medications should be taken *prior* to exposure to allergen(s).
- Treatment is associated with improvement of nasal congestion, daytime fatigue and sleepiness, and general quality of life (Craig et al., 1998).
- **Intranasal steroids:** first-line treatment
  ⇒ Superior to nonsedating antihistamines in symptom control (Weiner et al., 1998); fewer side effects and lower overall costs (Hadley, 1999).
  ⇒ Efficacy correlates with correct usage. Patients should be instructed to deliver the medication to the lateral portion of the nose, aiming the nozzle up and outward towards top of the ear.
- **Antihistamines**
  ⇒ New "nonsedating" antihistamines have a 7% incidence of significant drowsiness. Generally better tolerated and easier to administer than the first-generation agents, but are much more expensive (Corren, 2000).
  ⇒ First-generation antihistamines cause drowsiness, which improves with continued use (but persists in 15%). Anticholinergic effects are seen, especially in elderly.
  ⇒ Intranasal antihistamines offer no advantage in efficacy or side effects to oral antihistamines.
- **Decongestants**
  ⇒ Cause vasoconstriction and decrease edema in nasal tissue; can cause rebound nasal congestion (Corren, 2000).
  ⇒ Oral decongestants in combination with antihistamines are highly effective.
  ⇒ Nasal decongestants can potentiate efficacy of nasal steroids; use for 3 days or less to avoid rebound congestion.
  ⇒ Avoid in pregnancy during first trimester because of risk of infant gastroschisis (Corren, 2000).
- **Other medications**
  ⇒ Intranasal cromolyn sodium useful in some patients as a preventive medication prior to exposure to allergens (Corren, 2000).
  ⇒ Intranasal ipratropium blocks acetylcholine, thereby relieving rhinorrhea and postnasal discharge.
  ⇒ Local release of leukotriene during rhinitis episodes led to the investigation of the leukotriene antagonists as potential therapy. Loratadine and montelukast improve symp-

toms over 2 weeks; combination of both is more effective than either is alone (Meltzer et al., 2000).

⇒ Study comparing zafirlukast and intranasal steroids found significantly worse symptom control in zafirlukast and placebo groups vs. intranasal steroid group (Pullerits, et al. 1999). Further studies of these medications are needed prior to establishing therapeutic guidelines regarding their use.

Immunotherapy

- Immunotherapy offers the only long-lasting treatment option and should be considered for those not responsive to medical management. Improves quality of life and reduces symptoms even after therapy is discontinued (Durham et al., 1999; Walker et al., 2001).
- Once maintenance dose is achieved, patient receives allergy shots for 3 to 5 years (Corren, 2000).
- Approximately three-fourths of patients will develop a permanently diminished allergen response; the remainder require lifelong immunotherapy.

FUTURE DIRECTIONS

- Recombinant monoclonal IgG antibodies against Fc portion of IgE molecule reduce IgE levels, skin test reactions, and nasal symptoms (Adelroth et al., 2000).
- Soluble receptors for IL-4 and IL-5 receptor antagonists are under investigation (Kay, 2001).
- DNA vaccines: administration of CpG motifs either alone or with allergens or plasmid vectors that encode for allergens reduce inflammatory responses in animals (Kay, 2001).

SELECTED REFERENCES

1. Adelroth E, Rak S, Haahtela T, et al. Recombinant humanized mAb-E25, an anti-IgE mAb, in birch pollen induced seasonal allergic rhinitis. *J Allergy Clin Immunol* 2000;106:253–259.
2. Corren J. Allergic rhinitis: treating the adult. *J Allergy Clin Immunol* 2000;105:S610–S615.
3. Craig TJ, Teets S, Lehman EB, et al. Nasal congestion secondary to allergic rhinitis as a cause of sleep disturbance and daytime fatigue and the response to topical nasal corticosteroids. *J Allergy Clin Immunol* 1998;101: 633–637.
4. Durham SR, Walker SM, Varga EM, et al. Long-term clinical efficacy of grass pollen immunotherapy. *N Engl J Med* 1999;341:468.
5. Dykewicz MS, Fineman S, Nicklas R, et al. Joint Task Force algorithm and annotations for diagnosis and management of rhinitis. *Ann Allergy Asthma Immunol* 1998;8:469–473.
6. Hadley J. Evaluation and management of allergic rhinitis. *Med Clin North Am* 1999;83:13–25.
7. Irby B (ed.). Allergic rhinitis: current treatment options. *Drug Therapy* (an internal Massachusetts General Hospital publication). April 1998;8(4).
8. Kay AB. Allergy and allergic diseases (first of two parts). *N Engl J Med* 2001;344:30–37.
9. Kay AB. Allergy and allergic diseases (second of two parts). *N Engl J Med* 2001;344:109–113.
10. Meltzer EO, Malstrom K, Lu S, et al. Concomitant monteleukast and loratadine as treatment for seasonal allergic rhinitis: a randomized, placebo-controlled trial. *J Allergy Clin Immunol* 2000;105:917–922.
11. Pullerits R, Praks L, Skoogh BE, et al. Randomized placebo-controlled study comparing a leukotriene receptor antagonist and a nasal glucocorticoid in seasonal allergic rhinitis. *Am J Respir Crit Care Med* 1999;159: 1814–1818.
12. Skoner D. Complications of allergic rhinitis. *J Allergy Clin Immunol* 2000;105:S605–S609.
13. Sly M. Changing prevalence of allergic rhinitis and asthma. *Ann Allergy Asthma Immunol* 1999;82:233–252.
14. Von Mutius E. The environmental predictors of allergic disease. *J Allergy Clin Immunol* 2000;105:9–19.
15. Walker SM, Pajno GB, Torres Lima M, et al. Grass pollen immunotherapy for seasonal rhinitis and asthma: a randomized, controlled trial. *J Allergy Clin Immunol* 2001;107:87–93.
16. Weiner JM, Abramson MJ, Puy RM. Intranasal corticosteroids versus oral H1 receptor antagonists in allergic rhinitis: systematic review of randomised controlled trials. *BMJ* 1998;317:1624–1629.
17. Weiss KB, Sullivan SD. The health economics of asthma and rhinitis. I. Assessing the economic impact. *J Allergy Clin Immunol* 2001;107:3–8.

ASTHMA

INTRODUCTION

- Asthma is defined as chronic inflammatory disease of the tracheobronchial tree, characterized by hyperresponsiveness to various stimuli, mucous gland hypersecretion, and reversible narrowing of airways due to bronchospasm and edema.
- More than 14 million Americans are afflicted, with over 470,000 hospitalizations and more than 5,000 deaths annually.
- These rates have increased over the last decade, particularly among the medically underserved.

PATHOPHYSIOLOGY

- Airway inflammation (caused by both immunologic and nonimmunologic mediators) cyclically contributes to further airway hyperresponsiveness, leading to recurrent airflow limitation and airway wall remodeling.
- "Extrinsic" or atopic asthma, produced by environmental allergens, is distinguished from "intrinsic" asthma, which is triggered by nonspecific irritants (e.g., exercise, cold air, emotion).

DIFFERENTIAL DIAGNOSIS

- Heart disease, recurrent pulmonary embolism, upper/lower airway obstruction, vasculitis, immune deficiencies, vocal cord dysfunction, cystic fibrosis, gastroesophageal reflux disease (GERD), Churg-Strauss syndrome

EVALUATION

History

- Frequency, duration, and severity of symptoms including shortness of breath, nocturnal cough, chest tightness
- History of medical care (emergency room visits, hospitalizations, intubations, steroid tapers, use of inhalers)
- Precipitating factors including allergens (such as perfumes, detergents, odors, molds, smoke), infections, GERD, cold air, drugs, emotional stress, physical activity

Physical Exam

- Assess for tachypnea, wheezing, increased expiratory phase of respiration, hyperresonance with chest percussion, use of accessory muscles.
- Check for nasal polyps, atopy.

Pulmonary Function Tests (PFTs)

- All patients should have PFTs to make diagnosis and rate severity. True asthma will show decreased forced expiratory volume (FEV1), increased total lung capacity (TLC) and residual volume (RV) with coving of flow-volume loop.
- Home monitoring of peak expiratory flow rates (PEFR) is helpful for those with more severe asthma.

Stepwise Classification

- 1997 National Institutes of Health (NIH) National Asthma Education and Prevention Program (NAEPP) reclassified categories of ambulatory asthma severity into four categories: mild intermittent, mild persistent, moderate persistent, and severe persistent (see Table 12.1).

TABLE 12.1 STEPWISE APPROACH FOR MANAGING ASTHMA IN ADULTS*

Step	Symptoms	Nighttime Symptoms	Lung Function	Long-term Control
Step 1: Mild intermittent	• Symptoms 2 times/week • Asymptomatic and normal PEFR between exacerbations • Exacerbations brief; intensity varies	2 times a month	• FEV_1 or PEFR = 80% predicted • PEFR variability <20%	No daily medication needed. Nighttime β_2-agonist
Step 2: Mild persistent	• Symptoms >2 times a week but <1 time a day • Exacerbations may affect activity	>2 times a month	• FEV_1 or PEFR = 80% predicted • PEFR variability 20–30%	Daily medication: • Antiinflammatory: either inhaled corticosteroid (low dose) or cromolyn or nedocromil (children usually begin with trial of cromolyn or nedocromil) • Zafirlukast or zileuton may also be considered for patients under age 12, although their position in therapy is not fully established. • Sustained-release theophylline to serum concentration of 5–15 mcg/mL is an alternative.
Step 3: Moderate persistent	• Daily symptoms • Daily use of inhaled short-acting β_2-agonist • Exacerbations affect activity • Exacerbations = 2 times a week; may last days	>1 time a week	• FEV_1 or PEFR >60%–80% predicted • PEFR variability >30%	Daily medications, either • Antiinflammatory: inhaled corticosteroid (medium dose), or • Inhaled corticosteroid (low-medium dose) and add a long-acting bronchodilator, especially for nighttime symptoms; either long-acting inhaled β_2-agonist, sustained-release theophylline, or long acting β_2-agonist tablets. If needed • Antiinflammatory: inhaled corticosteroids (medium-high dose), and • Long-acting bronchodilator, especially for nighttime symptoms; either long-acting inhaled β_2-agonist, sustained-release theophylline, or long acting β_2-agonist tablets. • Consider antileukotriene agent.
Step 4: Severe persistent	• Continual symptoms • Limited physical activity • Frequent exacerbations	Frequent	• FEV_1 or PEFR = 60% predicted • PEFR variability >30%	Daily medications: • Antinflammatory: inhaled corticosteroid (high dose), and • Long-acting bronchodilator: either long-acting inhaled β_2-agonist, sustained-release theophylline, or long-acting β_2-agonist tablets, and • Corticosteroid tablets or syrup long term (generally do not exceed 60 mg per day). • Consider antileukotriene agent.

PEFR, peak expiratory flow rates; FEV_1, forced expiratory volume.
* *Source*: Adapted from the National Institutes of Health, Expert Panel Report 2: Guidelines for the Diagnosis and Management of Asthma.

- If quick-relief medication is necessary more than twice a week, patient should be moved up to next level of care; conversely, if good control is maintained for at least 3 months, a step-down in classification may be considered.

TREATMENT

Education

- Most common causes of asthma therapy failure are noncompliance and poor metered dose inhaler (MDI) techniques.
- NAEPP (National asthma education and prevention program) recommends PEFR monitoring for all patients with moderate-to-severe persistent asthma, measured daily (best of three maximal attempts) upon awakening before using MDI.

Long-Term Control Medications (Table 12.1)

- Cromolyn and mast cell stabilizers
  ⇒ Stabilize mast cell membranes; inhibit eosinophil/epithelial mediator release by interfering with chloride channel function, thereby blocking both early and late response to allergens. Trials of 4 to 6 weeks may be needed to see full benefit.
  ⇒ Useful as prophylaxis prior to exercise or exposure to allergen.
- Inhaled corticosteroids
  ⇒ The most effective antiinflammatory medication currently available. By inhibiting cytokine production and inflammatory cell taxis/activation, they block the late reaction and reduce airway hyperresponsiveness.
  ⇒ Primary agent in all but mild intermittent disease.
  ⇒ May produce cough, dysphonia, and oral thrush. Adrenal suppression is more common with fluticasone (Flovent) than with other inhaled steroids (Derom, 2000). All side effects are diminished by spacer use.
- Long-acting β2 agonists (salmeterol MDI)
  ⇒ Mechanism: Adenylate cyclase activation → increased cAMP → bronchodilation.
  ⇒ When used as adjunct to antiinflammatory medication, may provide more effective control than increasing dose of steroid inhaler (Nelson et al., 1998).
  ⇒ Asthma control is better with low-to-moderate dose inhaled steroids plus salmeterol than with high dose inhaled steroids alone (Greening et al., 1994).
  ⇒ Side effects: tachycardia, tremor, and hypokalemia
- Methylxanthines (theophylline)
  ⇒ Mechanisms (not well understood): Adenosine receptor antagonism plus phosphodiesterase (PDE) effect → increased cAMP level → bronchodilation. May inhibit both early and late asthmatic responses.
  ⇒ Useful for nocturnal symptoms as adjunct to steroid MDI.
  ⇒ Side effects: multiple dose-related toxicities (tachycardia, arrhythmias, nausea, vomiting, diarrhea, headache, insomnia)
- Antileukotrienes
  ⇒ LTD4/LTE4 receptor competitive inhibitors (zafirlukast and montelukast), and a 5-lipoxygenase inhibitor (zileuton).
  ⇒ Alternative to steroid MDI in mild persistent asthma; adjunctive treatment in more severe disease.
  ⇒ Drug of choice in aspirin-sensitive asthmatics (Nasser et al., 1994); may be useful in exercise-induced bronchoconstriction (Leff et al., 1998).
  ⇒ Side effects of zafirlukast include inhibition of warfarin metabolism, rare cases of Churg-Strauss syndrome. Zileuton side effects include reversible transaminitis and inhibition of metabolism of terfenadine, warfarin, and theophylline.
- Steroid-sparing antiinflammatory medications
  ⇒ Methotrexate, cyclosporine, and troleandomycin can be effective in severe steroid-dependent asthma.
  ⇒ A recombinant human murine monoclonal anti-IgE antibody (RhuMAb-E25) is under investigation for allergic asthma.

Quick Relief Medications

- Short-acting β_2 agonist MDIs
  - $\Rightarrow$ Relieves acute symptoms; prevents exercise-induced bronchospasm; to be used "as needed."
- Anticholinergics
  - $\Rightarrow$ Second-line agent for relief of acute symptoms; medication of choice for bronchospasm induced by beta-blockers
- Systemic corticosteroids
  - $\Rightarrow$ For use with moderate-to-severe exacerbations (see Table 12.1)
  - $\Rightarrow$ Side effects: glucose intolerance, edema, mood alteration, hypertension, osteoporosis, immunosuppression

Action Plan for Home Treatment

- Studies have demonstrated clinical improvement with use of formal action plan (see Fig. 12.1).

RESOURCE

- National Heart, Lung, and Blood Institute (NHLBI) asthma website: http://www.nhlbisupport.com/asthma/index.html.

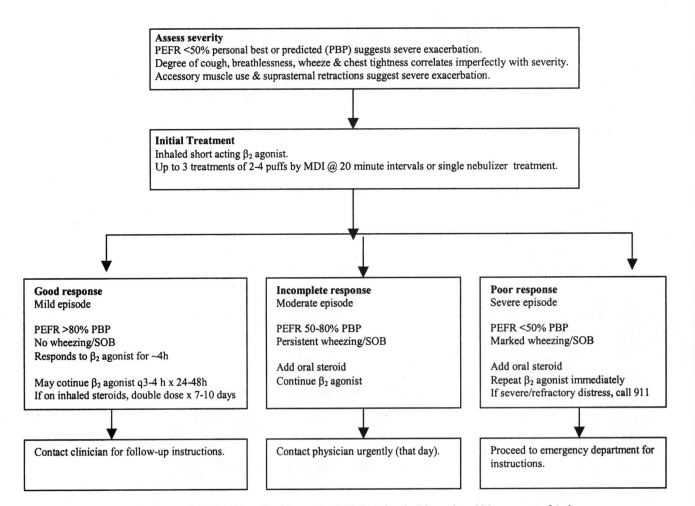

Assess severity
PEFR <50% personal best or predicted (PBP) suggests severe exacerbation.
Degree of cough, breathlessness, wheeze & chest tightness correlates imperfectly with severity.
Accessory muscle use & suprasternal retractions suggest severe exacerbation.

Initial Treatment
Inhaled short acting β_2 agonist.
Up to 3 treatments of 2-4 puffs by MDI @ 20 minute intervals or single nebulizer treatment.

Good response
Mild episode

PEFR >80% PBP
No wheezing/SOB
Responds to β_2 agonist for ~4h

May cotinue β_2 agonist q3-4 h x 24-48h
If on inhaled steroids, double dose x 7-10 days

Contact clinician for follow-up instructions.

Incomplete response
Moderate episode

PEFR 50-80% PBP
Persistent wheezing/SOB

Add oral steroid
Continue β_2 agonist

Contact physician urgently (that day).

Poor response
Severe episode

PEFR <50% PBP
Marked wheezing/SOB

Add oral steroid
Repeat β_2 agonist immediately
If severe/refractory distress, call 911

Proceed to emergency department for instructions.

*Source: National Institutes of Health. Expert Panel Report 2: Guidelines for the Diagnosis and Management of Asthma.

FIGURE 12.1: Management of asthma exacerbation (home action plan). (Adapted from the National Institutes of Health, Expert Panel Report 2: Guidelines for the Diagnosis and Management of Asthma.)

SELECTED REFERENCES

1. NIH Global Initiative for Asthma. Global Strategy for Asthma Management and Prevention. *NHLBI/WHO Workshop Report,* March 1993.
2. Derom E, Van Schoor J, Verhaeghe W, et al. Systemic effects of inhaled fluticasone propionate and budesonide in adult patients with asthma. *Am J Respir Crit Care Med* 1999;160(1):157–161.
3. Drazen JM, Israel E, O'Byrne PM, et al. Treatment of asthma with drugs modifying the leukotriene pathway. *N Engl J Med* 1999;340(3):197–206.
4. Drazen JM, Israel E, Boushey HA, et al. Comparison of regularly scheduled with as-needed use of albuterol in mild asthma. *N Engl J Med* 1996;335(12):841–847.
5. Evans DJ, Taylor DA, Zetterstrom O, et al. A comparison of low-dose inhaled budesonide plus theophylline and high-dose inhaled budesonide for moderate asthma. *N Engl J Med* 1997;337:1412–1418.
6. Greening AP, Ind PW, Northfield M, et al. Added salmeterol versus higher-dose corticosteroids in asthma patients with symptoms on existing inhaled corticosteroids. *Lancet* 1994;344(8917):219–224.
7. Laviolette M, Malmstrom K, Lu S, et al. Montelukast added to inhaled beclomethasone in treatment of asthma. *Am J Respir Crit Care Med* 1999;160(6):1862–1868.
8. Leff JA, Busse WW, Pearlman D, et al. Montelukast, a leukotriene-receptor antagonist, for the treatment of mild asthma and exercise-induced bronchoconstriction. *N Engl J Med* 1998;339:147–152.
9. Nasser SM, Bell GS, Foster S, et al. Effect of the 5-lipoxygenase inhibitor ZD2138 on aspirin-induced asthma. *Thorax* 1994;49(8):749–756.
10. Nelson JA, Strauss L, Skowronski M, et al. Effect of long-term salmeterol treatment on exercise-induced asthma. *N Engl J Med* 1998;339(3):141–146.
11. O'Byrne PM, Israel E, Drazen JM. Antileukotrienes in the treatment of asthma. *Ann Intern Med* 1997;127(6):472–480.

CHRONIC OBSTRUCTIVE PULMONARY DISEASE

INTRODUCTION

- Chronic obstructive pulmonary disease (COPD) is a progressive respiratory disorder characterized by some combination of cough, sputum production, dyspnea, airflow obstruction, and impaired gas exchange.
- COPD affects more than 10% of U.S. adults over age 55 and is the fourth leading cause of death in the United States.

PATHOPHYSIOLOGY/CLINICAL PRESENTATION

- Chronic bronchitis ("blue bloater"): Productive cough that lasts for 3 months in each of 2 successive years with other causes excluded
- Emphysema ("pink puffer"): Pathologic definition involving abnormal permanent enlargement of airspaces distal to terminal bronchioles, accompanied by destruction of their walls, without obvious fibrosis
- Cigarette smoking accounts for 80% to 90% of risk of developing COPD.
  - ⇒ Only 15% of smokers develop clinically significant COPD.
  - ⇒ Rate of forced expiratory volume (FEV_1) decline is directly related to age, number of pack-years, and number of cigarettes currently smoked; inversely related to initial FEV_1 and FEV_1/FVC (forced vital capacity).
  - ⇒ Age of starting, total pack-years, and current smoking status are directly predictive of COPD mortality. From time of initial diagnosis, 10-year mortality rate exceeds 50%.
  - ⇒ Once smokers have quit, their rate of FEV_1 decline returns to normal.
- Homozygous alpha-1-antitrypsin (AAT) deficiency accounts for less than 1% of COPD cases in the United States.
- Occupational exposures, such as cadmium, silica, dusts, and fumes, may increase risk.

EVALUATION

History

- Assess smoking history, family history, extent and triggers of dyspnea, functional status.

Physical Exam

- Useful findings include wheezing, barrel chest, decreased cardiac dullness, hyperresonant lungs, rhonchi (Hollerman and Simel, 1995).

Radiologic Data

- Specific chest x-ray (CXR) features: right dome of the diaphragm at or below seventh rib, retrosternal air space greater than 4.4 cm, cardiac diameter less than 11.5 cm (Burki, 1980).

- High-resolution chest CT (HRCT) is more sensitive and specific than CXR.
- Obstruction is diagnosed by an FEV_1/FVC ratio below fifth percentile (less than 0.7 in most adults), then graded by FEV_1. Symptoms often begin when FEV_1 drops below about 1.5 liters.

TREATMENT
Pharmacotherapy (Figure 13.1)

- **Anticholinergics** (ipratropium bromide)
  ⇒ Regular use for daily symptoms. Maximal doses of β_2-agonists produce same degree of bronchodilation (Easton et al., 1986).
  ⇒ Recommended dose (2 puffs four times daily) may be suboptimal; can be doubled or tripled without increased side effects.

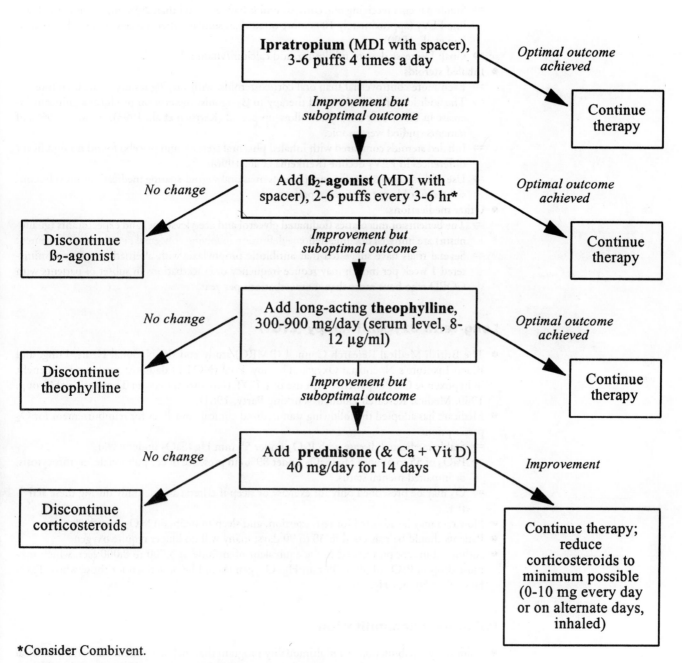

*Consider Combivent.

FIGURE 13.1. Typical chronic obstructive pulmonary disease (COPD) regimen. (Adapted from Ferguson G, Cherniack R. Management of COPD. *N Engl J Med* 1993;328:1017–1022.)

- β_2-agonists (albuterol)
  - ⇒ Appropriate initial nighttime inhaled therapy for patients with intermittent symptoms; should be used as second-line therapy to anticholinergics.
  - ⇒ Little evidence that regular use is more beneficial than PRN ("as occasion requires") use (Boueri and Make, 1999). Faster onset (5 to 15 minutes) than anticholinergics makes these better PRN medications.
- **Theophylline**
  - ⇒ Adding theophylline can result in additional benefit (Karpel, 1994). Consider for those without optimal clinical response.
  - ⇒ Monitor serum levels; discontinue if no symptomatic or spirometric benefit. Be cautious of drug interactions.
- **Corticosteroids**
  - ⇒ Role of systemic and inhaled therapy in stable COPD is controversial.
  - ⇒ Stable patients receiving oral corticosteroids have a greater than 20% improvement in baseline FEV_1 (approximately 10% more often than similar patients receiving placebo) (Callahan et al., 1990).
  - ⇒ Goal: Decrease dose to minimum, add calcium/vitamin D.
- **Inhaled steroids**
  - ⇒ Even more controversial than oral corticosteroids, with varying results in the literature.
  - ⇒ The addition of inhaled steroid therapy to β_2-agonist medication produces significant increase in FEV_1 over a 2.5-year follow-up period (Kertsjen et al., 1993). However, 56% of patients studied were atopic.
  - ⇒ Inhaled steroids compared with inhaled plus oral steroids and placebo found no significant differences in FEV_1 decline (Renkema et al., 1996).
  - ⇒ Use of these agents in refractory patients or as oral steroid-sparing medications must be considered until larger studies are performed.
- **Other medications**
  - ⇒ The benefits of mucolytics (iodinated glycerol and acetylcysteine) and expectorants (guaifenesin) are not well documented.
  - ⇒ Several trials have suggested that antibiotic prophylaxis with alternating agents administered 1 week per month may reduce frequency of exacerbations in subset of patients with COPD who have more than 4 exacerbations per year.

Long-Term Oxygen Therapy (LTOT)

- The British Medical Research Council (BMRC) study and the National Heart, Lung, and Blood Institute's Nocturnal Oxygen Therapy Trial (NOTT) demonstrated survival benefit in hypoxemic COPD patients with use of LTOT (Nocturnal Oxygen Therapy Trial Group, 1980; Medical Research Council Working Party, 1981).
- Medicare has adopted the following standardized clinical guidelines for reimbursement for O_2 prescription:
  - ⇒ Stable medicated disease with PaO_2 under 55 mm Hg (SaO_2 under 88%).
  - ⇒ PaO_2 of 55 to 59 mm Hg (SaO_2 under 89%) in presence of cor pulmonale, erythrocytosis, or impaired mental status.
  - ⇒ O_2 may be prescribed only for exercise or sleep if criteria are met only during these activities.
- Flow rate may be adjusted for rest, exertion, and sleep to maintain SaO_2 over 90%.
- Patients should be reassessed in 30 to 90 days; many will no longer require oxygen.
- Airline cabins are pressurized to the equivalent of altitude of 5,000 to 8,000 feet, which may cause drop in PaO_2 of 30 to 35 mm Hg. Oxygen should be prescribed for those whose PaO_2 falls below 50 mm Hg.

Pulmonary Rehabilitation

- Pulmonary rehabilitation is a multimodality program that includes patient education, medical care, respiratory/physical/occupational therapy, nutritional aid, exercise, and psychosocial assistance.

- Studies show improvement in objective scores of quality of life and health status, enhanced activities of daily living, improved psychological function, and fewer hospitalizations in year following rehabilitation. Survival studies have variable results.
- Cardiac and pulmonary stress testing should precede entry into program.

Surgery

- For select patients, bullectomy, lung-volume reduction surgery (LVRS), and lung transplantation may be considered.
- Lung-transplantation for appropriate patients is ultimate treatment for severe COPD. Single-lung transplantation is recommended in most cases as it improves FEV_1 by 20% to 50% with only slightly less gain in exercise performance than double-lung surgery.
- Preoperative evaluation should include the following:
  - ⇒ Stage II/III patients should be admitted 24 hours before surgery for maximal medical management.
  - ⇒ The further the incision from the diaphragm, the lower the risk.
  - ⇒ For abdominal surgery, patients with FEV_1 less than 1 liter are at increased risk.
  - ⇒ Steroids given after postoperative day 3 should not delay wound healing.
  - ⇒ Smoking cessation should precede surgery by at least 8 weeks.

COPD Exacerbation

- Triggers include viral or bacterial infections, airborne irritants, aspiration, pneumothorax, intercurrent illness, undermedication, sedatives, and cardiopulmonary events. Studies suggest viral etiology in 20% to 30% of flares.
- β_2-agonists and anticholinergics are useful. However, no data support practice of administering both. Ipratropium bromide and metaproterenol are equivalent in bronchodilation, but no further improvement occured when patients crossed over to other agent (Karpel, 1994).
- Systemic steroid administration should be used.
  - ⇒ Significant reduction in hospital stay and higher FEV_1 by 0.10 in treated group by 1 day after enrollment (Niewoehner et al., 1999).
  - ⇒ Maximal benefit with oral steroids achieved at 2 weeks; treating for 8 weeks has more side effects without additional benefit.
  - ⇒ Lower rate of treatment failure in steroid group at 30 days.
- Antibiotics during flares are controversial, but appear to be beneficial.
  - ⇒ While some studies have found no significant improvement, others have demonstrated statistically significant shortening of flare symptoms with antibiotic therapy (Anthonisen et al., 1982).
  - ⇒ A metaanalysis of nine trials found a small but statistically significant overall summary effect size of 0.22 supporting antibiotic therapy for flares (Saint et al., 1994).
- Theophylline has no demonstrated role for acute COPD flares (in contrast to its proven role in stable outpatient regimens).

FUTURE DIRECTIONS

- Tiotropium bromide produces significant improvement in airflow and symptom relief in COPD.
- Other drugs aimed at interfering with the cytokine inflammatory chain such as leukotriene B_4 (LTB_4) inhibitors, chemokine antagonists, matrix metalloproteinase (MMP) inhibitors, and NF-kB antagonists are still in development.

SELECTED REFERENCES

1. Anthonisen NR, Manfreda J, Warren CPW, et al. Antibiotic therapy in exacerbations of chronic obstructive pulmonary disease. *Ann Intern Med* 1982;106:196–204.
2. Boueri F, Make B. Current concepts in pharmacologic management of COPD. *Seminars in Respiratory and Critical Care Medicine* 1999;20(4):279–288.

3. Burki NK. Correlation of pulmonary function with the chest roentgenogram in chronic airway obstruction. *Ann Rev Respir Dis* 1980;121:217–223.
4. Callahan C, Dittus R, Katz B. Oral corticosteroid therapy for patients with stable chronic obstructive pulmonary disease. *Ann Intern Med* 1990;114:216–220.
5. Easton P, Jadue C, Dhinera S, et al. A comparison of the bronchodilating effects of a beta-2 adrenergic agent (albuterol) and an anticholinergic agent (ipratropium bromide), given by aerosol alone or in sequence. *N Engl J Med* 1986;315:735–739.
6. Ferguson G, Cherniack R. Management of COPD. *N Engl J Med* 1993;328:1017–1022.
7. Holleman D, Simel D. Does the clinical examination predict airflow limitation? *JAMA* 1995;273:313–319.
8. Karpel JP. Bronchodilator responses to anticholinergic and beta-adrenergic agents in acute and stable COPD. *Chest* 1994;99:871–874.
9. Kertsjens HA, Brand PL, Hughes MD, et al. A comparison of bronchodilator treatment with or without inhaled corticosteroid therapy for obstructive airway disease. *N Engl J Med* 1992;327:1413–1419.
10. Medical Research Council Working Party. Long term domiciliary oxygen therapy in chronic hypoxic cor pulmonale complicating chronic bronchitis and emphysema. *Lancet* 1981;1:681–686.
11. Niewoehner DE, Erbland ML, Deupree R, et al. Effect of systemic glucocorticoids on exacerbations of chronic obstructive pulmonary disease. Department of Veterans' Affairs Cooperative Study Group. *N Engl J Med* 1999;340:1941–1947.
12. Nocturnal Oxygen Therapy Trial Group. Continuous or nocturnal oxygen therapy in hypoxemic chronic obstructive lung disease: a clinical trial. *Ann Intern Med* 1980;93:391–398.
13. Renkema TE, Schouten JP, Koeter GH, et al. Effects of long-term treatment with corticosteroids in COPD. *Chest* 1996;109:1156–1162.
14. Saint S, Bent S, Vittinghoff E, et al. Antibiotics in COPD exacerbations. *JAMA* 1994;273:957–960.

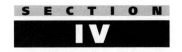

INFECTIOUS DISEASE

UPPER RESPIRATORY INFECTIONS: COMMON COLD, INFLUENZA, PHARYNGITIS, AND SINUSITIS

COMMON COLD

Introduction

- Common cold affects the average U.S. adult two to four times a year, and the average child five to seven times a year.
- Colds account for seven lost workdays per adult per year and have an estimated annual U.S. economic burden of $5 billion.

Pathogenesis

- Viral etiology: rhinoviruses (more than 110 serotypes; responsible for 30% to 40% of colds), respiratory syncytial virus (RSV), coronavirus, adenovirus, parainfluenza, influenza. Protective immunity is short-lived or absent, with multitude of viruses and serotypes (hence, development of a vaccine is unlikely).
- Rhinoviruses use intracellular adhesion molecule-1 (ICAM-1) to enter host cells. Infection begins in adenoidal area and spreads to nasal epithelium. Cytokine levels in nasal secretions, including interleukin-1 (IL-1), interleukin-6 (IL-6), and tumor necrosis factor (TNF), dramatically increase in first 24 hours of symptomatic infection.
- Direct hand-to-hand contact transmits infection most effectively; large aerosolized particles occasionally transmit virus. Wet feet and chill do not increase experimental transmission.
- Incubation is 24 to 72 hours; shedding lasts up to 14 days; symptoms generally resolve in 7 days (though cough may linger longer).
- Uncommon bacterial complications (less than 2%) include otitis media, sinusitis, pneumonia (sinus involvement typically viral and self-limited); a more common complication is exacerbation of reactive airway disease.
- Symptom complex: nasal congestion/drip; sneezing; sore, scratchy throat; laryngitis; ear/sinus discomfort; malaise; headache; fever.

Treatment (Table 14.1)

- Prevention of colds involves hand-washing and avoiding aerosol/mucous exposures. Neither vitamin C nor zinc prevents colds. Evidence suggests Echinacea taken at onset of symptoms may shorten duration of upper respiratory infections (URI), but efficacy for prevention not demonstrated (Melchart et al., 2000).
- Treatment for the cold is purely symptomatic. Antibiotics have been found to have no benefit.

TABLE 14.1 TREATMENT OF THE COMMON COLD

Treatment	Dose/Specifics	Mechanism/Evidence	Comments
Decongestants: Reduce secretions	Pseudoephedrine Afrin (nasal spray use for more than 3 days may cause rebound symptoms)	Alpha-adrenergics, vasoconstrict to reduce secretions	Phenylpropanolamine removed from market in 2000 (risk of hemorrhagic CVA)
Anticholinergics: Reduce secretions	Nasal ipratropium 0.06% qid × 4 days	RCT showed improved rhinorrhea/sneezing (Hayden et al., 1996)	
Expectorants/Steam: Loosen thick secretions	Guaifenesin Steam/hot soup/liquids	No benefit to guaifenesin, but steam/hot soup with subjective improvement/increased nasal patency	Risk-free and inexpensive
Antihistamines: Dry secretions	Chlorpheniramine Diphenhydramine	Systemic review without improvement in overall symptom score (Luks et al., 1996)	May be beneficial at night for sedating effects. May thicken secretions without changing volume.
Analgesics/NSAIDs	Tylenol Ibuprofen	For headache, fever, myalgias; no consistent effect on nasal secretions	
Cough suppressants	Codeine Dextromethorphan	More useful in long-term cough than acute viral URI; some studies show benefit	Cough may respond to bronchodilators (airway hyper-reactivity) or decongestants (postnasal drip)
Vitamin C	High dose, 1000 mg qd	Small studies suggested benefit, but not held up in metaanalyses. Recent systemic reviews suggest it may shorten sympton duration by half a day	Likely minimal effect as either treatment or prevention
Zinc	Cold-eez lozenges	Metaanalysis showed shortened symptom duration in 3 out of 6 trials (Jackson et al., 1997)	Limited usefulness given bad taste, nausea, need for frequent
Echinacea	300 mg PO tid (dried powder capsules)	Proposed immune stimulation properties and traditional use for URI have spurred trials; most studies small and methodologically flawed.	Possible efficacy as treatment, but not as prophylaxis; lozenges/teas/drinks likely not useful due to low dose.
Antibiotics/antivirals		No role for antibiotics, regardless of purulent sputum: rising drug resistance due to inappropriate use.	Interferon effective, but many local side effects and not used clinically

CVA, cerebrovascular accident; qid, four times daily; RCT, randomized controlled trial; NSAIDs, nonteroidal antiinflammatory drugs; URI, upper respiratory infection; qd, every day; po, by month; tid, three times a day.

INFLUENZA

Introduction

- Influenza is prevalent during winter months, primarily from December to early March.
- Influenza accounts for 20,000 deaths per year, especially among elderly (over age 65) and those with chronic illness.
- Vaccination remains the priority: prevention is far superior to treatment.

Pathogenesis

- Influenza A and B both epidemics and are transmitted person-to-person by aerosolization and oral mucous membrane contact. Both infect upper and lower respiratory epithelium.
- Influenza A is responsible for 80% of cases and more serious complications. It undergoes rapid antigenic drift of surface antigens (hemagglutinin, neuraminidase), requiring yearly changes in the vaccine, whereas influenza B does not. Antibody immunity to surface antigens reduces likelihood of infection and severity of illness if infection does occur.
- Abrupt onset of febrile illness with respiratory symptoms characterizes influenza; symptom constellation includes cough, sore throat, myalgia, headache, nasal congestion, and fatigue.

- Complications of influenza include primary pneumonia and secondary bacterial pneumonia (strep pneumonia most common, but *Staphylococcus aureus* seen with increased frequency); myositis; rhabdomyolysis (rare); Reye's syndrome (seen in children; associated with aspirin use; rare); central nervous system (CNS) disease (unusual).

Evaluation

- Diagnosis by one of three methods:
  - ⇒ **Culture** of nasal washing is the gold standard. Used early in season for public health reasons (that is, tracking epidemics and developing future vaccines).
  - ⇒ **Rapid antigen assay** of Dacron nasal swab. Highly sensitive and specific for both influenza A and B.
  - ⇒ **Clinical diagnosis** once flu is proven to exist in the community. Predictive value 70% by clinician for "influenza-like illness," defined by CDC as: fever (temperature over 100°F) plus cough *or* sore throat.

Treatment and Prevention

- Vaccination/prophylaxis (see Table 14.2):
  - ⇒ Vaccines contain inactivated influenza A and B viruses, which have been grown in chicken eggs, that are selected annually to provide the best antigenic match to the year's predicted epidemic. The actual fit varies yearly.
  - ⇒ It takes approximately 2 weeks to develop antibodies; vaccine should be given starting in late October.
  - ⇒ Vaccines prevent infection in 80% of healthy young people. In elderly nursing home residents, it is 50% to 60% effective in preventing hospitalization and 80% effective in preventing death from influenza.
  - ⇒ Adverse effects include: local tenderness (25% of adults, lasting up to 48 hours); systemic symptoms (rare, particularly in adults); delayed-type hypersensitivity to thimerosal. Risk of Guillain-Barré is low: only 1 additional case per million vaccinations, far lower than the risk of severe influenza in all age groups.
  - ⇒ Contraindications to vaccination include: allergy to egg or to the vaccine previously; previous Guillain-Barré; persons with an acute febrile illness (minor colds are not a contraindication).
  - ⇒ Live attenuated vaccine given intranasally is safe and effective; FDA approval is pending.

TABLE 14.2 TARGET GROUPS FOR ANNUAL INFLUENZA VACCINATION

People at high risk for complication(s) of influenza
People over age 50
Residents of long-term care facilities
Adults/children with chronic pulmonary or CV disease (including asthma)
Adults/children requiring care for chronic metabolic disease, renal dysfunction, hemoglobinopathy, or immunosuppression (including HIV)
Children (6 months to 18 years old) receiving long-term ASA therapy (risk for Reye's syndrome)
Women who will be in the second or third trimester of pregnancy during the influenza season (December to March)
People who can transmit influenza to those at high risk
Healthcare personnel
Employees of long-term care facilities
Employees of residences for people at high risk
Providers of home care to people at high risk
Household members (including children) of people at high risk
Groups to consider for vaccination
People at high risk traveling to areas where influenza virus may be circulating
People providing essential community services
Students and others in institutional settings
Any person wishing to reduce risk of influenza infection

CV, cardiovascular; ASA, aspirin.
Source: Adapted from Couch RB. Preventioin and treatment of influenza. *N Engl J Med* 2000;343: 1778–1787.

- Antiviral agents (see Table 14.3):
  - ⇒ Indications for chemoprophylaxis:
    1. Institutional outbreaks in places that house people at high risk, vaccinated or not (additive protective effects with vaccine). Continue until one week after outbreak.
    2. High-risk patients who are unvaccinated, or vaccinated less than 2 weeks prior to exposure.
    3. Immunodeficient patients (with a potential inadequate response to vaccination).
  - ⇒ Note: Most cases of influenza respond well to symptomatic treatment [rest, fluids, nonsteroidal antiinflammatory drugs (NSAIDs), cough suppressants], with symptom resolution by one week, and improvement in 2 to 5 days.
  - ⇒ Indications for treatment:
    1. High-risk patients who develop influenza, or patients with severe influenza.
    2. Early in illness course for those wishing to shorten duration of infection.
  - ⇒ A five-day course of amantadine/rimantadine started within 48 hours of symptoms shortens illness duration by approximately 1 day; do not use for treatment of index case and prophylaxis of contacts, as resistant strains develop in 25% to 35% of treated patients (Couch, 2000).
  - ⇒ Neuraminidase inhibitors (oseltamivir and zanamivir) block viral penetration of host cell surfaces. A five-day course initiated within 48 hours decreases symptoms by 1 to 1.5 days, and reduces frequency of complications (14% vs. 46%) and antibiotic use (14% vs. 38%) (MIST Study Group, 1998). Resistance is rare with oseltamivir (1.5%) and not reported with zanamivir.
  - ⇒ Selection of the "best" agent remains controversial. Although neuraminidase inhibitors are expensive and less cost-effective for prophylaxis, they are preferred for treatment because of fewer side effects, efficacy against both influenza A and B, minimal resistance, and evidence of decreased complication rate.

TABLE 14.3 ANTINFLUENZAL AGENTS

	Prophylaxis	Efficacy/Cost Per 5d	Dose	Metabolism	Adverse Effects
Amantadine	Prevents 50% of infections, 70%–90%, of illnesses	Influenza A only $1.72 generic	100 mg bid, 100 mg qd if over age 65 or CrCl under 50	Renal	CNS (13% delerium, nervousness, seizures), GI
Rimantadine	Prevents 50% of infections, 70%–90% of illnesses	Influenza A only $18.87	100 mg bid, 100 mg qd if over age 65 CrCl under 10, or hepatic dysfunction	Hepatic metabolism, renal clearance	CNS (6%, less than amantadine), GI
Oseltamivir (Tamiflu)	Prevents 50% of infections, 80% of illnesses	Influenza A and B $53.00	150 mg, decrease for CrCl under 30	Renal	N/V, relieved if dosed with food
Zanamivir (Relenza)	FDA approval pending (efficacy good)	Influenza A and B $44.40	10 mg inhaler bid (qd for prophylaxis in studies)	Inhaled, little bioavailable	Possible bronchospasm

bid, twice daily; qd, every day; CrCl, creatinine clearance; CNS, central nervous syndrome; GI, gastrointestinal; N/V, nausea and vomiting.

PHARYNGITIS

Introduction

- The bacterial agent of concern is group A β-hemolytic streptococcus (GABHS, *S. pyogenes*), the causative agent in 5% to 15% of adult cases.
- For GABHS, antibiotics shorten duration of symptoms and prevent suppurative complications (e.g., peritonsillar abscess) and rheumatic fever (the primary reason for treatment). Antibiotics do not prevent scarlet fever; controversy exists over their role in preventing poststreptococcal glomerulonephritis.

Differential Diagnosis (Table 14.4)

TABLE 14.4 DIFFERENTIAL DIAGNOSIS OF ACUTE PHARYNGITIS

GABHS	Group A β-Hemolytic Streptococcus (*S. pyogenes*)
Viral (25% of pharyngitis)	"Mononucleosis syndromes" (EBV, CMV), adenovirus, rhinovirus, parainfluenza, HSV, echovirus, coxsackievirus, HIV-1 acute retroviral syndrome
Other bacterial (non-GABHS)	*Chlamydia, gonococcus, mycoplasma. tularemia, diphtheria, yersinia* group C and G β hemolytic streptococcus
Fungal	Candida (rare consider in immunocompromised hosts)
Peritonsillar/retropharyngeal abscess	Caused by strep or other organisms

EBV, Epstein-Barr virus, CMV, cytomegalovirus; HSV, herpes simplex virus.

Evaluation

- History/physical exam:
  ⇒ Exposures: sick children, documented strep throat or mononucleosis contacts, oral sex [chlamydia, gonorrhea (GC), herpes simplex virus (HSV)], HIV risk factors (consider diagnosis of acute HIV).
  ⇒ Group A strep: typically presents in winter and early spring, most frequently in patients 5 to 15 years old.
  ⇒ Group A strep symptoms: sudden onset sore throat, odynophagia, fever, headache, nausea and vomiting (especially in children). Unusual symptoms include coryza, cough, and hoarseness (more indicative of viral etiology).
  ⇒ Group A strep signs: tonsillopharyngeal erythema/exudate, soft palate petechiae, anterior cervical adenopathy. Scarlet fever: concurrent scarlatiniform (sandpaper) rash on the trunk, groin, and axillae.
  ⇒ Infectious mononucleosis: classic pentad of fatigue, fever, pharyngitis, anterior and posterior cervical lymphadenopathy (50% have splenomegaly), and leukopenia with atypical lymphocytosis.
  ⇒ Primary HIV symptoms: acute onset, little to no tonsillar hypertrophy, maculopapular rash in 70%, occasional mucosal ulcers, arthralgias, myalgias, lethargy. Incubation 3 to 5 weeks.
- Diagnostic testing:
  ⇒ **Throat culture:** the gold-standard. Sensitivity is greater than 90%, specificity is 75% to 99% when culture collected properly (wipe tip of swab around back wall of pharynx, then roll down side of each tonsil). Preliminary results at 24 hours, final results at 48 hours.
  ⇒ **Rapid strep test:** an ELISA test looking for Group A strep antigen by extraction, with results in less than 1 hour. Median sensitivity of various products is 78%, median specificity is 97%. Given the relatively low sensitivity, controversy exists over the need to follow all negative rapid strep tests with a culture, particularly in adults where incidence of rheumatic fever is low.
  ⇒ **Clinical diagnosis:** poor, despite the use of multiple clinical criteria and algorithms. Most helpful in excluding those with a very low likelihood of strep.
  ⇒ Further studies if clinical suspicion: heterophile antibody (infectious mononucleosis); RNA polymerase chain reaction (PCR) for viral load with baseline enzyme-linked immunosorbent assay (ELISA) HIV antibody (primary HIV); Dacron swab for chlamydial and GC culture, mycoplasma PCR, HSV culture (unroof vesicle and swab base); fungal culture (Candida).
- Antibiotics (see Fig. 14.1):
  ⇒ A recent literature review argues that risk of excessive antibiotics for acute pharyngitis outweighs the fairly minimal risk of group A strep complications (Cooper et al., 2001). The goal of treatment is to exclude the large majority of patients who do not need antibiotics. Note that rheumatic fever is preventable even with a treatment delay of up to 9 days.
  ⇒ GABHS is universally sensitive to penicillin (PCN): regimen is PCN V 500 mg twice daily or 250 mg four times daily for 10 days.

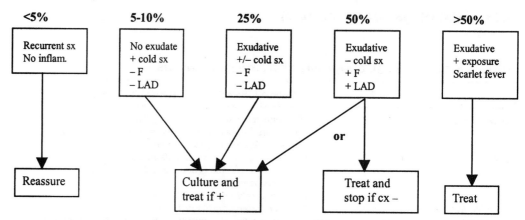

FIGURE 14.1. Potential decision-analysis for diagnosis and treatment of group A β-hemolytic streptococcus (GABHS) based on history and physical exam.

⇒ For noncompliant patients: single intramuscular (IM) injection of PCN (1.2 million units IM of PCN G).

⇒ For PCN allergic patients, a macrolide (erythromycin 500 mg twice daily for 10 days) may be used as a second-line agent. Recent studies of shorter course macrolides or cephalosporins show equal or superior efficacy, but are not standard given cost and resistance issues.

⇒ Analgesics and antipyretics should be recommended to all patients with pharyngitis.

ACUTE SINUSITIS

Introduction

● Sinusitis is classified as acute (less than 4 weeks) or chronic (more than 12 weeks), and infectious (viral, bacterial, fungal) or noninfectious (allergic, vasculitic, toxic).

Pathogenesis

● 87% of common colds include sinus inflammation (acute viral rhinosinusitis), which differs from acute sinusitis with ostial obstruction and infected fluid collection. Ciliated epithelia quickly denude, making it difficult to clear the infection. Bacterial sinusitis follows only 0.5% of all colds.

● Obstruction typically occurs at the osteo-meatal complex (OMC), the drainage area for the maxillary/frontal/anterior ethmoid sinuses, most commonly from viral or allergic rhinitis.

● Bacterial agents: *S. pneumoniae* (34%), *H. influenzae* (23%), gram-negative rods (GNRs) (9%), *M. catarrhalis* (2%), *S. pyogenes* (2%), *S. aureus* (4%) and anaerobes (6%). Fungal agents are much less common.

Evaluation and Diagnostic Testing

● Patients may have fever, ear pressure, halitosis, dental pain and fatigue, but classically present with: facial pain, headache, nasal congestion, purulent nasal discharge.

● **Sinus puncture:** Aspiration and culture of purulent secretions is the gold standard, but impractical in regular office practice.

● **Clinical diagnosis:** Symptoms which suggest bacterial processes include: symptoms lasting longer than 7 days; purulent nasal discharge; maxillary tooth/facial pain (particularly when unilateral); unilateral maxillary sinus tenderness; worsening of symptoms after initial improvement (Hickner et al., 2001).

● **Laboratory tests:** Helpful only if considering a systemic process (Wegener's, sarcoid, cystic fibrosis, immunodeficiency)

● **Imaging:** Although not usually indicated, consider sinus computed tomography (CT) if: the initial diagnosis is in question; symptoms persist after 10 to 14 days of initial medical treatment (rule out obstructive lesions); there have been recurrent episodes (more than 4 in a year).

Treatment

- Decongestants (oral preferred to intranasal): Effective in shrinking edema without overdrying secretions, helps open ostia and improve drainage. Drainage alone often clears infection. Expectorants, steam, intranasal saline, and NSAIDs also may relieve symptoms.
- Intranasal steroids are not recommended unless acute allergic component is obvious. Likewise, antihistamines are not recommended as they may thicken secretions and prevent drainage.
- Antibiotics: Add if symptoms persist for more than 7 days without improvement, particularly with the above constellation of findings. Start immediately for severe rhinosinusitis symptoms.
- Evidence-based regimens: penicillin or amoxicillin 500 mg orally three times a day for 10 days; Bactrim 1 double strength tablet orally twice daily for 10 days (Williams et al., 2000). No data show superior outcomes with newer, more expensive antibiotics, but quinolones and macrolides are well tolerated and at least equally efficacious.
- Rare complications of bacterial sinusitis include periorbital cellulitis, cortical vein and cavernous sinus thrombosis, subdural empyema, intracranial abscesses, and meningitis. Patients with symptoms suggestive of a complication require emergent intravenous antibiotics, imaging, lumbar puncture, and neurosurgical and ears, nose, throat (ENT) evaluation.
- Indications for referral to subspecialist:
  ⇒ Four courses of antibiotics within a year for recurrent sinusitis.
  ⇒ Persistent symptoms for more than 3 months while on therapy.

SELECTED REFERENCES

1. Adam D, Scholz H, Helmerking M, et al. Short-course antibiotic treatment of 4782 culture-proven cases of group A Streptococcal tonsillopharyngitis and incidence of post streptococcal sequelae. *J Infect Dis* 2000;182:509–516.
2. Bisno AL. Acute pharyngitis. *N Engl J Med* 2000;344:205–211.
3. Cooper RJ, Hoffman JR, Bartlett JG, et al. Principles of appropriate antibiotic use for acute pharyngitis in adults: background. *Ann Intern Med* 2001;134:509–517.
4. Couch RB. Prevention and treatment of influenza. *N Engl J Med* 2000;343:1778–1787.
5. Gonzales R, Bartlett JG, Besser RE, et al. Principles of appropriate antibiotic use for treatment of nonspecific upper respiratory tract infections in adults: background. *Ann Intern Med* 2001;134:490–494.
6. Guarderas JC. Rhinitis and sinusitis: office management. *Mayo Clin Proc* 1996;71:881–888.
7. Gwaltney JM Jr. Acute community-acquired sinusitis. *Clin Infect Dis* 1996;23:1209–1225.
8. Hayden FG, Atmar RL, Schilling M, et al. Use of the selective oral neuraminidase inhibitor oseltamivir to prevent influenza. *N Engl J Med* 1999;341:1336–1343.
9. Hayden FG, Diamond L, Wood PB, et al. Effectiveness and safety of intranasal ipratropium bromide in common colds. A randomized, double-blind, placebo-controlled trial. *Ann Intern Med* 1996;125:89–97.
10. Hayden FG, Gubareva LV, Monto AS, et al. Inhaled zanamivir for the prevention of influenza in families. *N Engl J Med* 2000;343:1282.
11. Hayden FG, Osterhaus AD, Treanor JJ, et al. Efficacy and safety of the neuraminidase inhibitor zanamivir in the treatment of influenza A virus infections. *N Engl J Med* 1997:874–878.
12. Hickner JM, Bartlett, JG, Besser RE, et al. Principles of appropriate antibiotic use for acute rhinosinusitis in adults: background. *Ann Intern Med* 2001;134:498–505.
13. Jackson JL, Peterson C, Lesho E. A meta-analysis of zinc salt lozenges and the common cold. *Arch Intern Med* 1997;157:2373.
14. Lorber B. The common cold. *J Gen Intern Med* 1996;11:229–236.
15. Luks D, Anderson MR, et al. Antihistamines and the common cold. *J Gen Intern Med* 1996;11:240–244.
16. Melchart D, Linde K, Fischer P, et al. Echinacea for preventing and treating the common cold. *Cochrane Database Syst Rev* 2000;(2):CD000530.
17. MIST (Management of Influenza in the Southern Hemisphere) Study Group. Randomized trial of efficacy and safety of inhaled zanamivir in treatment of influenza A and B virus infection. *Lancet* 1998;352:1877–1881.
18. Monto AS, Robinson DP, Herlocher ML, et al. Zanamivir in the prevention of influenza among healthy adults: a randomized controlled trial. *JAMA* 1999;282:31–35.
19. Nichol KL, Mendelman PM, Mallon KP, et al. Effectiveness of live, attenuated intranasal influenza virus vaccine in healthy, working adults. *JAMA* 1999;282:137.
20. Perkins A. An approach to diagnosing the acute sore throat. *Am Fam Prac* 1997;55:131–138.
21. Williams JW Jr, Aguilar C, Makela M, et al. Antibiotics for acute maxillary sinusitis. *Cochrane Database Syst Rev* 2000;2:CD000243.

BRONCHITIS AND PNEUMONIA

ACUTE BRONCHITIS

Introduction

- More than 10 million annual primary care visits for acute cough.
- The term "acute bronchitis" is often used for patients without underlying lung disease who present with acute cough but no clinical evidence of pneumonia.

Pathophysiology/Clinical Presentation

- Defining feature: infection and inflammation of trachea and bronchial tree up to distal respiratory bronchioles
- Predominant causes: respiratory viruses (rhinovirus, coronavirus, adenovirus, parainfluenza, respiratory syncytial virus, enteroviruses) and nonviral agents (*Mycoplasma pneumoniae*, *Chlamydia pneumoniae*, *Bordetella pertussis*)
- Unclear role of common respiratory flora (*Streptococcus pneumoniae*, *Haemophilus influenzae*, *Moraxella catarrhalis*)

Differential Diagnosis

- Diagnosis of exclusion. Consider other causes of cough:
    ⇒ Sinusitis: fever, headache, purulent nasal discharge, facial pain
    ⇒ Influenza: abrupt onset of systemic symptoms including fever, chills, headache, myalgias, malaise
    ⇒ Pneumonia: fever, dyspnea, pleuritic pain, chills
    ⇒ Asthma: wheezing, dyspnea, nocturnal cough, eczema, asthma, family history, exercise intolerance
    ⇒ Allergic rhinitis: seasonal variation in symptoms, rhinorrhea, eczema, watery eyes
    ⇒ Reflux esophagitis: heartburn, sour taste in mouth

Evaluation

- History: Acute cough, often initially accompanied by nasal congestion, rhinorrhea, or sore throat. Cough may persist and/or progress for 1 to 3 weeks, despite resolution of other symptoms after 3 to 4 days. Sputum production occurs in 50% of cases. Sputum purulence and color is neither sensitive nor specific for bacterial infection. Fever may or may not be present.
- Lung exam: Generally reveals clear lungs or diffuse wheezes/rhonchi from bronchospasm.
- Diagnostic testing: In nontoxic-appearing patients without clinical evidence of pneumonia, evaluation should be limited to complete blood count (CBC)/differential. In patients with productive cough, consider sputum gram stain/culture.

Treatment

- Antibiotics: Despite common viral etiology, antibiotics are prescribed for up to 75% of ambulatory patients. A metaanalysis by Fahey and colleagues (1998) (number of patients = 515) found antibiotics not to resolve productive cough vs. placebo after 1 to 2 weeks of therapy.

- Bronchodilators: Cough associated with tracheobronchial tree infection may result from bronchospasm. Small studies have found albuterol inhaler superior to placebo in relieving cough.
- Other symptomatic treatments: Expectorants, antihistamines, cough suppressants, hydration. Dextromethorphan (30 mg by mouth every 6 hours) is usually sufficient to suppress cough.

COMMUNITY-ACQUIRED PNEUMONIA

Introduction

- Defined by American Thoracic Society as pneumonia acquired outside the hospital setting, including those acquired in nursing homes or chronic care facilities.
- 4 million annual cases, 600,000 hospitalizations. Overall mortality 1% to 5%, but approaches 25% in patients admitted to hospitals.

Pathophysiology/Clinical Presentation

- Pneumonia results when bacteria reach the lower respiratory tract/alveoli and proliferate.
- Most common organism is *S. pneumonia*. Other common causes are *M. pneumoniae, C. pneumoniae, L. pneumophila.*
- Etiology not identified in 50% of patients despite extensive testing. Studies show etiology cannot be determined based on clinical presentation (thus, the typical vs. atypical pneumonia distinction is largely artificial). Up to 30% of patients without identified cause (sputum culture, blood culture, serology) have pneumococcal pneumonia, as detected by transthoracic needle aspiration (see Table 15.1).

TABLE 15.1 PATHOGENS IN COMMUNITY-ACCQUIRED PNEUMONIA AND MORTALITY RISK

Under Age 60, Without Comorbid Illnesses*	Age 60 or Older, with Comorbid Illnesses	Hospitalized, Illnesses not Severe	Hospitalized, ICU
S. pneumoniae	*S. pneumoniae*	*S. pneumoniae*	*S. pneumoniae*
M. pneumoniae	Resiratory viruses	*H. influenzae*	Legionella species
Resiratory viruses	*H. influenzae*	Polymicrobial (including anaerobic bacteria)	Aerobic GN bacilli
C. pneumoniae	Aerobic GN bacilli	Aerobic GN bacilli	*M. pneumoniae*
H. influenzae	*S. aureus*	Legionella species	Respiratory viruses
Legionella species	*Moraxella catarrhalis*	*S. aureus*	*H. influenzae*
S. aureus	Legionella species	*C. pneumoniae*	*M. tuberculosis*
M. tuberculosis	*M. tuberculosis*	Resiratory viruses	Endemic fungi
Endemic fungi	Endemic fungi	*M. pneumoniae*	
Aerobic GN bacilli		*Moraxella catarrhalis*	
		M. tuberculosis	
		Endemic fungi	
Mortality: 1%–5%	Mortality: less than 5%	Mortality: 5% to 25%	Mortality: up to 50%

* Comorbid illnesses include chronic obstructive pulmonary disease, diabetes mellitus, chronic renal insufficiency congestive heart failure, ICU intensive care unit; GN, gram negative.
Source: Adapted from American Thoracic Society. Guidelines for the initial management of adults with community-acquired pneumonia: diagnosis, assessment of severity, and initial antimicrobial therapy. *Am Rev Respir Dis* 1993;48:1418–1426.

- Nursing-home acquired pneumonia is not categorized separately because location is less important than age or coexisting disease. Methicillin-resistant *Staphylococcus aureus, Mycobacterium tuberculosis,* and influenza are more common in this population.
- As severity increases, so does the incidence of gram-negative bacilli, *Legionella,* and polymicrobial infections (aspiration of oropharyngeal secretions).
- Aspiration pneumonia refers to aspiration of gastric contents ± bacteria-laden upper respiratory secretions. Risk factors for developing pneumonia from aspiration include: stroke history, neuromuscular disease, sedation, obtundation, alcoholism, dysphagia, intubation, or chronic illness.

Evaluation

History

- Common symptoms include fever, chills, pleuritic pain, dyspnea, cough with purulent sputum.
- 10% to 30% of patients complain of headache, nausea, vomiting, abdominal pain, diarrhea, myalgias, arthralgias.
- Patients over age 65 may present with confusion or tachypnea only.
- Consider place of residence, comorbid illness, recent hospitalization, prior pneumonia episodes, recent antibiotic use, steroids/immunosuppressive agents, HIV risk factors, absence of spleen, occupational history, travel history, animal/bird exposure, immunization status, ill contacts.

Physical Exam

- Check vital signs, work of breathing (accessory musculature use, flaring nostrils). Rule out effusion (dullness to percussion, decreased tactile fremitus, decreased breath sounds). Rule out consolidation (dullness to percussion, increased tactile fremitus, crackles, bronchial breath sounds).

Diagnostic Testing

- Chest radiograph: X-ray showing infiltrate is the diagnostic "gold standard."
- Blood cultures: Two sets are recommended for hospitalized patients (prior to antibiotics if possible).
- Sputum gram stain/culture: Although controversial, a quality specimen (defined as fewer than 10 epithelial cells, more than 25 neutrophils, and more than 10 organisms per 100x field) is valuable towards therapy selection.
- *Legionella* urinary antigen: 70% to 90% sensitive for *L. pneumophila* serogroup 1 (responsible for 70% of *Legionella* infections).
- *Mycoplasma* cold agglutinins: Titer greater than or equal to 1:128 suggests infection.
- DNA-based assays: *Mycoplasma pneumoniae* polymerase chain reaction (PCR) and *Chlamydia pneumoniae* PCR are now available at many laboratories.
- Other serologies: Consider electrolytes, blood urea nitrogen (BUN), creatinine, CBC/differential, serum glutamic oxaloacetic transaminase (SGOT), alkaline phosphatase, bilirubin (may aid risk stratification).

PORT scores: Prognosis and Indications for Hospitalization

- Calculation of PORT (Pneumonia Patient Outcomes Research Team) score assists with risk stratification (based on validated instrument described by Fine et al.), and may help guide decision to hospitalize vs. to treat as outpatient (see Tables 15.2 and 15.3).
- Limitations: Higher level care may be warranted for patients with medical or psychosocial contraindications to outpatient therapy (intractable vomiting; situations limiting compliance such as alcoholism, intravenous drug abuse, severe psychiatric disorders; concomitant conditions such as immunosuppression or neuromuscular disease).

TABLE 15.2 ASSIGNMENT OF POINTS FOR PORT SCORE CALCULATION

Demographics	Comorbidities	Physical Exam	Laboratory
Male (+ age in years)	Neoplasm (+ 30)	Change MS (+ 20)	pH <7.35 (+ 30)
Female (Age − 10)	Liver disease (+ 20)	RR >30 (+ 20)	BUN >30 (+ 20)
Nursing home (+ 10)	CHF (+ 10)	SBP <90 (+ 20)	Sodium <130 (+ 20)
	CVA + 10)	T <35 or >40 (+ 15)	Glucose >250 (+ 10)
	Renal disease (+ 10)	HR >125 (+ 10)	PaO_2 <60 or SaO_2 <90 (+ 10)
			Pleural effusion (+ 10)

PORT, Pneumonia Patient Outcomes Research Team; CHF, congenital heart failure; CVA, cerebrovascular accident; MS, mental status; RR, respiratory rate; SBP, systolic blood pressure; T, Patient Outcomes Research Team; HR, heart rate; BUN, blood urea nitrogen (Fine et al. 1997).

TABLE 15.3 MORTALITY AND SUGGESTED TRIAGE BASED ON PORT SCORE

PORT Score	Class	Mortality	Suggested Triage
Age <50, no comorbidities	I	0.1%–0.4%	Outpatient
Score ≤70	II	0.6%–0.7%	Outpatient
Score 71–90	III	0.9%–2.8%	Outpatient/inpatient observation
Score 91–130	IV	8.2%–9.3%	Inpatient
Score >130	V	27.0%–31.1%	Intensive care unit

PORT, Pneumonia Patient Outcomes Research Team (Fine et al. 1997).

Treatment

- Duration: Consensus statements suggest 7 to 10 days of therapy. *M. pneumoniae* and *C. pneumoniae* may require 10 to 14 days; *Legionella* requires 14 days; immunosuppressed patients require up to 21 days (see Table 15.4).

TABLE 15.4 THERAPY RECOMMENDATIONS

Under Age 60 AND no Comorbid Illness (Oral Therapy)	Age 60 or Older OR Comorbid Illness (Oral Therapy)	Hospitalized, Not Severe (Intravenous Therapy)	Hospitalized, ICU (Intravenous Therapy)
Macrolide (erythromycin, clarithromycin, azithromycin) OR **Tetracycline** (doxycycline)	**Cephalosporin** (second generation OR Amoxicillin-clavulanate OR **Bactrim*** OR Newer **Fluoroquinolone** (levofloxacin, grepafloxacin)	**Cephalosporin** (second or third generation: cefuroxime, ceftriaxone, cefotaxime) ± Macrolide (if *Legionella* is a concern) OR **Ampicillin-sulbactam** ± macrolide OR **Bactrim + macrolide** (in penicillin-allergic patients)	**Third-generation cephalosporin** with antipseudomonal activity (ceftazidime) + macrolide OR **Imipenem†** OR **Levofloxacin + macrolide†**

* Note: Add macrolide if *Legionella* is a concern.
† Note: Add gentamicin to all above regimens for first few days of therapy.
Sources: Based on guidelines from the American Thoracic Society, the Canadian Community Acquired Pneumonia Consensus Conference Group, and The Medical Letter.

- *S. pneumonia:* Antibiotic recommendations in the 2000 Infectious Disease Society of America guidelines have been made for organisms with susceptibility to penicillin (parenteral penicillin G or oral amoxicillin), intermediate susceptibility (parenteral penicillin or parenteral amoxicillin), and high-level resistance (intravenous vancomycin or fluoroquinolone).

SELECTED REFERENCES

1. American Thoracic Society. Guidelines for the initial management of adults with community-acquired pneumonia: diagnosis, assessment of severity, and initial antimicrobial therapy. *Am Rev Respir Dis* 1993;48:1418–1426.
2. Abramowicz M, ed. The choice of antibacterial drugs. *Med Lett Drugs Ther* 1998;40:33–42.
3. Bartlett JG, Breiman RF, Mandell LA, et al. Community-acquired pneumonia in adults: guidelines for management. *Clin Infect Dis* 1998;26:811–838.
4. Bartlett JG, Mundy LM. Community-acquired pneumonia. *N Engl J Med* 1995;333:1618–1624.
5. Fahey T, Stocks N, Thomas T. Quantitative systematic review of randomised controlled trials comparing antibiotic with placebo for acute cough in adults. *BMJ* 1998;316:906–910.
6. Fine MJ, Auble TE, Yealy DM, et al. A prediction rule to identify low-risk patients with community-acquired pneumonia. *N Engl J Med* 1997;336:243–250.
7. Gwaltney JM Jr. Rhinoviruses. In: Evans AS, ed. *Viral infections in humans: epidemiology and control,* 3rd ed. New York: Plenum, 1989:593–615.

8. Hueston WJ. Albuterol metered-dose inhaler in the treatment of acute bronchitis. *J Fam Pract* 1994;39:437–440.

9. Mainous AG, Zoorob RJ, Hueston WJ. Current management of acute bronchitis in ambulatory care: The use of antibiotics and bronchodilators. *Arch Fam Med* 1996;5:79–83.

10. Marrie TJ. Community-acquired pneumonia. *Clin Infect Dis* 1994;18:501–515.

11. Metlay JP, Stafford RS, Singer DE. National trends in the management of acute cough by primary care physicians. *J Gen Intern Med* 1997;12(suppl):77.

12. Napolitano LA, Swartz MN. Community-acquired pneumonia. In: Lee BW, Hsu SI, Stasior DS, eds. *Quick consult manual of evidence-based medicine.* Philadephia: Lippincott-Raven, 1997:586.

13. Oeffinger KC, Snell LM, Foster BM, et al. Diagnosis of acute bronchitis in adults: A national survey of family physicians. *J Fam Pract* 1997;45:402–409

14. Ruiz-Gonzalez A, Falguera M, Nogues A, et al. Is *Streptococcus pneumoniae* the leading cause of pneumonia of unknown etiology? A microbiologic study of lung aspirates in consecutive patients with community-acquired pneumonia. *Am J Med* 1999;106:385–390.

15. Bartlett JG, Dowell SF, Mandell LA, et al. Practice guidelines for the management of community-acquired pneumonia in adults. *Clin Infect Dis* 2000;31:347–382.

PPD TESTING AND LATENT TUBERCULOSIS INFECTION

INTRODUCTION

- PPD is a 0.1 mL intradermal injection of "purified protein derivative" containing five tuberculin units, typically placed in the volar forearm. Results are read 48 to 72 hours after placement. Reactions remain positive for up to one week.
- PPD tests measure induration, not erythema.
- PPD response becomes positive within 1 to 10 weeks of tuberculosis (TB) infection.

EVALUATION

- Screening the general population is not recommended. The Centers for Disease Control and Prevention (CDC) recommends screening people with:
  ⇒ **High risk of TB exposure:** Close contact with TB-infected person; intravenous drug use; born in country where TB is common and living in the United States less than 5 years; residents and employees of long-term care facilities, prisons, homeless shelters; health care workers; some medically underserved, low-income populations, and high-risk ethnic groups.
  ⇒ **High risk of progressing to active TB once infected:** Known or suspected HIV; substance abuse; *M. tuberculosis* infection within past 2 years; diabetes mellitus; silicosis; prolonged corticosteroid therapy (equivalent of prednisone 15 mg per day for 1 month); other immunosuppressive therapy; cancer of the head or neck; hematologic or reticuloendothelial diseases (leukemia/Hodgkin's); end-stage renal disease; intestinal bypass/gastrectomy; chronic malabsorption; weight 10% below ideal.
- Classifying tuberculin reactions:
  ⇒ **5 mm** induration is considered positive in patients with known/suspected HIV; recent contact with TB-infected person; chest x-ray (CXR) suggestive of previous TB (Ghon's complex, upper-lobe scarring) but inadequate or no past treatment; immunosuppressant therapy.
  ⇒ **10 mm** induration is considered positive in patients at high risk for TB exposure and/or high risk for progression to active TB once infected (see above); children under 4 years old; adults who received bacille Calmette-Guérin (BCG) as infant. (Typically, BCG is given once to infants. Only 50% develop a positive PPD as infants, and 20% by age 2. The PPD reaction in patients with prior BCG is usually less than 10 mm, but can be up to 18. If greater than 20 mm, it's unlikely to be due to BCG.)
  ⇒ **15 mm** induration is considered positive in persons with no known risk factors for TB.
- Anergy testing ("placing controls"): Up to 60% of AIDS patients are anergic. However, the CDC no longer recommends anergy testing for HIV+ persons because: standardization/reproducibility of candida and mumps antigen tests are lacking; diagnosis of anergy is not associated with higher risk of TB vs. nonanergic populations; TB preventive therapy in HIV+ anergic patients is not beneficial. Utility of anergy testing overall has been questioned; not recommended by many experts.

- False negatives may occur with: severe febrile or chronic illness, administration of cortico-steroids/immunosuppressive drugs; measles/other viral infections; Hodgkin's disease; sarcoidosis; live-virus vaccination; age over 55 years. Up to 25% of all patients with active TB and 50% with miliary TB have negative PPD before initiating treatment; PPD may not become positive until 1 to 10 weeks after infection.
- False positives may be caused by infection with nontuberculous mycobacteria or BCG vaccination.
- Booster phenomenon: Delayed hypersensitivity to tuberculin may wane with time (particularly if over 55 years old), leading to false negative PPD. Subsequent testing "boosts" response due to immunologic recall (erroneously suggesting acquisition of TB). Booster response should be tested in patients receiving annual PPD, or if over age 55 and high risk. Booster dose is administered 1 to 4 weeks after initial negative PPD.

TREATMENT OF LATENT TUBERCULOSIS INFECTION (LTBI)

General Principles

- Goals are to (a) reduce risk of progression to active disease and (b) control or eliminate TB in the United States.
- Before starting LTBI treatment, rule out active TB with thorough history, physical exam, and CXR. Signs/symptoms of infection or CXR evidence of active disease (consolidations/parenchymal fibrosis, but not pleural thickening/granulomas) require induced sputum 3 times prior to treatment. Consider baseline laboratory testing [serum glutamic oxaloacetic transaminase (SGOT/AST), serum glutamate pyruvate transaminase (SGPT/ALT), bilirubin] if high risk for hepatotoxicity (chronic liver disease, regular alcohol use, pregnant women within 3 months of delivery, HIV+).
- CDC recommends treatment for:
  ⇒ Persons 35 years old with positive PPD and no active disease.
  ⇒ Persons over 35 years old with positive PPD in following high-risk groups: Converted to positive PPD in past 2 years (assume prior unknown PPD status to be negative); known/suspected HIV infection; close contact with known TB-infected person; CXR suggestive of prior TB; intravenous drug/substance abuse; diabetes mellitus; silicosis; prolonged immunosuppressant/corticosteroid therapy (equivalent of prednisone greater than or equal to 15 mg per day for 3 weeks); cancer of head/neck; hematologic/reticuloendothelial disease (leukemia, Hodgkin's); end-stage renal disease; intestinal bypass/gastrectomy; chronic malabsorption; weight 10% or more below ideal.
- In general, do not treat patients over 35 years old who are neither recent converters nor high risk, because danger of isoniazid-related hepatitis may outweigh benefits. However, therapy may be reasonable in selected patients based on clinical judgment.
- Pregnant women with positive PPD should begin preventive therapy after delivery. However, if likely recent infection or in high-risk group (especially HIV), therapy should begin immediately.
- Nursing is not a contraindication to isoniazid (INH).
- Likely noncompliant patients (e.g., some homeless persons) should be educated about TB and advised to seek medical evaluation immediately if symptoms of active TB develop. Many states now offer directly observed therapy (DOT) for LTBI.

Drug Therapy

- "Treatment completion" is based on total number of doses administered, not on duration of therapy alone. Regimens include:
  ⇒ INH 300 mg per day for 9 months is preferred regimen (regardless of HIV status). Clinical trials have supported altering prior recommendations of 12 months for HIV+ and 6 months for HIV−. Twice weekly INH 15 mg per kg (usually 900 mg) is an acceptable alternative (always with DOT). INH for 6 months provides significant protection, is superior to placebo in HIV−, and may be more cost-effective than 9-month regimen (not recommended in children, HIV+, or with CXR evidence of prior TB).

⇒ **Rifampin (RIF) and pyrazinamide (PZA)** daily for 2 months is similar in efficacy and safety to 12-month INH regimen in HIV+ (insufficient data in HIV−). Considered first-line in HIV+ and second-line in HIV−. Use for exposure to INH-resistant, RIF-susceptible TB. May substitute rifabutin for rifampin in HIV+ taking protease inhibitors. Twice weekly RIF and PZA has not been compared to 9- or 12-month INH, and is recommended only when alternative regimens cannot be used (always with DOT).

⇒ **Rifampin (RIF)** daily for 4 months is recommended when cannot tolerate INH or PZA. Randomized trial results for HIV− with silicosis showed daily RIF for 3 months equivalent to daily INH for 6 months [4 rather than 3 months is recommended because study patients had high annual rate (4%) of active TB].

⇒ **Alternatives:** For TB resistant to INH and RIF in HIV−, observation without preventive therapy is recommended because only INH and RIF have been evaluated in trials. In HIV+, a regimen with 2 or more drugs to which the organism is susceptible should be used. Potential alternatives include daily ethambutol and PZA for 6 months, or PZA plus a quinolone for 6 months [associated with adverse gastrointestinal (GI) effects].

Adverse Effects

- **INH:** Hepatotoxicity is most common; incidence peaks during first 3 months, is age related (0% in patients under 20 years old; 0.3% in ages 20 to 35; 1.2% in ages 35 to 49; 2.3% in those over age 50), and is fourfold higher in daily alcohol drinkers; deaths from hepatotoxicity have been reported rarely. Peripheral neuropathy occurs rarely: pyridoxine (25 to 50 mg per day) is recommended as an adjunct to INH in patients at risk for developing neuropathy (diabetes, uremia, alcoholism, HIV, malnutrition), pregnancy, over age 55, seizure disorder (it is not unreasonable to give pyridoxine to all patients receiving INH).
- **RIF and PZA** are potentially hepatotoxic, and are frequently associated with low-severity adverse reactions which result in drug discontinuation (GI distress, arthralgias, rash).
- Contraindications to INH or PZA include active hepatitis and end-stage liver disease.

Follow-up

- Regular office evaluations: Monthly (for INH or RIF alone) or at weeks 2, 4, and 8 (for RIF and PZA). Evaluate adherence, symptoms of hepatitis (nausea and vomiting, anorexia, dark urine, jaundice, malaise, fever, right upper quadrant tenderness), neurotoxicity/paresthesias.
- Monthly liver enzymes are not recommended, unless known liver disease, abnormal baseline values, HIV+, or high-risk for adverse reactions. Approximately 15% of patients on INH have mild, asymptomatic elevation of liver enzymes, which resolve even if INH is continued. INH should be stopped if measurements exceed 3 times the upper limit of normal with symptoms, or exceed 5 times the upper limit of normal without symptoms.

RESOURCES

- CDC TB sites: www.cdc.gov/nchstp/tb/pubs/corecurr/ and http://www.cdc.gov/nchstp/tb/pubs/mmwrhtml/maj_guide.htm

SELECTED REFERENCES

1. Centers for Disease Control and Prevention. Core curriculum on TB: *What the clinician should know,* 4th ed. 2000.
2. Centers for Disease Control and Prevention. Division of Tuberculosis Elimination. Major TB guidelines: http://www.cdc.gov/nchstp/tb/pubs/mmwrhtml/maj_guide.htm.
3. Gordin F, Chaisson RE, Matts JP, et al. Rifampin and pyrazinamide vs isoniazid for prevention of tuberculosis in HIV-infected persons: an international randomized trial. *JAMA* 2000;283:1445–1450.
4. Halsey NA, Coberly JS, Desormeaux J, et al. Randomised trial of isoniazid versus rifampicin and pyrazinamide for prevention of tuberculosis in HIV-1 infection. *Lancet* 1998;351(9105):786–792.
5. Hong Kong Chest Service, Tuberculosis Research Centre, Madras, and British Medical Research Council. A double-blind, placebo-controlled clinical trial of three antituberculosis chemoprophylaxis regimens in patients with silicosis in Hong Kong. *Am Rev Respir Dis* 1992;145:36–41.

6. International Union Against Tuberculosis Committee on Prophylaxis. Efficacy of various durations of isoniazid preventive therapy for tuberculosis: five years of follow-up in the IUAT trial. *Bull World Health Organ* 1982;60:555–564.

7. Mwinga A, Hosp M, Godfrey-Faussett P, et al. Twice weekly tuberculosis preventive therapy in HIV infection in Zambia. *AIDS* 1998;12(18):2447–2457.

8. Pape JW, Jean SS, Ho JL, et al. Effect of isoniazid prophylaxis on incidence of active tuberculosis and progression of HIV infection. *Lancet* 1993;342(8866):268–272.

9. Targeted tuberculin testing and treatment of latent tuberculosis infection. *Am J Respir Crit Care Med* 2000; 161:S221–S247.

10. Whalen CC, Johnson JL, Okwera A, et al. A trial of three regimens to prevent tuberculosis in Ugandan adults infected with the human immunodeficiency virus. *N Engl J Med* 1997;337(12):801–808.

URINARY TRACT INFECTIONS

INTRODUCTION

- Women have 50% lifetime chance of more than one urinary tract infection (UTI).
- More common in sexually active (especially women), postmenopausal, pregnant, benign prostatic hypertrophy (BPH) (men), bladder catheterization, incomplete bladder emptying (neurogenic, obstruction), structural abnormalities (incompetent vesicoureteral valve, reflux). Most common source of bacteremia in the elderly.
- Uncomplicated cystitis: UTI in nonpregnant adult without structural/neurological dysfunction
- Complicated UTI: involves upper tract, children, men, pregnancy, or structural/neurological abnormalities

PATHOGENESIS

- Uncomplicated cystitis involves bacteria that adhere to urothelium (adhesins on fimbriae), typically *Escherichia coli* (80% to 90%) or *Staphylococcus saprophyticus* (5% to 15%); less frequently *Klebsiella* or *Proteus* (5%).
- Complicated UTIs may involve *Enterococcus, Enterobacter, Serratia,* or *Pseudomonas.*
- Male UTIs occur with BPH/partial bladder outlet obstruction or persistent prostatitis. 20% of men with pyelonephritis or prostatitis have gram-negative bacteremia.
- Acute pyelonephritis involves ascending infection from bladder more than hematogenous seeding.
- Antibiotic resistance: estimated outpatient rates for *E. coli* isolates are 30% to amoxicillin, 15% to trimethoprim and sulfamethoxazole (TMP/SMX), greater than 5% to fluoroquinolones (Gupta et al., 1999). Risk factors for TMP/SMX resistance include recent TMP/SMX, current use of any antibiotic, diabetes, recent hospitalization (Wright et al., 1999).

EVALUATION

Symptoms

- Uncomplicated cystitis: increased frequency, dysuria, pyuria (greater than 10 white blood cells per high power field), positive leukocyte esterase/nitrites. Acute pyelonephritis: fever, flank pain.

Diagnostic Testing

- Consider urine culture (UCX) for recurrent infections (see Table 17.1), atypical features, or absence of pyuria. For suspected pyelonephritis, look for white blood cell (WBC) casts on urinalysis (UA), obtain UCX, blood cultures (15% to 20% positive), consider urine gram stain to guide therapy; if fevers last over 72 hours, repeat culture and consider abdominal computed tomography (CT) to rule out perinephric abscess; hospitalization not mandatory if otherwise stable (Mombelli et al., 1999). In men, evaluate for anatomical abnormalities if more than one UTI.

TABLE 17.1 URINALYSIS AND URINE CULTURE

Leukocyte esterase	Sensitivity 75%–96%; specificity 94%–98%; PPV 50%.
Nitrite detection	Sensitivity 35%–85%; specificity 92%–100%. False negatives with bacteria that do not produce nitrate reductase *(Staphylococcus, Enterococcus, Pseudomonas).*
Squamous cells	Common finding, does not indicate contamination.
Culture	10^5 colony-forming units (CFU) is significantly positive, although 10^2 is valid in symptomatic women. Polymicrobial growth suggests contamination (or rarely GI/GU fistula).

PPV, positive predictive value; GI, gastrointestinal; GU, genitourinary.

TREATMENT

- **Uncomplicated UTI:** 3-day regimens more effective than 1-day regimens, and fewer side effects than 7-day regimens. The Infectious Disease Society of America recommends starting with TMP/SMX (unless recently prescribed or known resistance). Other options are fluoroquinolones or nitrofurantoin (rare pulmonary fibrosis).
- **Complicated UTI:** regimen of 7 days or more
- **Acute pyelonephritis:** Optimal regimen/duration poorly defined. Recent study found 7 days of oral ciprofloxacin (Cipro) superior to TMP/SMX for 14 days due to *E. coli* resistance to TMP/SMX (18%) vs. Cipro (0%); adverse effects were equal (Talan et al., 2000).
- **Recurrent UTI:** Found in 25% of young women, mostly from reinfection. Obtain UCX; if more than three times per year and related to intercourse, consider postcoital prophylaxis with single dose of TMP/SMX, nitrofurantoin, or fluoroquinolone. May consider daily single strength TMP/SMX. Consider evaluation for urologic abnormalities or infectious focus.
- **Pregnancy:** Treat promptly (7% develop asymptomatic bacteriuria, 30% of which progress to pyelonephritis if untreated). Screen at initial prenatal visit and at 28 weeks. Antibiotics safe in pregnancy include sulfonamides until the third trimester, amoxicillin, cephalexin, nitrofurantoin. Treat for 7 days and document cure with UCX one week later.
- **Men:** If workup reveals prostatitis, recommend TMP/SMX or fluoroquinolone for 4 to 12 weeks.
- **Chronic indwelling catheters:** Bacteriuria and pyuria are universal and should not prompt reflexive treatment. Prophylactic antibiotics promote resistant organisms and do not prevent symptomatic UTI. For signs/symptoms of pyelonephritis/bacteremia or persistent fever without other source, treat for 10 to 14 days (requires UCX).
- **Nonpharmacologic therapies:**
  ⇒ Cranberry juice: No study convincingly demonstrates ability to prevent UTI. The aggregate of favorable evidence combined with plausible biological mechanism (interference with adhesion of *E. coli* to uroepithelium) does tend to support the claim, despite poor methodological quality of nearly all studies. The effective dose and duration has not been determined (Avorn et al., 1994; Jepson et al., 2001).
  ⇒ Postcoital voiding shown not to help (Hooton et al., 1996).
  ⇒ Estrogen replacement not shown effective for postmenopausal women with recurrent UTIs (Oliveria et al., 1998).
  ⇒ Acupuncture recently shown to reduce recurrence of UTI in adult women by 50% (Aune et al., 1998).

SELECTED REFERENCES

1. Aune A, Alraek T, LiHua H, et al. Acupuncture in the prophylaxis of recurrent lower urinary tract infection in adult women. *Scand J Prim Health Care* 1998;16:37–39.
2. Avorn J, Monane M, Gurwitz JH, et al. Reduction of bacteriuria and pyuria after ingestion of cranberry juice. *JAMA* 1994;271:751–754.
3. Bacheller CD, Bernstein JM. Urinary tract infections. *Med Clin North Am* 1997;81:719–730.
4. Gupta K, Scholes D, Stamm WE. Increasing prevalence of antimicrobial resistance among uropathogens causing acute uncomplicated cystitis in women. *JAMA* 1999;281:736–738.
5. Hooton TM, Scholes D, Hughes JP, et al. A prospective study of risk factors for symptomatic urinary tract infection in young women. *N Engl J Med* 1996;335:468–474.

6. Jepson RG, Mihaljevic L, Craig J. Cranberries for preventing urinary tract infections. *Cochrane Database Syst Rev* 2000;2:CD001321.
7. McCarty JM, Richard G, Huck W, et al. A randomized trial of short-course of ciprofloxacin, ofloxacin, or trimethoprim/sulfamethoxazole for the treatment of acute urinary tract infection in women. *Am J Med* 1999; 106:292–299.
8. Mombelli G, Pezzoli R, Pinoja-Lutz G, et al. Oral vs intravenous ciprofloxacin in the initial empirical management of severe pyelonephritis or complicated urinary tract infections: a prospective randomized clinical trial. *Arch Intern Med* 1999;159:53–58.
9. Oliveria SA, Klein RA, Reed JI, et al. Estrogen replacement therapy and urinary tract infections in postmenopausal women aged 45–89. *Menopause* 1998;5:4–8.
10. Orenstein R, Wong ES. Urinary tract infections in adults. *Am Fam Physician* 1999;59:1225–1234.
11. Stamm WE, Hooton TM. Management of urinary tract infections in adults. *N Engl J Med* 1993;329:1328–1334.
12. Talan DA, Stamm WE, Hooton TM, et al. Comparison of ciprofloxacin (7 days) and trimethoprim-sulfamethoxazole (14 days) for acute uncomplicated pyelonephritis in women: a randomized trial. *JAMA* 2000; 283:1583–1590.
13. Wright SW, Wrenn KD, Haynes ML. Trimethoprim-sulfamethoxazole resistance among urinary coliform isolates. *J Gen Intern Med* 1999;14:606–609.

SEXUALLY TRANSMITTED DISEASES: VAGINAL DISCHARGE/VAGINITIS, PELVIC INFLAMMATORY DISEASE, GENITAL ULCERS

INTRODUCTION

- The United States has 15 million sexually transmitted disease (STD) cases each year, majority in individuals between ages 15 and 25.
- Many cases are asymptomatic, identified only by screening tests.
- Women suffer worse complications, including ectopic pregnancy, infertility, cervical cancer.
- Patients with one STD should be counseled/screened for all STDs (syphilis, gonorrhea, chlamydia, HIV, hepatitis).
- Genital ulcers, urethritis, cervicitis may increase risk of HIV transmission.

ABNORMAL VAGINAL DISCHARGE/VAGINITIS

Pathogenesis

- Caused by change in vaginal flora: menses/pH change, vaginal infection, sexual contact, multiple partners, antibiotics, oral contraceptive pills (OCPs), pregnancy, diabetes mellitus, HIV/immunocompromised, abnormal uterine bleeding, smoking. Higher rates in low socioeconomic status.

Differential Diagnosis

- Common causes are yeast, bacterial vaginosis, trichomonas (see Table 18.1).
- Rule out cervicitis: remove vaginal discharge with cotton swab and swab cervical os. If gram stain reveals more than 10–30 white blood cells (WBC) without epithelial cells, most likely cervicitis.

TABLE 18.1 EVALUATION AND TREATMENT OF ABNORMAL VAGINAL DISCHARGE

Infection	Pathogens	Symptoms	Physical Exam	Diagnosis	Treatment	Recurrence/ Complications
Yeast infection (candida)	*C. albicans* (most common), *tropicalis, glabrata*	Pruritis	Fissures, labial rash. Discharge: thick, white to yellow, "cottage cheese." No odor.	KOH wet prep → hyphae, culture, and sensitivity. pH <4.5.	**Nonpharmacologic:** Daily intake 8 oz yogurt containing live *Lactobacillus acidophilus* may decrease candidal colonization/vaginitis (Hilton et al. 1992)	Recurrence is common. If more frequent than every 2–3 months, reexamine for other pathogens,

(continued)

TABLE 18.1 *(continued)*

Infection	Pathogens	Symptoms	Physical Exam	Diagnosis	Treatment	Recurrence/ Complications
					Pharmacologic: OTC vaginal preparations (miconazole, clotrimazole) are more or less equally effective. Shorter courses promote compliance but are associated with higher recurrence. Terconazole vaginal preparation (0.4% cream, 80 mg suppositories × 7 days) is more effective. Diflucan 150 mg po once.	consider fungal culture, changing or discontinuing OCPs, obtaining HIV or diabetes testing.
Bacterial vaginosis	*Gardnerella vaginalis, Mycoplasma hominis, Mobiluncus* sp., *Prevotella* sp.	50% asymptomatic	Discharge: thin, white to gray, homogeneous. Fishy odor.	Three of four criteria: homogeneous discharge, positive Whiff test, pH >4.5, clue cells.	Metronidazole 500 mg po bid × 7 days (cure rate 80% to 90%); clindamycin 300 mg po bid × 7 days; metronidazole gel 0.75% intravaginally bid × 5 days (fewer systemic reactions than oral pills); clindamycin gel 2% intravaginally qhs × 7 days; metronidazole 2 g po × 1 (alternative regimen). No benefit shown from treating sexual partner. Oral regimens preferable in pregnant women at risk for low birth weight infant.	In pregnancy may cause PROM, preterm labor, chorioamnionitis, endometritis. Increases likelihood of abnormal Pap smear (particularly atypical squamous cells). Possible association with PID.
Trichomonas infection	*Trichomonas vaginalis* (motile protozoan with four flagella)	Pruritis, often asymptomatic	Strawbery cervix. Discharge: profuse, green, watery. With or without odor.	NS wet prep → trichomonads; culture for trich. pH>4.5.	Metronidazole 2 g po × 1 (patient and partner). Resistance is increasing. If resistance is suspected: metronidazole 2 g po qD × 2–5 days, 2–2.5 g po × 7–10 days, or 3 g po × 14–21 days +/− metronidazole gel intravaginally. Rescreen for other STDs. Phenobarbital and phenytoin may decrease effectiveness of metronidazole.	Risk factor for pelvic inflammatory disease, PROM, neonatal respiratory tract infection.

KOH, potassium hydroxide; OTC, over the counter; OCP, oral contraceptive pills; po, by mouth; bid, twice daily; qhs, every night; PROM, premature rupture of membranes; PID, pelvic inflammatory disease; NS, normal saline; qd, every day; STD, sexually transmitted disease (Carr et al. 1998).

CERVICITIS/URETHRITIS

Epidemiology

- *Neisseria gonorrhea:* more than 1 million cases per year. *Chlamydia trachomatis:* 3 to 4 million cases per year. Incidence increasing in adolescents and inner city populations.
- Complications include pelvic inflammatory disease (PID), infertility, bartholinitis, epididymitis, prostatitis, Reiter's syndrome, Fitz-Hugh and Curtis syndrome, penile edema, urethral stricture, infection of neonate.
- Risk factors include multiple sexual partners, HIV/immunocompromised, coinfection with other sexually transmitted disease.

Differential Diagnosis

- Pathogens include *Neisseria gonorrhea, Chlamydia trachomatis, Lymphogranuloma venereum* (citrachomatis serotypes L1–3), *Ureaplasma urealyticum* (see Table 18.2).

Evaluation

Screening

- Screening is cost-effective. Screen all women under 20 years old at any pelvic exam.
- Screen all men and women if new sexual partner in last 3 months or since last screened, if barrier contraceptives not used consistently; if pregnant [including therapeutic abortion (TAB)]; if symptomatic.

History

- Cervicitis is usually asymptomatic. Vaginal discharge, vaginal bleeding, postcoital bleeding, abdominal pain, irregular/heavy menses, rectal pain, tenesmus, urethritis may occur.
- Men and women with urethritis may experience dysuria, discharge, anorectal symptoms (pruritus, rectal discharge). Pharyngitis, conjunctivitis, and disseminated disease may occur.
- 5% of men with gonococcal urethral infection are asymptomatic. Forty-five percent of men with *C. trachomatis* urethritis are asymptomatic.

Physical Exam

- Most women have normal exam, although mucopurulent discharge, with or without friable/edematous cervix, may occur.

Diagnosis

- Cervicitis: Gram stain of cervical swab reveals more than 10 to 30 WBC without epithelial cells.
- Urethritis: Gram stain of urethral swab reveals more than 4 WBC per high-power field (HPF).

TABLE 18.2 DIAGNOSIS AND TREATMENT OF CERVICITIS OR URETHRITIS

Pathogen	Diagnosis	Treatment	Comment
N. gonorrhea	Intracellular gram negative diplococci on urethral/cervical gram stain. Confirmatory culture on Thayer Martin medium or chocolate agar. Consider DNA probe, amplification test (LCR).	Uncomplicated urethritis/cervicitis: ceftriaxone 125 mg IM × 1 (safe in pregnancy); fluroquinolone × 1. For disseminated disease: ceftriaxone 1g IV × 7 days, may change to oral on day 3 (cefixime 400 mg bid or Cipro 500 mg bid).	Must treat for Chlamydia as well. Treat all partners. Safe sex counseling.
C. trachomatis	Culture from rotated swab, or direct monoclonal antibody staining, ELISA, amplification test (LCR), DNA probe.	Azithomycin 1 g po × 1 or doxycycline 100 mg bid, tetracycline 500 mg qid, ofloxacin 300 mg bid × 7 days. In pregnancy: erythromycin 500 mg po qid × 7 days (drug of choice) or amoxicillin 500 mg tid × 7 days.	Common cause of nongonococcal urethritis in men and silent PID in women. Remind patient not to have sex for 7 days after treatment. Treat all partners. Safe sex counseling.
Lymphogranuloma venereum	Serologies with CF >1:64, or increasing 4-fold.	Tetracycline 500 mg qid or doxycycline 100 mg bid or erythromycin 500 mg qid × 3 weeks.	Can cause cervicitis, urethritis, proctitis, or genital ulcers. May progress to ulcerations or fistulas. Treat all partners. Safe sex counseling.

IM, intramuscular; IV, intravenous; bid, twice daily; ELISA, enzyme-linked immunosorbent assay; LCR, ligase chain reaction; po, by mouth; qid, four times daily; tid, three times a day; PID, pelvic inflammatory disease; CF, complement fixation.

PELVIC INFLAMMATORY DISEASE (PID)

Pathogenesis

- Caused by gonococci (GC) or chlamydia. *Mycoplasma hominis* may be previously unrecognized cause.
- 20% long-term complications: infertility, ectopic pregnancy, chronic pain.

Differential Diagnosis

- Consider ectopic pregnancy, tubo-ovarian abscess, appendicitis, inflammatory bowel disease.

Evaluation

Symptoms

- Lower abdominal pain (unilateral/bilateral), worse with intercourse/Valsalva maneuver.
- Vaginal discharge, bleeding may or may not be present.
- Chlamydia PID may be asymptomatic.

Physical Exam

- Pelvic/adnexal/cervical motion tenderness, fever, vaginal discharge.

Diagnostic Tests

- Erythrocyte sedimentation rate (ESR)/C-reactive protein (CRP), GC/chlamydia cultures.
- Human chorionic gonadotropin (HCG) to rule out ectopic pregnancy; pelvic ultrasonography. to rule out ectopic/tubo-ovarian abscess.
- Laparoscopy if concern for adnexal mass or if diagnosis is in question.

Treatment

- Ofloxacin 400 mg by mouth twice daily plus Flagyl 500 mg by mouth four times daily for 14 days (first line), or ceftriaxone one 250 mg intramuscular dose plus doxycycline 100 mg by mouth twice daily for 14 days.
- Begin before diagnosis is established, reexamine after 48 hours.
- Consider inpatient treatment/intravenous antibiotics if diagnosis uncertain, pelvic abscess, pregnancy, concern for compliance (adolescent), HIV+, severe signs/symptoms, poor response to therapy.
- Treat partner(s).

GENITAL ULCERS/LESIONS

Differential Diagnosis

- Consider herpes simplex virus (HSV) 1 and 2, human papilloma virus (HPV), syphilis, chancroid (see Table 18.3). Other causes include granuloma inguinale, trauma, fixed drug reactions, Behcet's syndrome, neoplasm.
- Screen all patients for syphilis; repeat serology in 1 and 3 months if negative initially.

TABLE 18.3 DIAGNOSIS AND TREATMENT OF GENITAL ULCERS AND LESIONS

Pathogen	Signs/symptoms	Diagnosis	Treatment
Herpes simplex virus (HSV 1 and 2)	**Primary:** prodrome of malaise, headache, fever, myalgias, genital paresthesias. Painful/pruritic lesions +/− tender inguinal adenopathy, dysuria, vaginal/urethral discharge. Shedding up to 2 weeks. Lesions may take 3 weeks to resolve. **Recurrence:** Prodrome of pruritis, tingling, dysesthesias in 50%. Lesions crust over in 4–5 days, resolve in approx. 2 weeks. Asymptomatic shedding common (2%–28% of days).	Up to 20% in United States may have HSV-2 (2/3 unaware of infection). **Viral culture:** Unroof vesicle and obtain sample fluid from base of lesion onto Dacron applicator. **Tzanck smear:** Rapid detection (70%) but unable to differentiate HSV/VZV **DFA:** Distinguishes HSV 1/2 in 24 hours. **Serology:** not helpful. Rule out syphilis.	**Primary:** Acycolovir 200 mg 5x/day or 400 mg tid; famciclovir 250 mg TID or valacyclovir 1000 mg po bid × 7 days or until lesions resolve. For proctitis/HIV+: Acyclovir 400 mg 5x/day or until symptoms resolve. Therapy decreases symptom duration/severity, decreases shedding (no effect on recurrence frequency/likelihood). **Suppression:** For frequent/complicated recurrence (reduces frequency 75%, no effect on shedding). Acyclovir 200 mg tid or 400 mg po bid; famciclovir 250 mg bid, valacyclovir 500 mg bid or 1 g qd × 1 year.
Human papilloma virus (HPV)	Lesions 1–6 months after exposure (frequently unnoticed). Localized or throughout genital tract. In women, most common on vulva/perineum/intravaginal (introitus or fornices). In men, most common on penile shaft/under foreskin.	3%–5% acetic acid to lesion × 5 minutes makes tissue turn white (not specific for HPV). Colposcopy or biopsy if uncertain. DNA probes distinguish genotypes. Hybrid II capture assay may soon complement Pap smears as screen.	**Goal:** Eliminate lesion (virus may remain in nearby skin/mucosa, lesions may recur). **Cryotherapy:** Liquid nitrogen to lesion every 1–2 weeks until resolution (not intravaginal). **Trichloroacetic acid:** Effective for small lesions; possible increased recurrence rate. **Podophyllum:** Can be used by patient at home; possible increased recurrence rate (contraindicated in pregnancy). **Imiquimod:** 5% cream 3x/week up to 16 weeks; 50% cure. **Other:** Laser ablation or loop electrosurgery (for large lesions or if scarring a concern; 40%–50% cure); interferon α (intralesional injections; 50% cure rate). Close gynecological follow-up for genital warts/if partner with genital warts (several genotypes linked to cervical cancer).
Syphilis (*Treponema pallidum*)	**Primary:** 9–90 day incubation. Painless indurated ulcer(s) with surrounding induration, internal or external or extragenital, heals in approx. 6 wks. +/− inguinal adenopathy. **Secondary** (50%): 2–8 weeks after primary, +/− arthralgias, meningitis, uveitis, lymphadenopathy, hepatosplenomegaly, alopecia, mucocutaneous lesions, rash (maculopapular palms/soles, plaque-like, papular), lasts 2–10 weeks. **Early latent:** within 1 year, possible secondary symptoms, still contagious. **Late latent:** After 1 year, 33% progress to tertiary. **Tertiary:** End organ damage including aortic aneurysm, aortic insufficiency, neurosyphilis (meningitis, paresis, tabes dorsalis), deafness, ocular involvement, gummas (skin, upper respiratory tract, GI, liver).	**Serologic:** VDRL or RPR (nontreponemal), confirmed with fluorescent treponemal Ab absorption (FTA-Abs) or micro hemagglutination assay (MHA-TP) (remain positive for life). Nontreponemal tests may be negative early on (insensitive for 1–4 weeks after chancre forms). If negative, repeat in 3–4 weeks. **Microscopy:** Direct visualization of treponemes in lesion fluid (insensitive for 1–4 weeks after chancre forms), if negative, repeat in 3–4 weeks.	**Primary, Secondary, early latent:** Penicillin G 2.4 mu IM every week x2, or doxycycline 100 mg po bid × 14 days, or tetracycline 500 mg po qid × 14 days (if PCN allergic). Follow nontreponemal titers q6 months × 2 years. **Late latent, tertiary unknown duration:** Penicillin G 2.4 mu IM every week × 3 weeks, or doxycycline 100 mg po bid or tetracycline 500 mg qid × 28 days (if PCN allergic). LP if treatment with doxycycline or tetracycline. **Neurosyphilis:** Penicillin G 2.4 mu IV every 4 hours × 10–14 days. **In pregnancy:** PCN (if allergic, consider skin testing/desensitization). Evaluate/treat partner(s). **HIV + patients:** LP before treatment for latent syphilis.
Chancroid (*Haemophilius ducreyi*)	Rare in United States. Associated with transmission of HIV.	Painful, indurated papule, ragged edges, grey/yellow exudates, painful local adenopathy (may suppurate), ulcerates over 1–2 days. GNR tracking in pairs on GS of lesion edge, can culture.	Ceftriaxone 250 mg IM × 1, or azithromycin 1 g po × 1, or erythromycin 500 mg po qid × 7 days, or Ciprofloxacin 500 mg po bid × 3 days (not in pregnancy/pediatrics). Longer treatment if HIV+. Ulcers generally heal in 3–7 days. Treat partner(s).

tid, three times a day; po, by mouth; bid, twice daily; qd, every day; GI, gastrointestinal; VDRL, Venereal Disease Research Laboratory (test for syphilis); RPR, rapid plasma reagin; IM, intramuscular; qid, four times daily; PCN, penicillin; IV, intravenous; GNR, gram-negative rods; GS, Gram stain.

RESOURCE

- Centers for Disease Control (CDC) website: http://www.cdc.gov/nchstp/dstd/dstdp.html

SELECTED REFERENCES

1. Carne C. Recent advances: sexually transmitted diseases. *BMJ* 1998;317:129–132.
2. Carr PL, Felsenstein D, Friedman RH.. Evaluation and management of vaginitis. *J Gen Intern Med* 1998;13: 335–346.
3. Centers for Disease Control. Guidelines for treatment of sexually transmitted diseases. *MMWR Morb Mortal Wkly Rep* 1998;47:1–116.
4. Hilton E, Isenberg HD, Alperstein P. Ingestion of yogurt containing *Lactobacillus acidophilus* as prophylaxis for candidal vaginitis. *Ann Intern Med* 1992;116(5):353–357.
5. Miller KE. Sexually transmitted diseases. *Primary Care Clinics* 1997;24:179–193.
6. Scholes D. Prevention of pelvic inflammatory disease by screening for cervical chlamydial infection. *N Engl J Med* 1996;334(21):1362–1366.
7. Holmes KK, et al, eds. Sexually Transuitted Diseases, Second Edition, New York: McGraw-Hill Book Co., 1990.

19

HIV MANAGEMENT

INTRODUCTION

- More than 36 million people worldwide are infected with HIV, two-thirds in Africa (UN-AIDS/WHO, 1998).
- 920,000 people in the United States have HIV, 44,000 new cases annually, rising incidence in African-Americans and women.
- Over 22 million deaths (most common cause of infectious-disease related mortality).
- "Highly active antiretroviral therapy" (HAART) prolongs survival; complications include immune reconstitution syndromes, metabolic abnormalities, viral resistance.

PATHOPHYSIOLOGY/CLINICAL PRESENTATION

- **Acute retroviral syndrome (ARS):** Period from initial infection to generation of HIV-1 specific antibodies. 80% of patients recall ARS symptoms (Table 19.1); but it often goes unrecognized by clinicians. More severe symptoms correlate with faster progression to AIDS (Henrard, 1995).
    - ⇒ High-level viremia occurs 4 to 11 days after initial infection, followed by activation of cellular and humoral immune responses over 7 to 21 days.
    - ⇒ Seroconversion occurs 21 to 28 days after exposure.
    - ⇒ Viremia decreases with specific anti-HIV-1 immune response and reaches a "set point" (characteristic for each individual without antiretroviral therapy). Magnitude of viral set point predicts long-term survival.
- **Early HIV disease (CD4 greater than 500/mm^3):** Usually asymptomatic. Lymphadenopathy (cervical, axillary, inguinal) is common and referred to as "persistent generalized lymphadenopathy" (PGL). Without therapy, risk of opportunistic infection (OI) or death within 18 to 24 months is less than 5%.
- **Intermediate HIV disease (CD4 200/mm^3 to 500/mm^3):** Without therapy, risk of OI or death in 18 to 24 months is 20% to 30%.
- **Late HIV disease/AIDS (CD4 50/mm^3 to 200/mm^3):** Centers for Disease Control (CDC) definition of AIDS is CD4+ count less than 200/mm^3 or development of OI/malignancy. Without therapy, risk of OI or death in 18 to 24 months is 70% to 80%. Prophylaxis for common OIs is recommended.
- **Advanced HIV disease (CD4 less than 50/mm^3):** Without therapy, high likelihood of OI or death within 18 to 24 months.
- **Terminal HIV disease:** Inability to control signs/symptoms of advanced HIV/OIs. Consider comfort measures and end-of-life care.

TABLE 19.1 ACUTE RETROVIRAL SYNDROME: ASSOCIATED SIGNS AND SYMPTOMS

Fever	Hepatosplenomegaly
Lymphadenopathy	Weight loss
Pharyngitis	Neurologic symptoms

(continued)

TABLE 19.1 *(continued)*

Rash	Neurologic Symptoms
• Erythematous maculopapular lesions on face, trunk, or extremities (including palms/soles) • Mucocutaneous ulcerations involving mouth, esophagus, or genitals Myalgia, arthralgia Diarrhea Headache	• Meningoencephalitis or aseptic meningitis • Peripheral neuropathy or radiculopathy • Facial palsy • Guillain-Barré syndrome • Brachial neuritis • Cognitive impairment or psychosis Nausea/vomiting

EVALUATION

- Office-based testing: Voluntary, requires informed consent. Schedule follow-up for potential counseling.
- Home testing: Federal Drug Administration (FDA) approved (Home Access Express Test mail-in finger-stick: 1-800-HIV-TEST)
- Rapid tests (reduced specificity): Consider when follow-up is uncertain, or for occupational exposure cases (Table 19.2).

TABLE 19.2 LABORATORY TESTING IN HIV INFECTION

Laboratory Assay	Comments
HIV-1 RNA	Detects HIV-1 RNA in plasma. Useful for detecting ARS and for following response to antiretroviral therapy.
ELISA for HIV-1 specific antibodies	Negative during ARS (antibodies develop in 1–12 weeks). Over 99% sensitive and specific. Positive tests usually repeated for confirmation, plus Western blot.
Western blot	Positive result: At least two major bands present from different regions of HIV genome. Indeterminate result: Single band or two bands from same region of genome. False positive are rare.

ARS, acute retroviral syndrome; ELISA, enzyme-linked immunosorbent assay.

- Initial evaluation of confirmed HIV patients: Assess for candidiasis, tuberculosis, varicella zoster virus (VZV), sexually transmitted diseases (STDs), herpes simplex virus (HSV), history of opportunistic infections, history of antiretroviral therapy, fever, weight loss, diarrhea, night sweats, dyspnea, cough, anorexia, depression, psychosocial situation, travel, pets (Table 19.3).

TABLE 19.3 LABORATORY EVALUATION OF PATIENTS WITH CONFIRMED HIV

Recommend	Consider
CBC with differential	Fasting lipids (if considering protease inhibitor)
Chemistry panel with renal/hepatic function	G6PD level
Syphilis serology	Testosterone (men)
CMV serology (IgG)	Baseline CXR
TB skin test	
CD4+ count	
Viral load (same assay type each time)	
Toxoplasmosis serology (IgG)	
Hepatitis serologies (A,B,C)	
Pap smear (women)	

CBC, complete blood count; CMV, cytomegalovirus; IgG, immunoglobulin G; TB, tuberculosis; G6PD, glucose-6-phosphate isomerase, CXR, chest x-ray.

- Follow-up evaluation for confirmed HIV patients: Office visit every 2 months. Increase frequency with changing CD4/HIV RNA or in late disease.
  ⇒ Annual purified protein derivative (PPD) if high-risk for exposure to tuberculosis (unless previously positive/treated)
  ⇒ Pap smears for females every 6 months initially during the first year, then annually if normal
  ⇒ Anal Pap smears if history of anal intercourse or warts [increased risk of human papilloma virus (HPV)-related anal dysplasia and squamous cell carcinoma]
  ⇒ Ophthalmologist exam annually; every 6 months for CD4 under $50/mm^3$ or for cytomegalovirus (CMV) positive patients with CD4 under $100/mm^3$
  ⇒ CD4 cell count every 6 months if over $500/mm^3$; every 3 to 6 months if under $500/mm^3$
  ⇒ Viral load every 3 to 4 months when undetectable/stable, and when therapy is altered

TREATMENT

Prevention Counseling

- **Sexual exposure:** Latex condoms should be used for all sexual intercourse. Oral exposure to feces should be avoided.
- **Injection drug use:** Counseling should focus on recovery. Counsel patients never to reuse or share needles, water, or drug preparation equipment; to use only sterile syringes; to use only sterile/boiled water to prepare drugs; to clean skin with new alcohol swabs before injections; and to dispose of used syringes safely.
- **Environmental/occupational exposure:** Childcare providers/parents/gardeners should wash hands frequently (risk of CMV, cryptosporidiosis). Patients should avoid cave exploring, raising dust from surface soil, chicken coops, bird roosting sites (risk of histoplasmosis, cocciodiomycosis).
- **Animal exposure:** Patients should avoid animals with diarrhea (cryptosporidiosis, *Salmonella, Campylobacter*); reptiles (salmonellosis); aquarium cleaning (*Mycobacterium marinum*); cats (toxoplasmosis, *Bartonella*, enteric infections).
- **Food/water related exposure:** Patients should avoid raw/undercooked eggs, meat, and seafood and unpasteurized dairy products; avoid water directly from lakes or rivers (cryptosporidiosis, giardiasis). Boiling water for 1 minute eliminates risk of cryptosporidiosis.

Vaccinations

- May cause transient increase in viral load; more likely to induce immune response when CD4 greater than 100 cells/μl; response may be improved if immunization is delayed until after initiation of antiretroviral therapy (Table 19.4).

TABLE 19.4 VACCINATION RECOMMENDATIONS IN HIV-INFECTED PATIENTS

Vaccine	Indication	Regimen	Comment
Routine vaccines	Same as HIV negative patients	Same as HIV negative patients	Live vaccines are generally contraindicated in HIV+ patients. Exception may be measles vaccine.
Pneumococcal	All HIV patients	0.5 ml IM	Risk of *S. pneumoniae* infection increased × 100 in HIV+. Vaccine efficacy in HIV+ not established. Antigenic response best when CD4 >350.
Influenza	All HIV+ during Oct. to Dec., if CD4+ counts >100 cells/mm³	0.5 ml IM	Influenza risk not clearly increased, but prevention may avoid diagnosis evaluation of flu-like complaints.
Hepatitis B	All HIV+ (unless already immune)	3 IM doses at 0, 1, and 6 months	HIV increases risk of chronic hepatitis B infection. HIV+ are less likely to clear hepatitis B DNA.
Hepatitis A	HIV+ plus HBV+/HCV+	1 ml IM at 0, 6–12 months	Patients with HIV plus HBV/HCV have increased risk of fulminant hepatitis from HAV infection.

Measles in HIV+ can be severe, so risk-benefit of measles vaccine should be determined for each patient, and is generally recommended. Considered safe if CD4 >100.
IM, intramuscular; HBV, hepatitis B virus; HCV, hepatitis C virus; HAV, hepatitis A virus.

Prophylaxis Against Opportunistic Infections (Tables 19.5 to 19.7)

- HAART has dramatically reduced the occurrence of opportunistic infections.
- CDC recommendations can be found at: http://www.cdc.gov/epo/mmwr/preview/mmwrhtml/rr4810a1.htm

TABLE 19.5 OPPORTUNISTIC INFECTIONS AT DIFFERENT STAGES OF HIV INFECTION

CD4+ T Cell Count/mm³	Opportunistic Infections	
200–500/μL	Oral hairy leukoplakia	Oral and esophageal candidiasis
	Recurrent vaginal candidiasis	Recurrent HSV
	Varicella zoster virus infection	Seborrheic dermatitis
	Tuberculosis	Kaposi's sarcoma
	Bacterial sinusitis	Bronchitis
	Pneumonia	Recurrent bacterial infections
	Folliculitis	Cryptosporidiosis
50–200/μL	Pneumocystis pneumonia	Lymphoma
	Bartonella henselae	Kaposi's sarcoma
	Toxoplasmosis	Histoplasmosis
	Cryptococcosis	Coccidiomycosis
<50/μL	Cytomegalovirus	MAC
	Aspergillosis (invasive)	Cryptococcal meningitis
	Progressive multifocal leukoencephalopathy	Disseminated histoplasmosis
	Disseminated bartonellosis	

HSV, herpes simplex virus; MAC, *Mycobacterium avium* complex.
Source: Adapted from Kovacs JA, Masur H. Prophylaxis against opportunistic infections in patients with human immunodeficiency virus infection. *N Engl J Med* 2000;342:1416–1429.

TABLE 19.6 PREVENTION OF OPPORTUNISTIC INFECTIONS: PRIMARY PROPHYLAXIS (FROM BARTLETT, 2001; KOVACS, 2000)

Disease	Indications	Preferred Regimen	Alternatives/Comments
Tuberculosis	PPD+(≥5 mm induration); prior positive PPD without INH prophylaxis; high-risk exposure	INH 300 mg/day + pyridoxine 50 mg/day × 9–12 months OR INH 900 mg 3x/week + pyridoxine 100 mg tiw × 9 months OR Rifampin 600 mg/day + pyrazinamide 20 mg/kg/day × 2 months	Directly observed therapy: INH 900 mg 2x/week (>76 doses) × 12 months; rifabutin may be preferred to rifampin due to interactions with PIs.
P. carinti pneumonia	Prior PCP; CD4 <200; thrush or FUO	TMP-SMX 1 DS/day	Efficacy established. Cost effective, reduces morbidity/mortality. Alternatives: TMP-SMX 1 SS/day or 1 DS 3X/week; dapsone 100 mg/day; dapsone 50 mg/day + pyrimethamine 50 mg/week + leucovorin 25 mg/week; atovaquone 1500 mg/day; aerosolized pentamidine 300 mg/month.
Toxoplasmosis	CD4 <100 plus positive toxoplasma serology (IgG)	TMP-SMX 1 DS/day	Alternative regimens (for TMP-SMX intolerance): dapsone 50 mg/day + pyrimethamine 50 mg/week + leucovorin 25 mg/week; dapsone 200 mg/week + pyrimethamine 75 mg/week + leucovorin 25 mg/week; atovaquone 1500 mg/day.
M. avium	CD4 <50	Clarithromycin 500 mg bid; Azithromycin 1200 mg/week	Alternative (less effective): rifabutin 300 mg/day.

PPD, purified protein derivative; INH, isoniazid; tiw, three times a week; PIs, protease inhibitors; FUO, fever of undertermined origin; TMP-SMX, trimethoprim and sulfamethoxazole; DS, double strength; SS, single strength; IgG, immunoglobulin G; bid, twice daily.
Source: Adapted from Kovacs JA, Masur H. Prophylaxis against opportunistic infections in patients with human immunodeficiency virus infection. *N Engl J Med* 2000;342:1416–1429.

TABLE 19.7 PREVENTION OF OPPORTUNISTIC INFECTIONS: SECONDARY PROPHYLAXIS/MAINTENANCE

Pathogen	Preferred Regimen	Alternatives	Comments
Pneumocystis carinii	TMP-SMX 1 DS/day or 1 SS/day	TMP-SMX 1 DS 3x/week; dapsone 50 mg bid or 100 mg/day; dapsone 50 mg/day + pyrimethamine 50 mg/week + leucovorin 25 mg/day; dapsone 200 mg/week + pyrimethamine 75 mg/week + leucovorin 25 mg/week; atovaquone 1500 mg/day; aerosolized pentamidine 300 mg/month	May safely stop if CD4 >200/mm³ × 3 months
Toxoplasma gondii	Sulfadiazine 500–1000 mg qid + pyrimethamine 25– 75 mg/day + leucovorin 10 mg/day	Clindamycin 300 mg qid; 450 mg tid + pyrimethamine 25–75 mg/day + leucovorin 10–25 mg/day	Lifelong (consider discontinuation if CD4 >200/mm³ × 3 months and VL <5000 c/mL)
M. avium complex	Clarithromycin 500 mg bid + ethambutal 15 mg/kg/day +/– rifabutin 300 mg/day	Azithromycin 500 mg/day + ethambutol 15 mg/kg/day +/– rifabutin 300 mg/day	Lifelong
Cytomegalovirus	Ganciclovir 5–6 mg/kg IV 5–7 days/week or 1000 mg po tid; foscarnet 90–120 mg/kg IV. For retinitis: Ganciclovir sustained-release implant every 6–9 months + ganciclovir 1000–1500 mg tid	Cidofovir 5 mg/kg IV every other week; fomivirsen 1 vial injected intravenously, repeated every 2-4 week; oral valciclovir (investigational)	Consider stopping if CD4>100/mm³ × 3–6 months, nonsight threatening lesion, adequate vision. Close follow-up recommended.
C. neoformans	Fluconazole 200 mg/day	Amphotericin B 0.6–1.0 mg/kg IV 1–3x/week; itraconzole 200 mg/day	Lifelong
H. capsulatum	Itraconazole 200 mg/bid	Amphotericin B, 1.0 mg/kg IV every week.	Lifelong
C. immitis	Fluconazole 400 mg/day	Amphotericin B, 1.0 mg/kg IV every week; itraconzole 200 mg bid	Lifelong
Salmonella species	Ciprofloxacin 500 mg/day x 6–8 months	None	Not well-defined
Herpes simplex virus	None; for severe cases consider acyclovir 200 mg tid or 400 mg bid	Famciclovir 500 mg bid; valacyclovir 500 mg bid	N/A
Candida	None; for severe cases consider fluconazole 100–200 mg/day	Itraconazole 200 mg/day	Optional or as needed

TMP-SMX, trimethoprim and sulfamethoxazole; DS, double strength; SS, single strength; bid, twice daily; qid, four times daily; tid, three times a day; VL, viral load; IV, intravenous; po, by mouth.
Source: Adapted from Kovacs JA, Masur H. Prophylaxis against opportunistic infections in patients with human immunodeficiency virus infection. *N Engl J Med* 2000;342:1416–1429.

Discontinuing Primary Prophylaxis

- *Pneumocystis carinii* pneumonia (PCP): Very low incidence after discontinuation of primary prophylaxis when CD4 is over 200/mm³. Consider discontinuation in stable patients on HAART.
- CMV: Consider discontinuing retinitis prophylaxis if CD4 remains above 100/mm3, lesions not sight-threatening, and adequate vision in contralateral eye with ophthalmologist follow-up.
- *Mycobacterium avium-intracellulare* (MAI): Consider discontinuing primary prophylaxis if CD4 remains over 100/mm³.
- Other: Data are preliminary for other pathogens (toxoplasmosis, cryptococcus); discontinuation not yet recommended.

Discontinuing Secondary Prophylaxis

- Initial data suggest discontinuation of secondary PCP and CMV prophylaxis in patients with rising CD4 and suppressed viral loads is safe.

Initiating Antiretroviral Therapy (Tables 19.8 and 19.9):

- Offer antiretroviral therapy to: patients with AIDS (CD4 under 200/mm³ or OI/malignancy); symptomatic patients; within 6 months of seroconversion.

- Goals of therapy: Maximal/durable suppression of viral load; restoration and preservation of immune function; improved quality of life; reduction in HIV-related morbidity and mortality.
- Balance guidelines with: patient's readiness to begin therapy; likelihood of adherence; assessment of risks/benefits of therapy; degree of immunodeficiency (CD4 count); risk of disease progression (viral load).
- Two approaches to initiation in asymptomatic patients:

  1. Early therapy: Begin treatment before development of significant immunosuppression, with goal to achieve undetectable viremia.
  2. Delayed therapy (more conservative): Delay treatment of low-level viremia if low risk of disease progression, despite CD4 count. (Due to risks of antiretroviral therapy, expert opinion is shifting toward this approach.)

- Some experts recommend viral resistance testing prior to therapy initiation.

TABLE 19.8 INDICATIONS FOR ANTIRETROVIRAL THERAPY INITIATION IN HIV INFECTED PATIENTS

Clinical Category	CD4+ Count/HIV RNA	Recommendation
Symptomatic (AIDS, severe symtoms, ARS)	Any value	Treat
Asymptomatic, AIDS	CD4+ <200/mm^3 AND any HIV RNA	Treat
Asymptomatic	CD4+ >200, but <350 AND any HIV RNA[†]	Although controversial, treatment is generally offered.
Asymptomatic	CD4+ >350 AND >30,000 (bDNA) or <55,000 (RT-PCR)	Some experts recommend initiating therapy, recognizing 3 year risk of AIDS if untreated is >30%. In absence of high HIV RNA, others recommend deferring therapy and monitoring CD4 and HIV RNA. Clinical outcomes data after initiating therapy are lacking.
Asymptomatic	CD4+ >350 AND <30,000 (bDNA) or <55,000 (RT-PCR)	Many experts would defer therapy and observe, recognizing that the 3 year risk of AIDS in untreated patients is <15%.

[†]Clinical benefit demonstrated at CD4+ ≤200/mm^3; many experts would offer therapy at CD4+ <350.
Source: Based on United States Public Health Service-Infectious Disease Society of America 1999 Guidelines: http://hivatis.org.

TABLE 19.9 RECOMMENDED ANTIRETROVIRAL AGENTS FOR TREATMENT OF ESTABLISHED HIV INFECTION

Strongly recommended: Strong evidence of clinical benefit and sustained suppression of plasma viral load. (One drug from column A and two from column B. Drugs are listed in random order.)

Column A	Column B
Indinavir	Zidovudine (ZDV) + didanosine (ddI)
Nelfinavir	Zidovudine (ZDV) + lamivudine (3TC)
Ritonavir and saquinavir[†]	Stavudine (d4T) + lamivudine (3TC)
Efavirenz	Stavudine (d4T) + didanosine (ddI)[¶]
Ritonavir and indinavir	
Ritonavir/lopinavir[±]	

Recommended alternative: Less likely to provide sustained virus suppression. (One drug from column A and two drugs from column B. Drugs are listed in random order.)

Abacavir**	Didanosine (ddI) + lamivudine (3TC)
Amprenavir	Zidovudine (ZDV) + zalcitabine (ddC)
Delavirdine or nevirapine***	
Nelfinavir + saqinavir	
Ritonavir	
Saquinavir[†]	

No recommendations: insufficient data
  Hydroxyurea in combination with antiretrovial drugs
  Ritonavir + amprenavir
  Ritonavir + nelfinavir

(continued)

TABLE 19.9 *(continued)*

Not recommended: evidence against use, virologically undesirable

All monotherapies**	Zalcitabine (ddC) + stavudine (d4T)
Zalcitabine (ddC) + didanosine (ddI)	Saquinavir-HGC[†]
Stavudine (d4T) + zidovudine (ZDV)	Zalcitabine (ddC) + lamivudine (3TC)

[†] Hard gel capsule of saquinavir (Invirase) not recommended due to poor biovailability, except in combination with ritonavir. Soft gel formulation (Fortovase) is prefered when using single protease inhibitor (and is less expensive).
** Virologic/immunologic endpoints for abacavir + ZDV +3TC similar to IDV + 3TC after 48 weeks (long-term data not available).
*** The only combination of 2NRTIs + 1NNRTI (with exception of efavirenz) shown to suppress viremia to undetectable levels is ZDV + ddI + nevirapine (studied in antiretroviral naive individuals).
# High-level resistence develops to 3TC with 2–4 weeks in partially suppressive regimens; optimal use in 3 drug antiretroviral combinations that reduce viral load to <500 copies/mL.
ZDV monotherapy may be considered for prophylactic use in pregnant women with low viral load and high CD4 (to reduce perinatal transmission).
¶ Pregnant women have increased risk of lactic acidosis and liver damage with combination of stavudine and didanosine. Use only if potential benefit outweighs risk.
± Coformulated as Kaletra.
Source: Based on United States Public Health Service-Infectious Disease Society of America 1999 Guidelines: http://hivatis.org.

Antiretroviral Therapy Efficacy Assessment

- HIV RNA levels: Levels should decrease one-$\log_{10}$ at 8 weeks and become undetectable at 4 to 6 months.
- Failure of therapy: May be due to nonadherence, inadequate potency/levels of antiretroviral drugs, or viral resistance. If therapy fails despite adherence, change regimen based on treatment history and drug resistance testing.

Antiretroviral Therapy Toxicity Assessment

- Assess drug toxicity twice during first month, then every 3 months.
- Protease inhibitors: associated with hyperglycemia (5% incidence), hypercholesterolemia (24%), hypertriglyceridemia (19%), and lipodystrophy (13%).
- Nucleoside reverse transcriptase inhibitors (NRTIs): Associated with lactic acidosis (possibly due to drug-induced mitochondrial dysfunction), hepatic steatosis, and hepatic failure.
- For tables of drug interactions, go to: http://www.hivatis.org.

Considerations During Pregnancy

- Therapy recommendations similar to nonpregnant adults. Some drugs require dosing changes. Effects on fetus unknown for many antiretroviral drugs.
- Discuss possibility of perinatal HIV transmission: 66% reduction of perinatal transmission with zidovudine given prenatally, perinatally, and postnatally.
- Consider delaying therapy until second trimester (after organogenesis) if no adverse outcome for mother is anticipated.
- Refer patient for high-risk obstetrical care.

RESOURCES

- CDC HIV website: http://www.cdc.gov/hiv/testing.htm
- Johns Hopkins HIV website: http://www.hopkins-aids.edu
- University of California, San Francisco (UCSF) HIV website: http://hivinsite.ucsf.edu
- HIV/AIDS Treatment Information Service (ATIS) website: http://hivatis.org

SELECTED REFERENCES

1. CDC. 1999 USPHS/IDSA guidelines for the prevention of opportunistic infections in persons infected with the human immunodeficiency virus. *MMWR Morb Mortal Wkly Rep* 1999;49(No. RR-10).

2. De Quiros JCLB, Miro JM, Pena JM, etal (Grupo de Estudio del SIDA 04/98). A randomized trial of the discontinuation of primary and secondary prophylaxis against *Pneumocystis carinii* pneumonia after highly active antiretroviral therapy in patients with HIV infection. *N Engl J Med* 2001;344:159–167.

3. Furrer H. Discontinuation of primary prophylaxis against *Pneumocystis carinii* pneumonia in HIV-1-infected adults treated with combination antiretroviral therapy. *N Engl J Med* 1999;340:1301–1306.

4. Kahn JO, Walker BD. Acute human immunodeficiency virus type 1 infection. *N Engl J Med* 1998;339:33–39.

5. Kirk O. Can chemoprophylaxis against opportunistic infections be discontinued after an increase in CD4-cells induced by highly active antiretroviral therapy? *AIDS* 1999;13:1647–1651.

6. Kovacs JA, Masur H. Prophylaxis against opportunistic infections in patients with human immunodeficiency virus infection. *N Engl J Med* 2000;342;1416–1429.

7. Henrard DR. Natural history of HIV-1 cell-free viremia. *JAMA* 1995;274:554–558

8. Ledergerber B, Mocroft A, Reiss P, et al. (Eight European Study Groups). Discontinuation of secondary prophylaxis against *Pneumocystis carinii* pneumonia in patients with HIV infection who have a response to antiretroviral therapy. *N Engl J Med* 2001;344:168–174.

9. MMWR Appendix. Recommendations to help patients avoid exposure to opportunistic pathogens. *MMWR Morb Mortal Wkly Rep* 1999;48(RR10):61–66.

10. Palella FJ. Declining morbidity and mortality among patients with advanced human immunodeficiency virus infection. *N Engl J Med* 1998;338:853–860.

11. Rosenberg ES, Caliendo AM, Walker BD. Acute HIV infection among patients tested for mononucleosis [letter]. *N Engl J Med* 1999;340:969.

12. Schneider MME. Discontinuation of prophylaxis for *Pneumocystis carinii* pneumonia in HIV-1-infected patients treated with highly active antiretroviral therapy. *Lancet* 1999;353:201–203.

13. Sperling RS, Shapiro DE, Coombs RW, et al. Maternal viral load, zidovudine treatment, and the risk of transmission of human immunodeficiency virus type 1 from mother to infant. Pediatric AIDS Clinical Trials Group Protocol 076 Study Group. *N Engl J Med* 1996;335:1621–1629.

14. Tsiodras S. Effects of protease inhibitors on hyperglycemia, hyperlipidemia, and lipodystrophy. *Arch Intern Med* 2000;160:2050–2056.

15. UNAIDS/WHO. Report on the global HIV/AIDS epidemic. June 1998 (www.unaids.org/hivaidsinfo/statistics/june98/global_report/data).

16. Vanhems P, Lambert J, Cooper DA, et al. Severity and prognosis of acute human immunodeficiency virus type 1 illness: a dose-response relationship. *Clin Infect Dis* 1998;26:323–329.

17. Weverling GJ. Discontinuation of *Pneumocystic carinii* pneumonia prophylaxis after start of highly active antiretroviral therapy in HIV-1 infection. *Lancet* 1999;353:1293–1298.

18. Whitcup SM. Discontinuation of anticytomegalovirus therapy in persons with HIV infection and cytomegalovirus retinitis. *JAMA* 1999;282:1633–1637.

PREVENTION OF BACTERIAL ENDOCARDITIS

INTRODUCTION

- Infective endocarditis (IE) is an infection of the endocardial surface, including infections of intracardiac foreign bodies and major vessels.
- Despite adequate treatment, IE has high mortality due to valve failure and recurrences.
- Incidence ranges from 1.5 to 4 per 100,000 people, with peak between the ages 60 and 80 (Karchmer, 1997).

PATHOPHYSIOLOGY/CLINICAL PRESENTATION

- IE can be classified into 3 major syndromes (see Table 20.1).

TABLE 20.1 CLASSIFICATION OF ORGANISMS ASSOCIATED WITH INFECTIVE ENDOCARDITIS IN ADULTS BY SYNDROME

Native Valve Endocarditis		Prosthetic Valve Endocarditis %			Endocarditis from IVDA‡	
Organism	%	Organism	Early†	Late†	Organism	%
Streptococci (viridans, bovis)	45–65	Coag-negative staphylococcus	35–40	20	S. aureus	50–60
S. aureus	30–40	S. aureus	20–30	30	Enterococci	10
Enterococci	5–8	Streptococci	<5	40	Streptococci	9
Gram-negative bacilli	4–8	Gram-negative bacilli	10–15	<5	Gram-negative bacilli	7
Coag-negative staphylococcus (S. lugdunesis)	3–8	Enterococci	5	10	Polymicrobial	6
Fungi (Candida, Aspergillus)	1	Fungi	5	<5	Fungi	5
Polymicrobial	1	Diptheroids	3	<5	Culture-negative*	3
Culture-negative*	3–10	Culture-negative*	<5	<5		

* Culture-negative: Nutritionally-deficient strep, HACEK (Haemophilus parainfluenzae & aphrophilus, Actinobacillus, Cardiobacterium, Eikenella, Kingella), Bartonella, Coxiella, Brucella, Legionella, Chlamydia.
† Early-onset infective endocarditis E: < 60 days post-op; intermediate-onset infective endocarditis: 60 days to 12 months post-op; late-onset infective endocarditis: >12 months post-op.
‡ IVDA*, intravenous drug abuse.
Sources: Adapted from Skillings J. Endocarditis and endocarditis prophylaxis. Lippincotis Prim Care Prac 1998; 2(5): 529–532; Karchmer AW. Infective endocarditis. In: Braunwald E, ed. Heart disease: a textbook of cardiovascular medicine, 5th ed. Philadelphia: W. B. Saunders Company, 1997; and Kaye DA. Infective endocarditis. In: Isselbacher KJ, et al., eds. Harrison's principles of internal medicine, 13th ed. New York: McGraw-Hill, 1994.

- **Native valves:** risk factors and incidence (Karchmer, 1997):
  ⇒ Rheumatic heart disease (RHD): 25% to 30%
  ⇒ Congenital heart disease (CHD): 10% to 20%
  ⇒ Mitral valve prolapse (MVP): 10% to 30%
  ⇒ Intravenous drug abuse (IVDA): 15% to 35%

⇒ Unknown cause: 25% to 45%

⇒ CHD and IVDA-related IE are more common in younger patients. As patients age, degenerative heart disease and prosthetic valve endocarditis (PVE) become more important as risks.

● Prosthetic valves: incidence (Strom, 1998):

⇒ Prosthetic valve IE accounts for 10% to 20% of IE cases.

⇒ Risk of IE is greatest during first year postop, and is 1% per year thereafter.

⇒ There is a greater than 5% chance of acquiring IE over the life of a valve.

TREATMENT (PROPHYLAXIS)

● American Heart Association (AHA) recommendations for prevention of bacterial endocarditis are based on case-control and animal studies, and represent consensus statements (www.americanheart.org/presenter.jhtml).

● Data on efficacy of antimicrobial prophylaxis is limited by the lack of prospective, randomized, double-blind trials.

● Previous studies suggest that antimicrobial prophylaxis using current guidelines, even if 100% effective, would prevent fewer than 10% of cases of IE due to viridans Streptococci or similar oral flora (Kaye, 1991).

● Majority of cases of bacterial endocarditis occur in patients with abnormal valves who have not had a recent procedure (Strom, 1998).

● Given the high morbidity and mortality associated with IE and the evidence that antibiotic prophylaxis can reduce incidence of procedure-related IE, consensus remains that prophylaxis is warranted for certain procedures in patients with moderate- or high-risk cardiac or arterial conditions, as outlined in Tables 20.2 through 20.6 (Horstkotte, 1987; van der Meer, 1992).

TABLE 20.2 TYPES OF LESIONS FOR WHICH ENDOCARDITIS PROPHYLAXIS IS RECOMMENDED

High Risk Lesions	Moderate Risk Lesions
Prosthetic valves (mechanical, bioprosthetic, and homograft)	Other uncorrected congenital heart disease (PDA, VSD, complicated ASD, aortic coarctation, and bicuspid aortic valve), surgically or device-repaired congenital defects within first 6 months after repair or with residual defect after 6 months.
Previous bacterial endocarditis	Acquired valve dysfunction (rheumatic heart disease)
Complex congenital heart disease (single ventricle, transposition, tetralogy of Fallot)	Hypertrophic cardiomyopathy
Surgically constructed systemic-pulmonary shunts	Mitral valve prolapse with murmur or regurgitation or evidence of regurgitation or thickened leaflets on echocardiogram.

PDA, patent ductus arteriosus; VSD, ventricular septal defect; ASD, atrial septal defect.
Sources: Adapted from Dajani AS. Prevention of bacterial endocarditis: recommendations by the American Heart Association. *JAMA* 1997; 277 (22): 1794–1801; and Zuckerman JM. Prevention of endocarditis in the dental patient. *Infections in Medicine* 2001;18:107–113.

TABLE 20.3 TYPES OF LESIONS FOR WHICH ENDOCARDITIS PROPHYLAXIS IS *NOT* RECOMMENDED

Negligible Risk Category (no greater risk than the general population)
Isolated ostium secundum ASD
Surgically or device-repaired ASD, VSD, PDA without residual defect more than 6 months post-op (Prophylaxis should be given for 6 months regardless of the presence or absence of a persistent defect.)
Previous coronary artery bypass grafting (CABG)

(continued)

TABLE 20.3 *(continued)*

Negligible Risk Category (no greater risk than the general population)

Mitral valve prolapse without regurgitation
Physiologic, functional, or innocent heart murmurs
Previous Kawasaki or rheumatic heart disease without valve dysfunction
Cardiac pacemakers and implanted defibrillators

ASD, atrial septal defect; VSD, ventricular septal defect; PDA, patent ductus arteriosus.
Source: Adapted from Dajani AS. Prevention of bacterial endocarditis: recommendations by the American Heart Association. *JAMA* 1997;277(22):1794–1801.

TABLE 20.4 RISK OF BACTEREMIA FOR DENTAL AND ORAL PROCEDURES

Significant Risk of Bacteremia	Negligible Risk of Bacteremia
Dental extractions	Restorative dentistry (operative and prosthodontic with or without retraction cord (including restoration of decayed teeth, filling cavities, replacement of missing teeth). Note: If significant bleeding occurs or is anticipated, antibiotic treatment is warranted.
Periodontal procedures	Local anesthetic injections (nonintraligamentary)
Dental implant placement and reimplantation of avulsed teeth	Intracanal endodontic treatment; post placement and buildup
Endodontic (root canal) instrumentation or surgery only beyond the apex	Placement of rubber dams
Subgingival placement of antibiotic fibers or strips	Postoperative suture removal
Initial placement of orthodontic bands but not brackets	Placement of removable prosthodontic or orthodontic appliances
Intraligamentary local anesthetic injections	Taking of oral impressions or radiographs
Prophylactic cleaning of teeth or implants where bleeding is anticipated	Fluoride treatments
	Orthodontic appliance adjustment
	Shedding of primary teeth

Source: Adapted from Dajani AS. Prevention of bacterial endocarditis: recommendations by the American Heart Association. *JAMA* 1997;277 (22):1794–1801.

TABLE 20.5 RISK OF BACTEREMIA FOR MEDICAL PROCEDURES

Type of Procedure	Significant Risk of Bacteremia for All Patients	Risk Warrants Optional Prophylaxis in High Risk Patients Only	Negligible Risk of Bacteremia for All Patients
Respiratory tract	Tonsillectomy and adenoidectomy Surgery involving respiratory mucosa Rigid bronchoscopy	Flexible bronchoscopy with or without biopsy	Endotracheal intubation Tympanostomy tube insertion
Gastrointestinal tract (optional for moderate-risk patients)	Sclerotherapy of esophageal varices Esophageal stricture dilation Endoscopic retrograde cholangiopancreatography (ERCP) in the setting of biliary obstruction Biliary tract surgery Surgery involving intestinal mucosa	Transesophageal echocardiography Endoscopy with or without biopsy	

(continued)

TABLE 20.5 *(continued)*

Type of Procedure	Significant Risk of Bacteremia for All Patients	Risk Warrants Optional Prophylaxis in High Risk Patients Only	Negligible Risk of Bacteremia for All Patients
Genitourinary tract	Prostatic surgery Cystoscopy Urethral dilation	Vaginal delivery Vaginal hysterectomy	Cesarean section Circumcision In uninfected tissue: urethral catheterization; uterine dilatation and curettage; therapeutic abortion; sterilization procedures; insertion or removal of intrauterine devices
Cardiac/other			Cardiac catherization and balloon angioplasty; implanted cardiac pacemakers, defibrillators, and coronary stents; incision or biopsy of surgically scrubbed skin

Source: Adapted from Dajani AS. Prevention of bacterial endocarditis: recommendations by the American Heart Association. *JAMA* 1997; 227 (22):1794–1801.

- Prophylaxis is most effective if given perioperatively in doses that are sufficient to ensure adequate antibiotic concentrations in the serum during and after procedure.
- If multiple procedures must be performed, minimize number of procedures and separate by 9 to 14 days to decrease the promotion of resistance to prophylactic antibiotics.
- Prophylaxis does not preclude procedure-related IE. Look closely for IE even in patients who receive proper prophylaxis.
- Prophylactic antibiotic choices are made to cover most common bacterial pathogens associated with procedure type.
  ⇒ Oral, dental, respiratory, and esophageal procedures predispose to viridans Streptococcal bacteremia.
  ⇒ Genitourinary and nonesophageal gastrointestinal procedures predispose to *Enterococcus faecalis* bacteremia.
  ⇒ Gram-negative bacilli are only rarely associated with endocarditis.
- If patient is chronically taking antibiotics used for prophylaxis, select drug from another class for use prior to procedure.
- Patients on chronic penicillin or amoxicillin for secondary prevention of RHD should be given clindamycin, azithromycin, or clarithromycin.

TABLE 20.6 AHA RECOMMENDED PROPHYLACTIC ANTIBIOTIC REGIMENS

Valve or Lesion Risk		Significant Risk Procedure		Risk Warrants Optional Prophylaxis	
		Dental, Oral, Respiratory Tract, or Esophageal	Nonesophageal GI and GU	Dental, Oral, Respiratory Tract, or Esophageal	Nonesophageal GI and GU
High risk	PCN nonallergic	Amoxicillin po or ampicillin IV	Ampicillin and gentamicin	Amoxicillin po or ampicillin IV	Ampicillin and gentamicin
	PCN allergic	Clindamycin, cephalexin, azithromycin, or clarithromycin po or cefazolin IV	Vancomycin and gentamicin	Clindamycin, cephalexin, azithromycin, or clarithromycin po or cefazolin IV	Vancomycin and gentamicin
Moderate risk	PCN nonallergic	Amoxicillin po or ampicillin IV	Amoxicillin po or ampicillin IV	Optional for esophageal: amoxicillin po ampicillin IV	Optional for GI: amoxicillin po ampicillin IV

(continued)

TABLE 20.6 *(continued)*

Valve or Lesion Risk	Significant Risk Procedure		Risk Warrants Optional Prophylaxis	
	Dental, Oral, Respiratory Tract, or Esophageal	Nonesophageal GI and GU	Dental, Oral, Respiratory Tract, or Esophageal	Nonesophageal GI and GU
PCN allergic	Clindamycin, cephalexin, azithromycin, or clarithromycin po or cefazolin IV	Vancomycin IV	No prophylaxis	No prophylaxis

AHA, American Heart Association; GI gastrointestinal; GU, genitourinary; PCN, penicillin; po, by mouth; IV, intravenous.
Source: Adapted from Dajani AS. Prevention of bacterial endocarditis: recommendations by the American Heart Association. *JAMA* 1997;227 (22):1794–1801.

SELECTED REFERENCES

1. Dajani AS. Prevention of bacterial endocarditis: recommendations by the American Heart Association. *JAMA* 1997;277(22):1794–1801.
2. Durack DT. Prevention of infective endocarditis. *N Engl J Med* 1995;332(1):38–44.
3. Horstkotte D. Contribution for choosing the optimal prophylaxis of bacterial endocarditis. *Eur Heart J* 1987; 8(supplJ):379.
4. Karchmer AW. Infective endocarditis. In: E Braunwald, ed. *Heart disease: a textbook of cardiovascular medicine,* 5th ed. Philadelphia: WB Saunders, 1997.
5. Kaye D, Abrutyn E. Prevention of bacterial endocarditis: 1991 [editorial]. *Ann Intern Med* 1991;114:803–804.
6. Kaye DA. Infective endocarditis. In: Isselbacher KJ, et al., eds. *Harrison's principles of internal medicine,* 13th ed. New York: McGraw-Hill, 1994.
7. Skillings JB. Endocarditis and endocarditis prophylaxis. *Lippincotts Prim Care Pract* 1998;2(5):529–532.
8. Strom BL. Dental and cardiac risk factors for infective endocarditis. A population-based case-control study. *Ann Intern Med* 1998;129(10):761–769.
9. Strom BL. Risk factors for infective endocarditis: oral hygiene and nondental exposures. *Circulation* 2000; 102(23):2842–2848.
10. van der Meer, JTM. Efficacy of antibiotic prophylaxis for prevention of native-valve endocarditis. *Lancet* 1992;339:135–139.
11. Zuckerman JM. Prevention of endocarditis in the dental patient. *Infect Med* 2001;18:107–113.

TRAVEL MEDICINE

INTRODUCTION

- One billion passengers travel by air annually; over 50 million visit the developing world from industrialized nations.
- Travelers should seek medical consultation more than 1 month before departure.

EVALUATION

- Consider underlying medical conditions: cardiopulmonary disease, thromboembolic disease, HIV and other immunocompromised states (such as with malignancy, corticosteroid use, chemotherapy), splenectomy (due to increased risk of babesiosis, encapsulated organisms; allergy to medications or vaccine components (e.g., eggs, gelatin, neomycin), pregnancy, diabetes, immunization history.
- Obtain details of planned journey: itinerary, length of stay, type of travel (rural, urban, business, backpacking), level of accommodation.
- Evaluate potential exposures/risks: freshwater bathing; sexual activity; scuba diving; mountaineering/climbing; contact with animals. Increased risk associated with backpacking; long-term travel; returning home of foreign-born travelers; health-care excursions; adventure trips.

TREATMENT

General Advice

- Travelers should carry a medical kit containing: thermometer, tweezers, bandages, sunscreen, insect repellant, topical antibiotic, acetaminophen, antimotility agent for diarrhea, personal medications (enough for trip carried in prescription bottles). If appropriate, also carry: oral rehydration therapy (ORT), iodine tablets (water sterilization), oral antibiotics (for diarrhea).
- Travelers should also carry a written list with medical information: allergies, medications (generic names, dosages), contact numbers, immunization documentation, recent electrocardiogram, blood type.
- Medical evacuation insurance should be purchased for high-risk or long-term travel.
- Identify risks associated with region/type of travel (see Tables 21.1 and 21.2).

TABLE 21.1 ILLNESSES ASSOCIATED WITH TRAVEL AND RECOMMENDATIONS

Condition	Pathogenesis/Recommendations
Traveler's diarrhea	• Common bacteria: enterotoxic *E. coli*, possibly enteroaggregative *E. coli*, campylobacter, shigella, salmonella. Viruses; rotavirus, norwalk-like viruses. • Symptoms: diarrhea, nausea, bloating, malaise for 3–7 days. Complications: reactive arthritis, postinfectious enteropathy, *C. jejuni*-associated Guillain-Barré.

(continued)

TABLE 21.1 *(continued)*

Condition	Pathogenesis/Recommendations
	• Prevention: Avoid contaminated food/water. Drink beverages made with boiled water, canned/bottled carbonated beverages, beer, wine. Disinfect potentially contaminated water with iodine/chlorine (kills most bacterial/viral pathogens, but protozoal cysts of *Giardia lamblia*, *Entamoeba histolytica* and oocysts of cryptosporidum may survive). Avoid raw food (salad, vegetables, and fruits unless peeled by self), unpasteurized milk, raw meat, shellfish. Immunocompromised patients should consider bringing water filtration devices.
	• Treatment: Fluid/electrolyte replacement antimotility agent (loperamide 4 mg, then 2 mg after diarrhea up to 16 mg/day), antibiotics (fluoroquinolone for 3 days, although not in women or children; resistance increasing; azithromycin is reasonable alternative). Seek medical attention if diarrhea is severe, bloody, lasts for more than 5–7 days, is accompanied by fever or chills, or unable to keep up with fluid loss.
Tuberculosis (TB)	• Risk of TB after more than 3 weeks in endemic countries is 7.9/1000 person-months/travel in health care workers and 2.8/1000 in all others (Coeblens et al., 2000). Consider PPD before and after travel.
Insect-borne illnesses: malaria, dengue fever, yellow fever, Japanese encephalitis (via mosquito); leishmaniasis (via sandfly)	• Prevention: Minimize exposure of skin day and night. On skin, use 10%–30% DEET-based products; on clothes, consider permethrin-based product. Consider netting over bed at night (fine mesh for sand flies, which are smaller than mosquitoes). Regular checks for ticks.
HIV, hepatitis B, hepatitis C	• High-risk behaviors: Sexual intercourse (vaginal, anal, orogenital); use of nonsterile needles (acupuncture, intravenous drug abuse, steroids/vitamins, medical/dental procedures, piercing, tattooing); tranfusions outside the United States, Australia, New Zealand, Canada, Japan, Western Europe.
	• Prevention: Avoid sharing razors/toothbrushes; travelers with hemophilia/Type 1 diabetes should bring sufficient syringes/needles/alcohol wipes; health care workers should consider bringing postexposure antiretroviral prophylaxis.
Sexually transmitted diseases	• Risk: ≥5% of short-term travelers engage in casual sex while abroad, and often do not use condoms.
	• Prevention: Abstinence/safe-sex practices (condoms). Avoid commercial sex workers.
Animal bites, envenomations	• Prevention: Consider rabies vaccine for long term/remote travel. Avoid petting/feeding animals (especially dogs and monkeys). Check bedding before use, check shoes before wearing; use covered footwear, consider reef shoes in water.

PPD, purified protein derivative (of tuberculin); DEET, diethyltoluamide.

TABLE 21.2 ENVIRONMENT-RELATED CONDITIONS AND RECOMMENDATIONS

Condition	Pathogenesis/Recommendations
Altitude/mountain sickness	• Symptoms: ≥25% of those who ascend rapidly to 2500 meters develop symptoms including headache, nausea, lightheadedness, insomnia.
	• Prevention: Ascend slowly; acclimatize 2–3 days at 2500–3000 meters, then 1–2 days per 1000 meters above that.
	• Treatment: Stop ascent; if symptoms worsen, descend immediately; drink fluids, avoid alcohol.
Freshwater, soil-borne risks	• Risk of schistosomiasis, leptospirosis in freshwater areas of prevalence. Walking barefoot on soil and beaches contaminated with human/canine feces may lead to cutaneous larva migrans, hookworm, or strongyloides.
Heat, humidity, sun-related illnesses	• Prevention: Drink fluids, avoid dehydration, rest frequently; wear light-colored, loose-fitting clothing; wear sunscreen with sun protection factor (SPF) ≥15 and wear hat and sunglasses.

Immunizations (Table 21.3)

- For current recommendations, see: http://www.cdc.gov/travel.
- Patients traveling to developing countries should be immunized to measles, mumps, rubella, tetanus, diphtheria, pertussis, varicella and *H. influenza* type B.
- Patients traveling to Asia or Africa should be immunized to poliovirus.
- If indicated, pneumococcal vaccine should be given.
- Patients at high risk for severe influenza traveling to tropics or with a large tour group (any time of year), or to southern hemisphere (April to September), should receive influenza vaccine.

TABLE 21.3 VACCINATIONS FOR ADULT TRAVELERS

Illness	Vaccine	Dose Schedule (for Nonimmune Adult Person)	Booster
Hepatitis A	Inactivated virus	2 doses at 0,12–18 months	≥10 years
	Immune globulin	1 dose 0.02 ml/kg is standard. For prolonged travel use 0.06 ml/kg.	3 months if 0.02 ml/kg 5 months if 0.06 ml/kg
Hepatitis B	Recombinant hepatitis B SAg vaccine	3 doses at 0, 1, and 6 months	Not routine
Influenza	Inactivated whole virus or subunit	1 dose	Annual
Japanese encephalitis‡	Inactivated mouse-brain derived vaccine	3 doses at 0, 7, 14 or 30 days	≥3 yr
Lyme disease‡	*B. burgdorferi* OspA vaccine	3 doses at 0, 1, and 12 months	Not establised; possibly annually
Measles	Live attenuated virus	2 doses at 0 and at least 4 weeks	As indicated
Meningococcal meningitis	Polysaccharide	1 dose	≥3–5 years
Mumps	Live attenuated virus	1 dose	None
Pneumococcal	Polysaccharide	1 dose	None if after age 65. After 5 years if <65.
Polio	Inactivated virus (eIPV)	3 doses at 0, 4, weeks, and 6–12 months	Immunize if >10 years since last immunization and traveling to Africa or Asia
Rabies	Cell-cultured derived vaccines: purified chick-embryo cell culture (PCEC); rabies vaccine adsorbed (RVA); human diploid cell vaccine (HDCV)	Preexposure 3 doses at 0, 7, 21, or 28 days	≥6–36 months
Rubella	Live attenuated virus	1 dose	None
Tetanus-diphtheria	Toxoid	Three doses at 0, 4 weeks and 6–12 months	10 years
Tick borne encephalitis‡	Inactivated whole-virus vaccines	Varies according to vaccine 0, 1–3 mos, and 9–12mos	≥3 years
Typhoid	Parenteral Vi capsular polysaccharide typhoid vaccine	1 dose	2 years
	Oral live attenuated *S. typhi* strain Ty21a vaccine	4 oral doses every other day	5 years
	Parenteral heat and phenol inactivated vaccine	2 doses ≥4 weeks apart or 3 doses 1 week apart (less effective) (unavailable)	3 years
Varicella	Live attenuated virus	2 doses at 0 and 4–8 weeks	None
Yellow Fever*	Live attenuated 17D viral strain vaccine	1 dose 10 days to 10 years before travel	10 years

‡ Not routinely given. Refer to specialist if considering Japanese encephalitis or tick-borne encephalitis vaccination (tick-borne encephalitis vaccine not available in United States).
* Refer to travel clinic for vaccination. Some countries require proof of vaccination for entry.

- Immunization special cases:
  ⇒ Pregnancy: Avoid live attenuated viruses (yellow fever, oral polio, measles, mumps, rubella, varicella). If travel cannot be deferred to areas of high risk for yellow fever, the potential benefit of immunization should be assessed. If not previously immunized against polio, advise two doses of vaccine before travel (at 0 and 1 month). If not measles immune, recommend deferring travel until after delivery.
  ⇒ Immunocompromised patients: Avoid live attenuated viruses (yellow fever, oral polio, measles, mumps, rubella, varicella).
  ⇒ HIV positive patients: Advise killed parenteral polio and typhoid vaccines if indicated (avoid live attenuated vaccines). Risks of live yellow fever vaccine not defined; those with

asymptomatic HIV who cannot avoid exposure to yellow fever should be offered immunization. In general, measles immunization may be given if CD4 higher than 100 (higher incidence of severe measles in HIV; benefits of vaccination may outweigh risks).

⇒ People who live with immunocompromised patients: Avoid oral polio vaccine.

Malaria Chemoprophylaxis (Table 21.4)

- Malaria (*Plasmodium falciparum, P. vivax, P. ovale, P. malariae*) is spread by female anopheles mosquito.
- Medical attention should be sought for signs/symptoms of malaria associated with travel to an endemic area (recurrent fever/chills, coma, acute renal failure, pulmonary edema, diarrhea).

TABLE 21.4 MALARIA CHEMOPROPHYLAXIS (FOR ADULTS)*

Usage	Drug	Adult Dose	Side Effects	Comments
Chloroquine sensitive areas*	Chloroquine phosphate	500 mg (300 mg base) by mouth each week. Start 1–2 weeks before travel, continue 4 weeks after.	Nausea; may worsen psoriasis.	Take on full stomach to limit nausea. Avoid if prolonged QT or porphyria.
Chloroquine resistant areas*	Mefloquine (Lariam) (Mefloquine resistant *P. falciparum* is found in western Cambodia, eastern Myanmar, and at Thailand-Myanmar and Thailand-Cambodia borders)*	250 mg (228 mg base) each week. Start 1–2 weeks before travel, continue 4 weeks after.	Nausea, headache, sleep disorder, QT-prolongation, depression, vivid dreams, psychosis (rare).	Not recommended if epilepsy, seizure, psychiatric disorder, cardiac conduction abnormality. Safe in second and third trimesters of pregnancy, likely safe in first trimester (controversial).
	Atovaquone/progaunil (Malarone) (effective in mefloquine resistant areas)*	One 250 mg/100 mg tablet daily. Start 1–2 days before travel, continue 7 days after.	Headache, myalgia.	Take with food or milk. Unknown risk in pregnancy/lactation.
	Doxycycline	100 mg by mouth daily. Start 1–2 days before travel, continue 4 weeks after.	Photosensitivity, nausea, vaginal yeast infection. May decrease efficacy of oral contraceptive pills.	Contraindicated in pregnancy/lactation.
Alternative	Primaquine	52.6 mg (30 mg base) by mouth daily. Start 1–2 days before travel, continue 7 days after.	Nausea; granulocyptopenia (uncommon in malaria doses).	Decreases relapse risk of *P. vivax* or *P. ovale*. Contraindicated in pregnancy and G6PD deficiency. Take with food.

* For current sensitivities, see: *http://www.cdc.gov/travel*.
† Atovaquone/proguanil (Malarone) is FDA approved for prevention/treatment of *P. falciparum* only, and may be less effective against other malaria species.

Specific medical conditions:

- Diabetics: Carry sufficient insulin, needles, syringes, snacks for trip (east-to-west travel may require changes in insulin dosing schedule).
- Pregnant travelers: Consider healthcare access/quality at destination to determine if travel is advisable. Travel is generally safest during second trimester (lower risk of spontaneous abortion or premature labor), but for most healthy women travel is acceptable earlier. Pregnant women planning trips to areas where live virus vaccines are required or where multidrug-resistant malaria is endemic should be referred for travel-clinic specialist advice.
- Pulmonary disease: If baseline PaO_2 is less than 70 mmHg, consider supplemental O_2 in flight (PaO_2 falls 10 mmHg during air travel). For chronic obstructive pulmonary disease (COPD), consider carrying antibiotics. Recommend influenza and pneumococcal vaccines if indicated.
- Anaphylactic allergic reaction history: Travelers should carry epinephrine pen.

SELECTED REFERENCES

1. Centers for Disease Control (CDC) guidelines: http://www.cdc.gov/travel
2. Coeblens FG, van Deutekom H, Draayer-Jansen IW, et al. Risk of infection with *Mycobacterium tuberculosis* in travelers to areas of high tuberculosis endemicity. *Lancet* 2000;356:461.
3. Cook GC, ed. *Manson's tropical diseases,* 20th ed. Philadelphia: WB Saunders, 1996.
4. Guerrant RL, Walker DH, Weller PF, eds. *Tropical infectious diseases: principles and practice.* Philadelphia: Churchill Livingstone, 1999.
5. Houweling H, Coutinho RA. Risk of HIV infection among Dutch expatriates in sub-Saharan Africa. *Int J STD AIDS* 1991;2:252–257.
6. Ryan ET, Kain KC. Health advice and immunizations for travelers. *N Engl J Med* 2000;342(23):1716–1725.
7. Strickland GT, ed. *Hunter's tropical medicine and emerging infectious diseases,* 8th ed. Philadelphia: WB Saunders, 1997.
8. Update on adult immunization: recommendations of the Immunization Practices Advisory Committee (ACIP). *MMWR Morb Mortal Wkly Rep* 1991;40(RR-12):1–5.

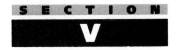

ENDOCRINE

OBESITY

INTRODUCTION

- Obesity affects 26% of U.S. adults.
- Number two cause of preventable death in the United States, contributing to 300,000 deaths per year (Calle et al., 1999).
- $100 billion per year spent on medical and disability costs; patients spend $45 billion per year on weight-loss programs and products (Wolf and Colditz, 1998).

PATHOPHYSIOLOGY

- The hypothalamus regulates body weight using information regarding food intake, body energy stores, and the environment.
- Leptin (product of obesity gene), secreted by adipocytes signals amount of body fat stores to the hypothalamus, inhibiting appetite and increasing energy expenditure in response to increasing fat stores. Leptin and related hormones are being investigated as possible antiobesity drugs.

DIFFERENTIAL DIAGNOSIS

- Hypothyroidism
- Cushing's syndrome
- Medications: steroids, insulin, citalopram, olanzapine, paroxetine, sulfonylureas, valproate

EVALUATION

- Classify patient's weight (see Table 22.1).
  $\Rightarrow$ Body mass index (BMI) = weight (kilograms)/(height in meters)^2 *OR* weight (pounds) $\times$ 704/(height in inches)^2

TABLE 22.1 BMI CLASSIFICATIONS

Classification	BMI
Underweight	<19
Goal weight	19–25
Overweight	26–30
Obesity class I	30–35
Obesity class II	35–40
Obesity class III	>40

BMI, body mass index.

- Evaluate for psychiatric conditions.
  $\Rightarrow$ 10% of patients with obesity meet formal Diagnostic and Statistical Manual of Mental Disorders, 4th ed. (DSM-IV) criteria for "binge eating disorder" (BED), defined as rapid in-

take of large amounts of food, often in private and beyond the point of comfortable fullness, at least two times per week.

⇒ Screen with the "CAGE" questions for BED:

Can't stop—unable to stop eating when desired
Amount—eats large amounts in a short period of time
Guilty/depressed—feeling after each episode
Eat healthier—patient determined to eat healthier or diet after each episode

  ⇒ Other psychiatric conditions such as depression also common; may contribute to overeating.
- Assess lifetime and family weight history:
  ⇒ Most nonobese Americans slimmest at age 18, gain 10% to 15% over baseline weight in adulthood, trend down slightly after age 70.
  ⇒ Determine onset of obesity and assess for family history of obesity.
- Elicit diet/exercise history:
  ⇒ Assess pattern of eating (amounts/types of foods).
  ⇒ Assess exercise habits.
  ⇒ Identify precipitants of eating, weight gain, and circumstances affecting diet (home and job schedules, financial constraints).

TREATMENT

Goals

- Achieve modest weight loss (10% initial body weight) and maintain that loss.
- Minimize obesity-related medical problems (see Table 22.2).

TABLE 22.2 HEALTH CONSEQUENCES OF OBESITY*

Metabolic	Anatomic	Neoplastic	Degenerative
Diabetes mellitus	OSA	Reproductive	CAD and PVD
Hypertriglyceridema	GERD	Breast	Osteoarthritis
Hypercholesterolemia	Venous stasis	Endometrial	Vertebral disc disease
Hypertension	Cellulitis	Ovarian	Lower back pain
Cholelithiasis	Pseudotumor cerebri	Prostate	
Steatohepatitis	Stress incontinence	GI	**Psychological**
Gout	Fungal skin infections	Colorectal	Anxiety
Central sleep apnea	Decubitus ulcers	Esophageal (adeno)	Depression
Reproductive dysfunction	Increased injury risk	Renal cell carcinoma	Binge eating disorder

*Modest weight reductions and prevention of weight gain have been shown to decrease rate of complications (Williamson et al., 2000).
OSA, obstructive sleep apnea; GERD, gastroesophageal reflux disease; GI, gastrointestinal; CAD, coronary artery disease; PVD, peripheral vascular disease.

Dieting

- Popular **diets** (Atkins, The Zone, Sugarbusters) work in short term for modest weight loss, but few people can maintain them long term. Balanced hypocaloric diets are more biological.
- Assess eating patterns and teach dieting skills (e.g., eat midafternoon snacks to avoid evening binges).
- Referral to dietitian or nutritionist is often helpful to reinforce dieting skills.
- A diet deficient by 500 calories a day will result in a 1 pound per week weight loss (assuming no compensatory decrease in energy expenditure).

Exercise

- Exercise improves maintenance of weight loss and decreases the cardiovascular risk and muscle loss associated with weight loss.
- Modest amounts of exercise are often sufficient.

- Those who have been sedentary with risk factors for coronary artery disease (CAD) should undergo exercise tolerance testing before initiating an exercise regimen.
- Referral to physical therapy can be helpful to draft a comprehensive exercise plan.

Cognitive Behavioral Approaches

- Long-term behavioral modifications are necessary to sustain eating and exercise patterns.
- Adjunctive therapies include self-monitoring (diaries), stimulus recognition and control, and self-reward.

Pharmacotherapy

- **Sibutramine (Meridia):** Norepinephrine and serotonin reuptake inhibitor; suppresses appetite and increases energy expenditure. May cause hypertension, which must be monitored and treated. Use cautiously with selective serotonin reuptake inhibitor (SSRI) antidepressants.
- **Phentermine and diethylpropion (Tenuate):** noradrenergic agents approved for short-term use.
- **Orlistat:** Pancreatic lipase inhibitor, causes 70% reduction in absorption of dietary fat. After one year, 55% of patients lost more than 5% of their body weight, and 25% lost over 10%, compared with 33% and 15%, respectively, in the placebo group (Davidson et al., 1999).
- **Recombinant leptin (SQ):** Shown to induce weight loss in one study (Heymsfield et al., 1999); may be effective in conjunction with other methods by preventing endogenous decrease in leptin that occurs with weight loss.
- **Fenfluramine and phentermine (Fen-Phen):** Combination of two serotonergic-agonist anorectics that produced short-term effects; withdrawn from the market because of association with pulmonary hypertension and valvular heart disease.

Surgical Therapy

- **Only proven method of long-term weight reduction.**
- Consider for patients with BMI over 35, who have failed more conservative approaches, and who suffer from medical complications of obesity.
- Roux-en-Y gastric bypass is most common procedure; activates the natural satiety pathways via mechanical distention with only a small amount of food and stimulation of intestinal satiety factors by funneling food directly into the jejunum.
    ⇒ Results in significant decreases in comorbidities: more than 90% of patients with Type II diabetes mellitus discontinue all drugs; hypercholesterolemia, sleep apnea, and nonalcoholic steatohepatitis (NASH) are greatly reduced.
    ⇒ Complications: perioperative mortality (0.3%), dumping syndrome (5%), anastomotic stenosis (10%), and B_{12}/iron/vitamin D deficiencies (5% to 10% for each).

SELECTED REFERENCES

1. Abenhaim L, Moride Y, Brenot F, et al. Appetite suppressant drugs and risk of primary pulmonary hypertension. *N Engl J Med* 1996;335(5):609–616.
2. Balsiger BM, Luque de Leon E, Sarr MG. Surgical treatment of obesity: Who is an appropriate candidate? *Mayo Clin Proc* 1997;72:551–558.
3. Bruce B, Wilfley D. Binge eating among the overweight population: a serious and prevalent problem. *J Am Diet Assoc* 1996;96:58–61.
4. Calle EE, Thun MJ, Petrelli JM, et al. Body-mass index and mortality in a prospective cohort of U.S. adults. *N Engl J Med* 1999;341:1097–1105.
5. Connolly HM, Crary JL, McGoon MD, et al. Valvular heart disease associated with fenfluramine-phentermine. *N Engl J Med* 1997;337:581–588.
6. Davidson MH, Hauptman J, DiGirolamo M, et al. Weight control and risk factor reduction in obese subjects treated for 2 years with orlistat. *JAMA* 1999;281(3):235–242.
7. Goldstein DJ. Beneficial effects of modest weight loss. *Int J Obes Relat Metab Disord* 1992;16:397–415.
8. Heymsfield SB, Greenberg AS, Fujioka K, et al. Recombinant leptin for weight loss in obese and lean adults: a randomized, controlled, dose-escalation trial. *JAMA* 1999;282:1568–1575.
9. Kuczmarski RJ, Flegal KM, Campbell SM, et al. Increasing prevalence of overweight among U.S. adults. *JAMA* 1994;272:205–211.

10. Manson JE, Willett WC, Stampfer MJ, et al. Body weight and mortality among women. *N Engl J Med* 1995; 333:677–685.
11. McGinnis JM, Foege WH. Actual causes of death in the U.S. *JAMA* 1993;270:2207–2210.
12. NIH Consensus Development Panel on Physical Activity and Cardiovascular Health. *JAMA* 1996;276:241–266.
13. Rosenbaum M, Leibel RL, Hirsch J. Obesity. *N Engl J Med* 1997;337:396–407.
14. Stevens J, Cai J, Pamuk ER, et al. Effect of age on association between BMI and mortality. *N Engl J Med* 1998; 338:1–7.
15. Stunkard AJ, Berthold HC. What is behavior therapy? A very short description of behavioral weight control. *Am J Clin Nutr* 1985;41:821–823.
16. Weissman NJ. Appetite suppressants and valvular heart disease. *Am J Med Sci.* 2001;321(4):285–291.
16. Wilding J. Science, medicine and the future: obesity treatment. *BMJ* 1997;315:997–1000.
17. Williamson DF, Thompson TJ, Thun M, et al. Intentional weight loss and mortality among overweight individuals with diabetes. *Diabetes Care* 2000;23(10):1499–1504.
18. Wolf AM, Colditz GA. Current estimates of the economic cost of obesity in the United States. *Obes Res* 1998; 6(2): 97–106.

DIABETES MELLITUS

INTRODUCTION

- Diabetes mellitus (DM) is a group of metabolic disorders characterized by hyperglycemia and defects in insulin secretion, action, or both.
- 15 million Americans have type 2 DM (600,000 new cases per year); 1 million have type 1.
- Of those with type 2 DM, only half are diagnosed.
- Type 2 DM is often accompanied by hyperlipidemia, hypertension, and marked excess risk for cardiovascular disease.

DIFFERENTIAL DIAGNOSIS (TABLE 23.1)

TABLE 23.1 DIFFERENTIAL DIAGNOSIS FOR DIABETES MELLITUS

Cushing's disease	**Drug effects:**
Cystic fibrosis	β-blockers
Gestational diabetes (4% of pregnancies)	Estrogen-containing products
Growth hormone excess	Furosemide
Hemochromatosis	Glucocorticoids
Pancreatic disease	Nicotinic acid
Pheochromocytoma	Thiazides

PATHOPHYSIOLOGY

- Type 1 DM [formerly insulin-dependent DM (IDDM)] is caused by absolute deficiency of insulin secretion.
- Type 2 DM [formerly noninsulin-dependent DM (NIDDM)] is caused by a combination of resistance to insulin action and inadequate compensatory insulin secretory response.
- Type 2 DM may develop 5 to 7 years prior to diagnosis, so both cardiovascular and microvascular (retinopathy, nephropathy, neuropathy) complications may already be present at time of diagnosis.

EVALUATION

- Elicit history of polyuria, polydipsia, polyphagia, obesity or recent weight loss, fatigue, nausea.
- According to the American Diabetes Association (ADA), screening should be done:
  ⇒ In all individuals age 45 or older. If normal, repeat every 3 years.
  ⇒ More frequent screening should be done in all patients if:
    - Overweight: 120% or over desirable body weight or body mass index (BMI) greater than or equal to 27
    - First-degree relative with DM (stronger genetic component in type 2 than type 1)
    - Member of high-risk ethnic population (African-American, Hispanic, Native American, Asian-American, Pacific Islander)
    - Have delivered a baby over 9 pounds, or have been diagnosed with gestational DM

- Hypertensive: blood pressure 140/90 or above
- High-density lipoproteins (HDLs) under 35 mg/dl and/or triglycerides above 250 mg/dl
- History of impaired glucose tolerance or impaired fasting glucose
- 1997 ADA criteria for diagnosis include any of following conditions on more than one occasion:
  ⇒ Fasting plasma glucose 126 mg/dl or above
  ⇒ Symptoms of diabetes (polyuria, polydipsia, weight loss) and random glucose 200 mg/dl or above
  ⇒ Two-hour plasma glucose 200 mg/dl or above (using standard oral glucose tolerance test)
- 1997 ADA criteria also define an abnormal (but not diabetic) state of impaired fasting glucose and an impaired response to glucose tolerance testing (40% progress to type 2 DM; morbidity of impaired fasting glucose not yet well understood).
  ⇒ Impaired fasting glucose: fasting blood glucose greater than or equal to 110 mg/dl and less than 126 mg/dl
  ⇒ Impaired glucose tolerance: two-hour plasma glucose greater than or equal to 140 mg/dl and less than 200 mg/dl

TREATMENT

Goals

- Correction of hyperglycemia and prevention of vascular complications (see Table 23.2)
- Intensive management of hyperlipidemia and hypertension

Patient Education

- DM requires long-term self-management.
- Patients may be advised to exercise daily, control their diet, check fingerstick blood sugars, check their feet daily, watch for symptoms of hypoglycemia (if on sulfonylureas or insulin), and adhere to often complex medical regimens.
- Consider a nutrition referral. A diet with 60% carbohydrate, 10% protein, and less than 30% fat is recommended.
- Aggressive attempts at smoking cessation are essential.

Aggressive Risk Factor Control

- Hypertension and lipid control reduces cardiovascular morbidity and mortality with greater absolute effect in diabetics than in nondiabetics.

Glucose Monitoring

- HgbA$_1$C every 3 to 6 months, with goal of less than 7% (normal is less than 6.4%).
- Self-monitoring of blood sugars is helpful when pursuing better control.

TABLE 23.2 OVERVIEW OF DIABETES MELLITUS COMPLICATIONS

Complication	Screening	Therapy
Hypoglycemia	Symptoms of autonomic hyperactivity; both sympathetic (tremulousness, tachycardia, diaphoresis), and parasympathetic (nausea).	Adjustment of therapy, patient education regarding symptoms of hypoglycemia and its management (eat simple carbohydrates).
Retinopathy[a] • Nonproliferative • Proliferative • Macular edema	Annual dilated eye exam with eye care professional (ophthalmologist or optometrist).	Intensive glycemic control. Laser photocoagulation.
Autonomic neuropathy • Postural hypotension • Gastroparesis, nocturnal diarrhea, constipation • Sexual dysfunction • Neurogenic bladder	History of dizziness on standing or syncope. Check for orthostasis. History of anorexia, early satiety, reflux. History of impotence. Increase in interval between voiding, dribbling, incomplete voiding, incontinence.	Lifestyle changes (stand up slowly); Florinef 0.1–1 mg/day (can lead to fluid overload). Metroclopromid 10 mg tid. Erectile supplements (e.g., sildenafil) remove offending drugs. Consider referral to urologist.

(continued)

TABLE 23.2 *(continued)*

Complication	Screening	Therapy
Peripheral neuropathy	Annual neurologic exam (include Semmes-Weinstein 5.07 monofilament touch test). History of dysesthesias, paresthesias, unsteadiness, ataxic gait.	Glycemic control. Amitriptyline 25–50 mg qd. Gabapentin 100 mg tid → 300 mg tid. Topical capsaicin.
Nephropathy	Annual spot urine for microalbumin and creatinine. Microalbuminuria: 30–300 μg/mg /Cr or 30–300 mg/24 hr. Clinical albuminuria: >300 μg/mg Cr or >300 mg/24 hr. Findings must be present on at least two occasions (fever, exercise and infection can cause false positive).	Glycemic control. Blood pressure. ACEI or ARB for microalbuminuria or albuminuria even if normotensive. No clear benefit of protein restriction.
Foot disease (50,000 lower extremity amputations/yr)	Semmes-Weinstein 5.07 monofilament touch test: Insensitivity to >80% of touches indicates high risk foot. Look for ulcers, calluses, assess vascularity. Charcot's joint (acute/chronic painless deformed joint, + neuropathy).	Regular foot self-examination. Custom-built shoes, change shoes often. Podiatry referral. Vascular surgery referral for PVD. Charcot's joint: Minimize weight-bearing.
Hypertension	Regular blood pressure checks.	ACEI as primary intervention, especially if micro or gross albuminuria present. β-blockers and thiazides are also evidence-based first-line agents. α-blockers are weak insulin sensitizers.
Dyslipidemia	Annual fasting lipid panel.	Calcium channel blockers are reasonable second-line agents. NCEP 2001 ATP3 recommendations for lipid management. LDL <100 for all diabetic patients.
Coronary artery disease	Consider electrocardiogram and/or ETT in older patients or those with CHO risk factors. Screen for and treat cardiac risk factors.	ASA, β-blockers (no ocular contraindications even if hemorrhage present). β-blockers prolong life and prevent recurrent coronary events in type 2 patients with heart disease. Patients with diabetes and one or more cardiac risk factor should be treated with an ACEI.
Hyperosmolar hyperglycemic nonketotic syndrome	Ask about recent infection, cardiac ischemia, dehydration, drugs (phenytoin, diuretics). Weakness, polyuria, lethargy, confusion.	Inpatient evalution, fluid replacement, insulin, potassium replacement.

[a]100% of individuals with type 1 diabetes mellitus and 60% of individuals with type 2 diabetes mellitus develop retinopathy after 20 years. Number one cause of blindness in United States.
tid, three times a day; qd, every day; ACEI, angiotensin-converting enzyme inhibitor; PVD, peripheral vascular disease; NCEP, National Cholesterol Education Program; LDL, low-density lipoproteins; ASA, aspirin; ARB, Angiotensin receptor blocker; ATP3, Adult Treatment Panel 3.

Pharmacologic Treatment (Tables 23.3 and 23.4; Figures 23.1 and 23.2)

- If glycemic goals are not met in 1 to 2 weeks, advance therapy.
- Many endocrinologists prefer insulin as first option, particularly in elderly patients.

TABLE 23.3 ORAL TREATMENT OPTIONS IN TYPE 2 DIABETES

Name	Mechanism of Action	Side Effects and Contraindications	Comments	Dose Starting/ Maximum	Cost/ Month	Comments
Sulfonylureas (SU) Glyburide (Micronase, DiaBeta)	Acute effects medicated through insulin release. ↑ number of insulin receptors. Potentiation of insulin action.	Hypoglycemia; SIADH; hyponatremia. Contraindicated in renal/hepatic insufficiency. Use with caution in the elderly.	Many patients do not respond. 3%–10% rate of secondary failure after many months. 50% failure at 5 yrs. Cause weight gain. ↓ in HgbA1c = 1–2.	2.5 mg qd/ 20 mg qd. Take 30 min preprandial.	$10.50	If total dose is >10 mg, dose bid.
Glipizide (Glucotrol)				5 mg qd/ 40 mg qd	$18.00	If total dose is >15 mg, dose bid.

(continued)

TABLE 23.3 *(continued)*

Name	Mechanism of Action	Side Effects and Contraindications	Comments	Dose Starting/ Maximum	Cost/ Month	Comments
Biguanides Metformin (Glucophage)	↑ muscle and fat glucose uptake. ↓ hepatic glucose production. ↑ HDL.	GI upset. Lactic acidosis: increased risk if Cr >1.5, in pts with severe CV or liver disease, and with IV contrast.	Consider in obese patients. No weight gain. No hypoglycemia. HgbA1c = 1–2.	500 mg bid/ 850 mg tid	$47.20	Can combine with insulin or SUs. Hold prior to IV contrast and for 48 hours after IV contrast.
Alphaglucosidase inhibitor Acarbose (Precose)	Inhibits cleavage of saccharides, delaying carbohydrate absorption.	GI upset: gas, bloating, anemia. Many patients cannot tolerate this drug because of GI side effects.	↓ in HgbA1c = 0.5. No hypoglycemia.	25 mg tid/ 100 mg tid	$41.05	May ↑ hypoglycemia risk if used with insulin or SUs. Avoid using with metformin.
Thiazolidinediones Rosiglitazone (Avandia) Pioglitazone (Actos)	Binds to peroxisome proliferator-activated receptor γ (PPAR-γ) in muscle, fat, and liver to decrease insulin resistance.	No risk of hypoglycemia. Contraindicated in patients with ALT >2x normal. Contraindicated in class III/IV heart failure due to expansion of plasma volume.	Consider adding to insulin in patients with high insulin requirements ↓ in HgbA1c = 0.5 No hypoglycemia ↓ in HgbA1c = 0.5; ↓ = 1–1.5 if used with insulin.	2 mg bid/ 4mg bid 15 mg qd/ 45 mg qd.	$75.00 $85.00	Can combine with SUs, metformin, or insulin. LFTs every 2 months for 1 yr, then perodically. Do not use in noncompliant patients.
Meglitinides Repaglinide, (Prandin) Nateglinide (Starlix)	Insulin secretagogue like the SUs. Fast onset, short duration of action for preprandial administration.	Hypoglycemia. Avoid in hepatic and renal insufficiency.	Importance of periprandial glucose regulation is subject of debate.	0.5 mg tid/4 mg tid 60 mg tid/ 120 mg tid before meals.	$77.10	Use with metformin, not with SUs.

SIADH, syndrome of inappropriate antidiuretic hormone secretion; HgbA1c, hemoglobin A,C; qd, every day; bid, twice daily; HDL, high-density lipoproteins; GI, gastrointestinal; CR, creatinine; CV cardiovascular; IV, intravenous; tid, three times a day; ALT, alanine transaminase.

TABLE 23.4 INSULIN PHARMACOKINETICS

Insulin	Onset in Hours	Peak in Hours	Duration in Hours
Lispro (Humulog)	1/4	1/2–11/2	2–6
Regular	1/2	3–5	6–8
NPH	1	5–12	24
Lente	2	7–15	24
Ultralente	4–8	10–30	>36
Glargine (Lantus)	2–5	No Peak	14–24

NPH, isophane insulin (neutral protamine Hagedorn).

Goals: Fasting glucose, 80-120; Pre-dinner glucose, 80-120; HbA1c <7%

METFORMIN

Pros: No risk of hypoglycemia, no weight gain, may help BP control, may increase HDL.

Cons: Risk of lactic acidosis in patient with contraindications (very rare in patients without contraindications), GI upset (usually resolved by increasing dose slowly).

Dosage: Start 500-850mg qd, increase to 850mg bid. Maximum dose is 850mg tid.

Contraindications:
- Creatinine >1.5
- Impaired liver function.
- Conditions that pre-dispose to lactic acidosis.
- Hold 24 hours prior to and 48-hour post IV contrast.

SULFONYLUREAS

Pros: Safe in patients with moderate CRI.

Cons: Risk of hypoglycemia (particularly in elderly), weight gain (3-4kg), drug interactions (including with EtOH). 10-20% primary failure, and 50% of pts who respond initially no longer respond after 5yrs.

Glyburide: Start 2.5mg qd. When dose >10 mg qd split to bid. No evidence for further improvement when dose >15mg qd.

Glipizide: Start 5 mg qd. When >15 mg qd split to bid. No evidence for further improvement when dose >20mg qd.

Contraindications: Severe liver disease, severe renal disease (for glyburide only), pregnancy. Use with caution in the elderly.

COMBINATION THERAPY:
- Consider a combination of sulfonylurea with Metformin.
- Keep first drug at current dose (usually at maximum dose).
- Start new drug at low dose and increase as needed.

INSULIN THERAPY: INDICATIONS
- Primary treatment at time of diagnosis in patients with ketonuria; significant weight loss or severe symptoms; and in pts with Type 1 DM.
- Secondary treatment in patients failing to achieve glycemic control despite maximal dose of combined sulfonylurea and Metformin.
- Primary treatment in patients with contraindications to oral agents after diet and exercise prove to be ineffective in improving blood sugars.

IF PATIENT REQUIRES HIGH DOSES OF INSULIN:
- Consider adding Rosiglitazone/Pioglitazone or Metformin. However, many endocrinologists prefer high dose insulin alone.
- Rosiglitazone/Pioglitazone: Less risk of liver toxicity (never reported, but new to market). No risk of hypoglycemia. Can lead to fluid retention and weight gain.

FIGURE 23.1. Achieving glycemic control in type 2 diabetes mellitus after failure of diet and exercise alone

---

Step I:
One Injection of NPH at Bedtime or Before Breakfast
(Many endocrinologists now prefer bedtime injection)

- Initial Dose: 0.2-0.3 units/kg. May need up to 1 to 1.5 unit/kg.
- Weekly adjustments in insulin dose based either upon self glucose monitoring or venous glucose monitoring.
- If unable to achieve optimal glycemic control with once daily injection, proceed to step 2.

Step II:
One Injection of NPH at Bedtime and one Before Breakfast

- Suggested starting dose for second injection: 0.2-0.3 units/kg.
- Alternative: Determine total amount of insulin required per day, give 2/3 in AM, 1/3 in PM.
- Weekly adjustments in insulin doses.
- If unable to achieve optimal glycemic control with once daily injection, proceed to step 3.

Step III:
Addition of Regular Insulin

- Monitor AM, pre-lunch and bedtime glucose levels.
- If only the pre-lunch values are high, add regular insulin to AM NPH.
- If only bedtime values are high (and bedtime is >2 hours after dinner), give regular insulin before dinner in addition to AM and bedtime NPH.
- If pre-lunch and bedtime blood glucose levels are both elevated, add regular insulin to AM NPH and give regular insulin before dinner.
- Start regular dose at 0.075 units/kg.
- Alternative: Add total insulin dose per day, give 2/3 total dose in AM and 1/3 total dose in PM
      Then, for both the AM and PM dose, give 2/3 NPH and 1/3 regular.

*Note that many different insulin regimens are effective and that few trials have compared different regimens in
Type 2 diabetes. This is one suggested approach to insulin dosing. Other approaches may be equally effective.

FIGURE 23.2. Stepwise approach to insulin therapy. (Note that many different insulin regimens are effective and that few trials have compared different regimens in type 2 diabetes. This is one suggested approach to insulin dosing. Other approaches may be equally effective.

- Blood sugar monitoring and adjustment:
  ⇒ Morning glucose level reflects nighttime isophane insulin (NPH or neutral protamine Hagedorn).
  ⇒ Prelunch glucose level reflects morning regular.
  ⇒ Predinner glucose reflects morning NPH.
  ⇒ Bedtime glucose reflects predinner regular.
- Rule of newer insulins (lispro, glargine) in type 2 DM remain undefined, but may be useful in some cases. Lispro is given with meals to control prandial glycemic surges. Glargine provides long-term basal insulin activity (do not mix with other insulins when injecting).

RESOURCES

- American Diabetes Association (ADA) website: http://www.diabetes.org/main/application/commercewf
- National Institute of Diabetes & Digestive & Kidney Diseases: http://www.niddk.nih.gov/
- Juvenile Diabetes Research Foundation International: http://www.jdf.org/

SELECTED REFERENCES

1. Colditz GA, Willett WC, Stampfer MJ, et al. Weight as a risk factor for clinical diabetes in women. *Am J Epidemiol* 1990;132:501–513.
2. Curb JD, Pressel SL, Cutler JA, et al. Effect of diuretic-based antihypertensive treatment on cardiovascular disease risk in older diabetic patients with isolated systolic hypertension. Systolic Hypertension in the Elderly Program Cooperative Research Group. *JAMA* 1996;276:1886–1892.
3. Diabetes Control and Complications Trial Research Group. The effect of intensive treatment of diabetes on the development and progression of long-term complications in insulin-dependent diabetes mellitus. *N Engl J Med* 1993;329:977–986.
4. Early Treatment Diabetic Retinopathy Study (ETDRS) Investigators. Aspirin effects on mortality and morbidity in patients with diabetes mellitus: Early Treatment Diabetic Retinopathy Study Report 14. *JAMA* 1992;268:1292–1300.

5. Haffner SM, Lehto S, Ronnemaa T, et al. Mortality from coronary heart disease in subjects with type 2 diabetes and in nondiabetic subjects with and without prior myocardial infarction. *N Engl J Med* 1998;339:229–234.

6. Hansson L, Zanchetti A, Carruthers SG, et al. Effects of intensive blood-pressure lowering and low-dose aspirin in-patients with hypertension: Principal results of the Hypertension Optimal Treatment (HOT) randomised trial. *Lancet* 1998;351:1755–1762.

7. Hansson L, Lindholm LH, Niskanen L, et al. Effect of angiotensin converting enzyme inhibition compared with conventional therapy on cardiovascular morbidity and mortality in hypertension: The Captopril Prevention Project (CAPP) randomised trial. *Lancet* 1999;353:611–616.

8. Heart Outcomes Study Investigators. Effects of angiotensin-converting-enzyme inhibitor, Ramipril, on cardiovascular events in high-risk patients. *N Engl J Med* 2000;342:145–153.

9. Helmrich SP, Ragland DR, Leung RW, et al. Physical activity and reduced occurrence of non-insulin-dependent diabetes mellitus. *N Engl J Med* 1991;325:147–152.

10. Hu FB, van Dam RM, Liu S. Diet and risk of type II diabetes: the role of types of fat and carbohydrate. *Diabetologia* 2001;44:805–817.

11. Lynch J, Helmrich SP, Lakka TA, et al. Moderately intense physical activities and high levels of cardiorespiratory fitness reduce risk of non-insulin-dependent diabetes mellitus in middle-aged men. *Arch Intern Med* 1996;156:1307–1314.

12. Pyorala K, Pedersen TR, Kjekshus J, et al. Cholesterol lowering with simvastatin improves prognosis of diabetic patients with coronary artery disease. A subgroup analysis of the Scandinavian Simvastatin Survival Study (4S). *Diabetes Care* 1997;20:614–620.

13. Sacks FM, Pfeffer MA, Moye LA, et al. The effect of pravastatin on coronary events after myocardial infarction in patients with average cholesterol levels. *N Engl J Med* 1996;335:1001–1009.

14. Steering Committee of the Physicians' Health Study Research Group. Final report on the aspirin component of the ongoing Physicians' Health Study. *N Engl J Med* 1989;321:129–135.

15. Tuomilehto J, Lindström J, Eriksson JG, et al. Prevention of type 2 diabetes mellitus by changes in lifestyle among subjects with impaired glucose tolerance. *N Engl J Med* 2001;344:1343–1350.

16. UK Prospective Diabetes Study Group. Intensive blood-glucose control with sulphonylureas or insulin compared with conventional treatment and risk of complications in-patients with type 2 diabetes (UKPDS 33). *Lancet* 1998;352:837–853.

17. UK Prospective Diabetes Study Group. Tight blood pressure control and risk of macrovascular and microvascular complications in type 2 diabetes (UKPDS 38). *BMJ* 1998;317:703–713.

18. UK Prospective Diabetes Study Group. Effect of intensive blood-glucose control with metformin on complications in overweight patients with type 2 diabetes (UKPDS 34). *Lancet* 1998;352:854–865.

THYROID DISEASE

HYPOTHYROIDISM

Introduction

- Hypothyroidism is predominantly due to failure of the thyroid gland to produce adequate amount of thyroid hormone, but in minority of cases it results from pituitary or hypothalamic disease.
- Most common cause in United States is chronic autoimmune, or Hashimoto's, thyroiditis.
- Prevalence: Overt hypothyroidism, 0.4% (1.5% to 2% of women); subclinical hypothyroidism, 9.1%, most of which is unrecognized (Canaris et al., 2000).

Evaluation

Signs and Symptoms

- Nonspecific (see Table 24.1).
- In the elderly, less specific changes including confusion, deafness, dementia, ataxia, depression, and hair loss are seen.

TABLE 24.1 SIGNS AND SYMPTOMS OF HYPOTHYROIDISM

Physical Findings	Symptoms
Goiter	Fatigue
Nonpalpable thyroid gland	Weakness
	Cold intolerance
Hoarseness	Weight gain
Edema	Dry skin
Bradycardia	Hoarseness
Slowed speech	Muscle cramps
Cool, dry skin	Joint pain
Delayed relaxation of deep tendon reflexes	Depression
	Mental impairment
	Irregular menses
	Menorrhagia
	Infertility

Screening

- Thyroid-stimulating hormone (TSH) is best screening test, but both TSH and free T4 should be measured if central hypothyroidism is suspected.
- If TSH is elevated, send repeat TSH, free T4, and antithyroid peroxidase antibody (anti-TPO, formerly known as antimicrosomal).
- In presence of low T4, if TSH is not sufficiently elevated, central hypothyroidism (pituitary or hypothalamic) must be ruled out. If present, pituitary-adrenal axis must be assessed before administering thyroid replacement therapy to avoid precipitating adrenal crisis if cortisol levels are marginal.

- If TSH is elevated and free T4 low, then patient has overt primary hypothyroidism.
- Patients with history of thyroid disease should be screened with TSH measurement yearly.
- Women over age 50 should be screened every 5 years because of high prevalence.
- TSH should also be checked in patients with autoimmune diseases, unexplained depression, cognitive dysfunction, or hypercholesterolemia.
- Subclinical hypothyroidism: Defined as elevated TSH (greater than 5) with normal free T4 and no hypothyroid symptoms (excluding other causes). 70% of patients with subclinical hypothyroidism and positive anti-TPO antibodies progress to clinical hypothyroidism in 20 years.

Treatment

- Thyroxine (T4), rather than triiodothyronine (T3), is drug of choice.
- Should be taken on empty stomach at least 4 hours after medications that interfere with absorption from gastrointestinal (GI) tract.
- Healthy adults generally require 1.6 mcg/kg per day for full replacement.
- Evaluate every 4 to 6 weeks; titrate dose until TSH level normalizes (and every 6 to 12 months thereafter); recheck TSH in 6 weeks if dose is adjusted or if change in brand of thyroid preparation.
- Patients with angina should begin with 25 mcg per day, then increase dose in 25 mcg increments. Patients who develop angina when starting thyroxine should stop the medication until the cardiac disease is fully evaluated.
- Drugs including phenytoin, phenobarbital, carbamazepine, and rifampin accelerate thyroxine metabolism, requiring higher dosing of thyroxine.
- Overreplacement is associated with increased risk of atrial fibrillation and decreased bone mineral content.
- Pregnant hypothyroid patients should have TSH checked each trimester because many require increased thyroxine doses as pregnancy progresses.
- Subclinical hypothyroidism:
  ⇒ Potential indications for treatment include TSH of 10 or above, elevated cholesterol, and presence of anti-TPO antibodies in high titer. If untreated, monitor with yearly TSH levels.
  ⇒ Treatment may improve lipid profile and cardiac contractility.

HYPERTHYROIDISM

Introduction

- Hyperthyroidism is defined as elevated serum levels of thyroid hormones (either T4 or T3).
- Prevalence: 4 to 20 individuals per 1000 (depending on sampling pool).
- Subclinical hyperthyroidism is more common.

Pathophysiology

- **Graves' disease** is most common cause of hyperthyroidism.
  ⇒ Thyroid-stimulating immunoglobulins (TSI) bind to the TSH receptor and stimulate overproduction.
  ⇒ 80% of patients have detectable TSI antibodies.
  ⇒ Anti-TPO and antithyroglobulin antibodies may be elevated (65% to 80%).
- **Autonomous toxic adenoma** (usually greater than 3 cm) can produce enough thyroid hormone to cause thyrotoxicosis.
  ⇒ Radioactive iodine uptake (RAIU) is relatively increased at site of adenoma but suppressed elsewhere.
- **Subacute thyroiditis:** transient destruction of thyroid tissue with release of preformed hormone resulting in a 6- to 12-week hyperthyroid phase, followed by recovery. The RAIU is less than 1% during the hyperthyroid phase.
  ⇒ Subacute granulomatous (de Quervain's) thyroiditis: secondary to viral infection; presents as enlarged, diffusely tender thyroid gland; treated with nonsteroidal antiinflammatory drugs (NSAIDs) and prednisone.

⇒ Subacute lymphocytic thyroiditis (silent or painless thyroiditis): autoimmune process that resolves spontaneously but may progress to chronic lymphocytic or Hashimoto's thyroiditis.

⇒ Radiation, palpation, and amiodarone can also cause subacute thyroiditis.

- **Other causes** of hyperthyroidism: (an elevated RAIU):
  ⇒ Trophoblastic disease and TSH-mediated hyperthyroidism (pituitary adenoma or resistance) have an elevated RAIU.
  ⇒ Struma ovarii or factitious ingestion of thyroid hormone have a low RAIU.
  ⇒ Pharmacologic amounts of iodine (radiocontrast, amiodarone) may cause hyperthyroidism in patients with goiter (Jod-Basedow phenomenon).
- **Subclinical hyperthyroidism**
  ⇒ Characterized by low TSH (under 0.5) with normal T4 and T3 (exclude other causes of low TSH).
  ⇒ Affects approximately 1.5% of women and 1% of men over age 60.
  ⇒ Associated with increased risk of atrial fibrillation, left ventricular hypertrophy, accelerated bone loss, development of overt hyperthyroidism.

Evaluation

History (Table 24.2)

- Exposure to iodine, current or prior thyroid hormone use, recent pregnancy, history of goiter, anterior neck pain, family history of thyroid disease
- In elderly, may present with less specific changes, particularly atrial fibrillation or congestive heart failure.

TABLE 24.2 SIGNS AND SYMPTOMS OF HYPERTHYROIDISM

Physical Findings	Symptoms
Hypertension	Decreased menstrual flow
Irregular rhythm	Diplopia (Graves')
Pretibial myxedema (Graves')	Exertional dyspnea
Proptosis (Graves')	Weight loss
Proximal muscle weakness	Eye irritation (Graves')
Tachycardia	Fatigue
Thyromegaly (diffuse or	Heat intolerance
nodular)	Irritability
Tremor	Increased frequency of
Weight loss	bowel movements
	Increased perspiration
	Muscle weakness
	Nervousness palpitations
	Sleep disturbance
	Tremor

Laboratory Data

- TSH under 0.5 and elevated free T4 or T3 (15% present with T3 toxicosis).
- If T4 is high but TSH is not suppressed, consider a TSH-producing pituitary adenoma or pituitary resistance to TSH (both rare).
- If hyperthyroidism is confirmed, check T3 level.
- The best test to distinguish among etiologies is the RAIU, which will be elevated in Graves' disease, low in subacute thyroiditis, and normal to elevated in toxic multinodular goiter.
- Not necessary to measure TSI (thyroid stimulating immunoglobulins), which are specific to Graves' disease.
- Anti-TPO antibodies may be measured as marker of autoimmune disease.

Treatment

General Principles

- Withhold treatment until cause is determined.
- Patients who are severely thyrotoxic or clearly have Graves' disease (proptosis, large goiter, high T3) may be treated with antithyroid drugs without radioactive iodine uptake test.
- Low uptake hyperthyroidism usually implies thyroiditis, which generally resolves on its own.
- Symptomatic relief can often be achieved with β-blockers (or calcium channel blockers).
- Steroids may ameliorate hyperthyroidism; iopanoic acid can be used to reduce T4 to T3 conversion.
- For Graves' disease: antithyroid drugs, radioactive iodine, and thyroid surgery.
- In elderly patients and patients with severe symptoms, use antithyroid drugs prior to iodine ablation to minimize risk of radioiodine-induced thyroiditis causing exacerbation of hyperthyroidism.
- Subclinical disease: Clinicians often do not treat TSH of 0.1 to 0.5 in low-risk patients (no cardiac disease, premenopausal women, postmenopausal taking hormone replacement therapy).

Antithyroid Drugs

- Initial doses are methimazole 10 to 40 mg every day (single or divided doses) or propylthiouracil (PTU) 50 to 150 mg three times a day, usually given for 1 to 2 years. Both drugs block thyroid hormone synthesis; propylthiouracil also blocks T4 $\rightarrow$ T3 conversion.
- Methimazole more effective than PTU, can be given as single daily dose, less serious toxicity.
- Adverse reactions: rash/hives, itching, arthralgias, hepatocellular necrosis (PTU) or cholestatic jaundice (methimazole), nausea/vomiting, agranulocytosis (0.3%).
- Follow-up: Check thyroid function tests (TFTs) initially at 4 to 6 week intervals.
- Once euthyroid, higher initial doses may be reduced to lower maintenance doses; monitor every 3–4 months.
- Evaluate at 2 weeks, then at 4 to 8 week intervals for first 3 to 4 months to assess possibility of remission after discontinuing drug.

Radioactive Iodine Therapy

- Most common treatment; generally necessitates lifelong thyroid hormone replacement therapy.
- Contraindications: pregnancy (exclude pregnancy in young women) and breast-feeding.
- Hypothyroidism generally occurs within first 6 to 18 weeks after radioiodine therapy, but can occur later.
- Start thyroxine when hypothyroidism develops.
- Once stable thyroxine dose is achieved, follow TSH yearly.

Surgery

- Thyroidectomy is reserved for large nodules, large goiters resistant to iodine, pregnant patients, patients allergic to antithyroid drugs, and patients with severe ophthalmopathy.
- Complications: hypoparathyroidism, recurrent laryngeal nerve injury.
- Follow TFTs 2 weeks postoperatively and again at 6 weeks to monitor for hypothyroidism.
- Start thyroxine postoperatively if: euthyroid preoperatively and had near-total thyroidectomy. If hyperthyroid preoperatively, wait until euthyroid before starting replacement since serum half-life of thyroxine is 7 days.
- Once euthyroid, follow TSH levels at yearly intervals.

TOXIC NODULAR GOITER

Pathophysiology

- Toxic nodular goiter is caused by single hyperfunctioning nodule or multiple such nodules.
- Radioiodine uptake and thyroid scan reveal hyperfunctioning nodules. If there are coexisting hypofunctioning nodules, perform fine needle aspiration to rule out thyroid carcinoma.
- Toxic nodular goiter is more common in elderly patients.

Treatment

- Treatment options include radioactive iodine therapy or surgery; antithyroid drugs may be administered prior to definitive therapy to attain euthyroid state.

THYROID NODULES

Introduction

- Very common (palpable nodule is present in 4% to 7% of population); most are benign; 5% are malignant.
- Prevalence using high-resolution ultrasound is greater than 25%, and on autopsies approaches 50%.
- Detecting cancerous, asymptomatic nodule benefits long-term mortality.
- Difficult to rule out or risk-stratify thyroid cancer based on history and exam.

Pathophysiology/Clinical Presentation

- **Adenomas** may be nonfunctional ("cold" on thyroid scan) or autonomously functioning ("hot").
  - ⇒ Nonfunctional adenomas are either follicular or colloid, usually grow slowly, have TSH receptors, and usually produce little or no thyroid hormone.
  - ⇒ Cysts seen on ultrasound are often adenomas that have outgrown their blood supply and have undergone necrosis.
- **Thyroid carcinoma** fails to take up iodine and therefore is "cold" on radioiodine uptake scan; 80% are solid on ultrasound.
  - ⇒ Risk factors include family history, history of childhood radiation exposure.
  - ⇒ *Papillary* and *mixed papillary/follicular* carcinoma: 70% of all thyroid cancers; solid or cystic-solid secondary to necrosis; best prognosis
  - ⇒ *Follicular* carcinomas (including Hürthle cell carcinomas): 15% with worse prognosis
  - ⇒ *Anaplastic* carcinomas: 10% to 12%; notable for poor prognosis
  - ⇒ *Medullary* carcinomas: 10%; arise from parafollicular cells of thyroid, produce calcitonin, may be associated with MEN II.
  - ⇒ Nodules in patients under age 30 or over age 60 are more likely to be malignant.
  - ⇒ Symptoms: hoarseness, dysphagia, obstructive symptoms
  - ⇒ Suspicious nodules are large, hard, fixed, or associated with lymphadenopathy.
  - ⇒ Thyroid cancer rarely affects thyroid function.
- **Hashimoto's thyroiditis** (chronic lymphocytic thyroiditis) is an autoimmune disease and is the major cause of goiter.
  - ⇒ Hashimoto's seen in 4% of general population.
  - ⇒ Anti-TPO (antimicrosomal) antibodies seen in 70% to 95% of patients.
- Multinodular goiter is polyclonal process causing focal growth and autonomy of follicular cell aggregates; associated with colloid cysts. On radioiodine scan, appearance is heterogeneous.

Evaluation (Figure 24.1)

- **Fine needle aspiration:** Sensitivity and specificity exceed 95%.
- **Radioisotope scanning** (thyroid scintigraphy) with iodine (I^{123}) or technetium pertechnetate (Tc_{99m}). I^{123} provides functional evaluation. Cancers are always "cold" on I^{123} scan, but some will trap technetium and appear "hot."
- **Ultrasonography:** High-resolution ultrasound is highly effective for detecting nodules but cannot distinguish malignant from benign. Microcalcifications may increase risk of malignancy to as high as 30%. Purely cystic lesions can still be malignant. 40% with one nodule on exam have multiple nodules on ultrasound. Indications include multiple thyroid nodules on palpation, history of thyroid cancer or neck irradiation, and difficulty with localization on blind fine needle aspiration.
- **Serum tests:** TSH is normal in malignant disease.
  - ⇒ Antimicrosomal antibodies increases likelihood that autoimmune disease is cause.

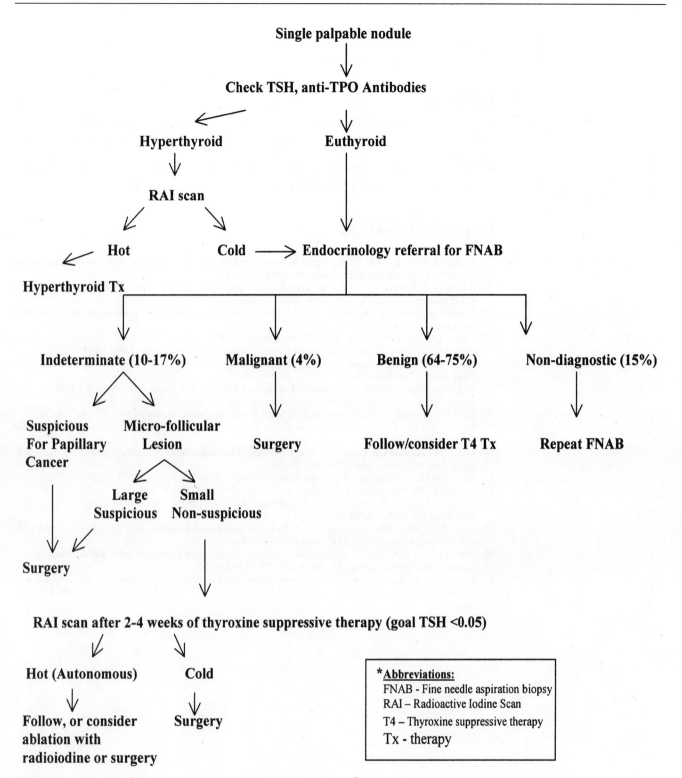

FIGURE 24.1. Algorithm for approach to a single palpable thyroid nodule.*

⇒ Elevated erythrocyte sedimentation rate (ESR) suggestive of subacute granulomatous thyroiditis.

⇒ Elevated calcitonin levels consistent with medullary carcinoma.

Treatment

- **Benign solitary nodule:** Reaspirate only if nodule grows, if initial biopsy is nondiagnostic, or if nodule is clinically suspicious but cytologically benign. Up to 33% of nodules regress spontaneously.

- **Autonomous nodules:** May be ablated with radioiodine or excised. After either treatment, patient should be monitored for hypothyroidism.

SELECTED REFERENCES

1. Brander A, Viikinkoski P, Tuuhea J, et al. Clinical versus ultrasound examination of the thyroid gland in the common clinical practice. *J Clin Ultrasound* 1992;20:37–42.
2. Bunevicius R, Kazanavicius G, Zalinkevicius R, et al. Effects of thyroxine as compared with thyroxine plus triiodothyronine in patients with hypothyroidism. *N Engl J Med* 1999;340:424–429.
3. Canaris GJ, Manowitz NR, Mayor G, et al. The Colorado thyroid disease prevalence study. *Arch Intern Med* 2000;160:526–534.
4. Cooper DS. Antithyroid drugs. *N Engl J Med* 1984;311:1353–1362.
5. Daniels GH. Thyroid nodules and nodular thyroids: a clinical overview. *Compr Ther* 1996;22:239–250.
6. Gharib H. Changing concepts in the diagnosis and management of thyroid nodules. *Endocrinol Metab Clin North Am* 1997;26:777–799.
7. Harjai KJ, Licata AA. Effects of amiodarone on thyroid function. *Ann Intern Med* 1997;126:63–73.
8. Helfand M, Crapo LM. Screening for thyroid disease. *Ann Intern Med* 1998;129:141–158.
9. Klein I, Ojamma K. Thyroid hormone and the cardiovascular system. *N Engl J Med* 2001;344:501–509.
10. Mandel SJ, Brent GA, Larsen PR. Levothyroxine therapy in patients with thyroid disease. *Ann Intern Med* 1993;119:492–502.
11. Marqusee E, Benson CB, Frates MC, et al. Usefulness of ultrasonography in the management of nodular thyroid disease. *Ann Intern Med* 2000;133:696–700.
12. Mazzaferri EL. Management of a solitary thyroid nodule. *N Engl J Med* 1993;328:553–559.
13. Sawin CT. Thyroid dysfunction in older persons. *Adv Intern Med* 1992;37:223–248.
14. Singer PA, Cooper DS, Levy EG, et al. Treatment guidelines for patients with hyperthyroidism and hypothyroidism. *JAMA* 1995;273:808–812.
15. Singer PA, Cooper DS, Daniels GH, et al. Treatment guidelines for patients with thyroid nodules and well-differentiated thyroid cancer. *Arch Intern Med* 1996;156:2165–2172.
16. Tan GH, Gharib H. Thyroid incidentalomas: management approaches to nonpalpable nodules discovered incidentally on thyroid imaging. *Ann Intern Med* 1997;126:226–231.
17. Zelmanovitz F, Genro S, Gross JL. Suppressive therapy with levothyroxine for solitary thyroid nodules: a double-blind controlled clinical study and cumulative meta-analyses. *J Clin Endocrinol Metab* 1998;83:3881–3885.

25

OSTEOPOROSIS

INTRODUCTION

- Osteoporosis is a skeletal disorder characterized by compromised bone strength and increased fracture risk.
- Leads to 1.3 million U.S. fractures per year; 30% to 50% of women over age 50 will experience osteoporotic fracture; costs over $13 billion per year.
- After sustaining hip fracture, one-third of patients regain prefracture level of function. Women who develop a vertebral fracture have 19% chance of additional fracture in next year.
- As of 1995, only 4 million of estimated 24 million Americans with osteoporosis had been diagnosed; half were treated with calcium alone; only 800,000 were on prescription medications.

EVALUATION

History

- Focus on factors that affect bone density (see Table 25.1).

TABEL 25.1 RISK FACTORS FOR DEVELOPMENT OF LOW BONE MINERAL DENSITY AND HIP FRACTURE

Risk Factors for Low Bone Mineral Density	Risk Factors for Hip Fracture
Age	Age
Female sex	Prior hip fracture or maternal history of hip fracture
Estrogen deficiency: postmenopausal status, amenorrhea, delayed puberty	Low bone mineral density
Low dietary calcium/vitamin D intake	Poor self-rated health
Family history of osteoporosis	Low physical function: slow gait, decreased quadriceps strength
European or Asian descent	Imparied cognition
Inactivity	Impaired vision
Smoking	Tall stature
Alcohol	Environmental factors, e.g., loose rugs
Low BMI	Hyperthyroidism
Glucocorticoid therapy	Tachycardia
Excess thyroid hormone	Current benzodiazepine use
Anticonvulsant therapy	Current anticonvulsant use
	Caffeine intake

BMI, body mass index.

- Asymptomatic unless it results in a fracture.
- Vertebral fractures occur with minimal stress. Pain begins suddenly and radiates to flanks and anteriorly.
- Secondary complications of hip fracture such as pulmonary embolus or infection carry mortality of 15% to 20%.

Diagnostic Testing

- Plain x-rays are insensitive for determining bone loss (30% to 40% of bone mass may be lost before x-rays show bone loss), but are useful to exclude conditions mimicking osteoporosis and to evaluate for fractures.

- Quantitative computed tomography (QCT) is most sensitive technique for detecting osteopenia but is more expensive, involves greater radiation exposure, and is less reproducible than other techniques.
- **Dual energy x-ray absorptiometry (DXA)** is preferred technique; rapid, accurate, highly reproducible, and involves minimal radiation exposure. Useful when serial scans are required to detect bone density changes over time.
  - ⇒ **T score:** Number of standard deviations (SD) the patient's value differs from mean values in 20- to 30-year-olds of same sex; used to define osteopenia/osteoporosis and to predict fracture risk. Normal bone density is T score between (−) 1 and (+) 2. For every SD below mean, there is two-fold increased risk of fracture.
    - ○ Osteopenia: T score between (−) 1 and (−) 2.5
    - ○ Osteoporosis: T score less than (−) 2.5
  - ⇒ **Z score:** Number of SDs that patient's value differs from mean values in age-matched patients of same sex. Z score below (−) 2 suggests that bone density is reduced beyond what is expected for patient's age and gender.
  - ⇒ A change in density of 0.03 g/cm^2 (lumbar spine) or 0.04 g/cm^2 (femoral neck) is clinically significant.
  - ⇒ Both proximal femur and lumbar spine predict cumulative risk for fractures equally well.
  - ⇒ Proximal femur is better predictor of hip fractures.
  - ⇒ Lumbar spine measurements are more sensitive, more reproducible, and better demonstrate changes over time.

Screening

- Recommended in:
  - ⇒ Postmenopausal women who present with fracture
  - ⇒ All women over age 65
  - ⇒ All women under age 65 with risk factors for osteoporosis (besides menopause)
  - ⇒ Women considering therapy for osteoporosis
  - ⇒ Men with a history of fractures induced by minimal trauma, low bone mass or vertebral fractures on radiographs, or conditions associated with osteoporosis (see Table 25.2).
- Screen for most common secondary causes of osteoporosis if bone density Z-score is less than (−) 2 SDs for reasons that are not apparent (see Table 25.2):
  - ⇒ Complete blood count (CBC), blood urea nitrogen (BUN)/creatinine, alkaline phosphatase, albumin, calcium, 25-OH vitamin D, thyroid-stimulating hormone (TSH), and parathyroid hormone (PTH)
  - ⇒ Serum testosterone in men with unexplained osteoporosis. Consider 24-hour urine cortisol and calcium, serum protein electrophoresis (SPEP).
- Biochemical markers of bone formation and resorption are currently under clinical investigation as possible means of detecting changes in bone remodeling before changes in bone density are evident.

TABLE 25.2 SECONDARY CAUSES OF OSTEOPOROSIS

Endocrine	Hematologic	Connective Tissue	Drugs	Gastrointestinal	Other
Hypogonadism	Multiple myeloma	Osteogenesis	Glucocorticoids	Malabsorption	Renal tubular
Hyperprolactinemia	Leukemia	imperfecta	Alcohol	Hepatobiliary	acidosis
Hyperthyroidism	Lymphoma	Ehlers-Danlos	Nicotine	disease	Immobilization
Primary	Hemolytic anemia	syndrome	Heparin	Gastrectomy	Rheumatoid
hyperparathyroidism	Polycythemia	Marfan's syndrome	Anticonvulsants		arthritis
Cushing's disease	Systemic mastocytosis	Homocystinuria	Methotrexate		Anorexia
Hypercalciuria		Scurvy	Cyclosporine		nervosa
Vitamin D deficiency			GnRH analogs		
Growth hormone			Suppressive doses		
deficiency			of thyroxine		
Amenorrhea					

GnRH, gonadotropin-releasing hormone.

TREATMENT

General Principles

- All women should be counseled about benefits of dietary calcium and vitamin D, weight-bearing exercise, and smoking cessation.
- The National Osteoporosis Foundation recommends treating:
  ⇒ Women with T scores less than (−) 2 without other risk factors for osteoporosis
  ⇒ Women with T scores less than (−) 1.5 with other risk factors for osteoporosis

Calcium and Vitamin D

- Both are necessary but not sufficient to prevent or treat osteoporosis.
- The average postmenopausal woman has daily calcium intake under 500 mg. The elderly are at risk for vitamin D deficiency because of low sunlight exposure, decreased synthesis, and low intake.
- The National Institutes of Health (NIH) Consensus Conference on Osteoporosis recommends daily calcium intake of 1000 mg (if estrogen-replete) and 1500 mg (if estrogen-deficient).

Bisphosphonates

- Bind to hydroxyapatite in bone and inhibit osteoclasts. Because bisphosphonates are incorporated into mineralized bone, reversal of their benefits upon discontinuation of treatment may be less than that after estrogen/selective estrogen-receptor modulator (SERM) withdrawal.
- **Etidronate**(Didronel) increases bone density and decreases vertebral fractures in women with osteoporosis when given for 2 to 3 years.
  ⇒ Given cyclically (400 mg daily for first 2 weeks of every 3-month period).
  ⇒ Side effects are rare.
  ⇒ Etidronate is not Food and Drug Administration (FDA) approved for treatment of osteoporosis and is usually reserved for patients who cannot tolerate more potent bisphosphonates.
- **Alendronate** (Fosamax): aminobisphosphonate; much more potent inhibitor of bone resorption than etidronate
  ⇒ FDA approved for prevention and treatment of osteoporosis. On average, alendronate increases bone density of hip (9%) and of spine (4% to 5%) over 3 years; reduces risk of vertebral, wrist, and hip fractures by 50% in patients with previous vertebral fractures.
  ⇒ 10 mg daily for treatment and 5 mg daily for prevention.
  ⇒ Weekly dosing (35 or 70 mg every week) is now FDA approved and seems to be as effective as daily dosing with less esophageal irritation.
- **Risedronate** (Actonel): newest bisphosphonate
  ⇒ Increases bone density at spine by 6% and at hip by 4% to 5% and reduces fractures by 50%.
  ⇒ Fewer gastrointestinal side effects than alendronate.
  ⇒ Dosing for prevention and treatment is 5 mg daily.
- Intravenous **pamidronate** (Aredia) for those who cannot tolerate oral bisphosphonates.
  ⇒ 30 mg every 3 months given over 2 to 4 hours; not FDA approved.

Estrogen replacement therapy (also see Chapter 26, Menopause and Hormone Replacement Therapy)

- Estrogen replacement therapy inhibits osteoclastic bone resorption.
- During the first 5 to 10 years of menopause there is accelerated loss of bone density at 2% to 4% per year that subsequently tapers off. Rapid bone loss resumes when estrogen is discontinued.
- Retrospective studies have reported fracture risk reduction but no large prospective trials have demonstrated such an effect. In the Heart and Estrogen/Progestin Replacement Study (HERS) (Cavley JA, et al. 2001) where women were not selected for osteoporosis, no statistically significant difference in nonvertebral fracture risk between treatment and placebo groups.

- The minimally effective daily doses to prevent bone loss are 0.625 mg of conjugated estrogens, 2 mg of estradiol, 20 μg of ethinyl estradiol, or 50 μg of transdermal estrogen.

Selective Estrogen-Receptor Modulators (SERMs)

- Raloxifene (Evista) has estrogen agonist effects on bone and serum lipids and antagonist effects on breast and uterus.
- Increases bone density and reduces risk of vertebral fractures by 50%.
- FDA approved for prevention and treatment.
- May reduce risk of breast cancer by 70%.
- The usual dosing of raloxifene is 60 mg daily. Side effects include hot flashes and leg cramps (both uncommon); increases risk for venous thromboembolism (like estrogen). Contraindicated in premenopausal women.

Calcitonin

- Inhibits osteoclastic bone resorption; FDA approved for treatment (not prevention) of osteoporosis.
- Evidence for fracture prevention is weak. May have analgesic effect; may be useful for patients with chronic pain related to fractures or skeletal deformity.
- Administered as nasal spray (Miacalcin), 200 IU (1 spray) daily. Side effects are uncommon.
- Not recommended if patients can tolerate other agents.

Orthopedic Management of Fractures

- Hip fractures: Early surgical management is associated with improved outcomes.
- Vertebral fractures: Open surgery is reserved for patients with unstable spines or neurologic deficits.

FUTURE DIRECTIONS

- While continuous infusion of PTH decreases bone density, intermittent administration of PTH increases bone density by stimulating more bone formation than resorption.
  - ⇒ PTH increases bone density more than any other available agent.
  - ⇒ PTH reduces the risk of vertebral fractures by nearly 70% and nonvertebral fractures by 55% without significant side effects (Neer, 2001).
  - ⇒ PTH is currently under review by the FDA for treatment of osteoporosis.
- An external hip protector can shunt the force of a fall away from the greater trochanter to the surrounding soft tissues.
- Statins block the same pathway as bisphosphonates and biochemical evidence suggests that they increase bone density.

SELECTED REFERENCES

1. Chesnut CH, Silverman S, Andriano K, et al. A randomized trial of nasal spray salmon calcitonin in postmenopausal women with established osteoporosis: The PROOF Study. *Am J Med* 2000;109:267–276.
2. Cummings SR, Black DM, Thompson DE, et al. Effect of alendronate on risk of fracture in women with low bone density but without vertebral fractures. Results from the FIT trial. *JAMA* 1998;280(24):2077–2082.
3. Delmas PD, Bjarnason NH, Mitlak BH, et al. Effects of raloxifene on bone mineral density, serum cholesterol concentrations, and uterine endometrium in postmenopausal women. *N Engl J Med* 1997;337(23): 1641–1647.
4. Eastell R. Drug therapy: treatment of postmenopausal osteoporosis. *N Engl J Med* 1998;338(11):736–746.
5. Ettinger B, Black DM, Mitlak BH, et al. for the MORE Investigators. Reduction of vertebral fracture risk in postmenopausal women with osteoporosis treated with raloxifene: results from a 3-year randomized clinical trial. *JAMA* 1999;282:637–645.
6. Finkelstein J. "Osteoporosis: etiology, diagnosis and treatment." Clinical Endocrinology review course, Harvard Medical School, 2000.
7. Harris ST, Watts NB, Genant HK, et al. Effects of risedronate treatment on vertebral and nonvertebral fractures in women with postmenopausal osteoporosis. *JAMA* 1999;282(14):1344–1352.

8. Hosking D, Chilvers CE, Christiansen C, et al. Prevention of bone loss with alendronate in postmenopausal women under 60 years of age. *N Engl J Med* 1998;338(8):485–492.

9. Hulley S, Grady D, Bush T, et al. Randomized trial of estrogen plus progestin for secondary prevention of coronary heart disease in postmenopausal women. *JAMA* 1998;280(7):605–613.

10. Kannus P, Parkkari J, Niemi S, et al. Prevention of hip fracture in elderly people with use of a hip protector. *N Engl J Med* 2000;343(21):1506–1513.

11. Liberman UA, Weiss SR, Broll J, et al. Effect of oral alendronate on bone mineral density and the incidence of fractures in postmenopausal osteoporosis. *N Engl J Med* 1995;333(22):1437–1443.

12. Lindsay R, Silverman SL, Cooper C, et al. Risk of new vertebral fracture in the year following a fracture. *JAMA* 2001;285(3):320–323.

13. McClung MR, Geusens P, Miller PD, et al. Effect of risdedronate on the risk of hip fracture in elderly women. *N Engl J Med* 2001;344(5):333–340.

14. Mortensen L, Charles P, Bekker PJ, et al. Risedronate increases bone mass in an early postmenopausal population: two years of treatment plus one year of follow-up. *J Clin Endocrinol Metab* 1998;83(2):396–402.

15. Neer RM, Arnaud CD, Zanchetta JR, et al. Effect of parathyroid hormone (1–34) on fractures and bone mineral density in postmenopausal women with osteoporosis. *N Engl J Med* 2001;344(19):1434–1441.

16. National Institutes of Health (NIH) Consensus Development Panel. Osteoporosis prevention, diagnosis and therapy. *JAMA* 2001;285(6):785–795.

17. PEPI Writing Group. Effects of hormone therapy on bone mineral density: results from the postmenopausal estrogen/progestin interventions (PEPI) trial. *JAMA* 1996;276(17):1389–1396.

18. Ravn P, Bidstrup M, Wasnich RD, et al. Alendronate and estrogen-progestin in the long-term prevention of bone loss: four-year results from the early postmenopausal intervention cohort study. *Ann Intern Med* 1999; 131:935–942.

19. Reginster J, Minne HW, Sorensen OH, et al. Randomized trial of the effects of risedronate on vertebral fractures in women with established postmenopausal osteoporosis. *Osteoporos Int* 2000;11:83–91.

20. Watts NB, Harris ST, Genant HK, et al. Intermittent cyclical etidronate treatment of postmenopausal osteoporosis. *N Engl J Med* 1990;323:73–79.

21. Thomas MK, Lloyd-Jones DM, Thadhani RI, et al. Hypovitaminosis D in medical inpatients. *N Engl J Med* 1998;338:777–783.

26

MENOPAUSE AND HORMONE REPLACEMENT THERAPY

INTRODUCTION

- Menopause is defined retrospectively as the absence of menses for 12 months.
- Median age: 51 years (range: 41 to 59 years).

PATHOPHYSIOLOGY/CLINICAL PRESENTATION

- Factors correlated with earlier age of menopause include cigarette smoking (menopause occurs 1 to 2 years earlier) and altitude (earlier menopause at higher altitude).
- Has short-term and long-term health effects:
  ⇒ Symptoms greatest within 5 years of menopause, most commonly hot flashes and sleep disturbance. 45% complain of vaginal dryness, which can lead to dyspareunia and decreased sexual function (Greendale et al., 1999).
  ⇒ Long-term consequences of estrogen deficiency include accelerated bone loss, worsening lipid profile, and increased risk of cardiovascular disease (CVD).
- At menopause, ovarian follicular function ceases, resulting in termination of menstruation.
- In perimenopausal transition, estrogen levels are erratic, leading to irregular, variable cycle lengths (both short and long) and periodic elevations in follicle-stimulating hormone (FSH).
- In menopause, follicular development ceases, estradiol levels fall, FSH rises, androgens decrease by 50%, and progesterone levels fall.

EVALUATION

- Diagnosis is made clinically based on age, cessation of menses with or without vasomotor symptoms.
- During perimenopausal period, FSH is not reliable diagnostic tool because levels vary.
- In menopause, it is not necessary to document elevated FSH (usually greater than 40) unless unusually young (under age 40).

TREATMENT

Symptoms (Table 26.1)

- Estrogen decreases episodes of hot flashes in a dose-dependent fashion.
  ⇒ 70% reduction with standard treatment; usually decrease naturally within 5 years of menopause.
- Clonidine has moderate efficacy, but causes side effects (dry mouth, constipation).
- Low-dose selective serotonin reuptake inhibitors (SSRIs) are effective for reducing hot flashes (McNagny, 1999).
- Oral or local delivery of estrogen is effective for vaginal dryness; can also use local moisturizing agents, including Astroglide and Gyne-moistrin (Greendale, 1999).

TABLE 26.1 ALTERNATIVES TO HORMONE REPLACEMENT THERAPY FOR MENOPAUSAL SYMPTOMS

Vasomotor Symptoms	Urogenital Symptoms
Clonidine 0.1–0.2 mg po bid or transdermal. Medroxyprogesterone acetate 10 mg po qd (irregular bleeding will occur in 40%). Counsel patients to avoid alcohol, caffeine, spicy, foods, and warm places. Paced breathing, relaxation techniques, and acupuncture shown to reduce hot flashes. Initial randomized trials show no benefit from dong quai; ginseng, soy, and black cohosh may reduce symptoms (safety not establised). Recent reports suggest low-dose SSRIs (Prozac, Effexor) reduce hot flashes.	Polycarbophil (Replens). Moisturizers: Astroglide, Gynemoistrin. Estring (estradiol 2 mg vaginal ring) delivers 7.5 mcg/day locally.

po, by mouth; bid, twice daily; qd, every day; SSRIs, selective serotonin reuptake inhibitors.

Cardiovascular Disease

- Observational studies suggest postmenopausal hormone replacement therapy (HRT) lowers risk of coronary events.
  ⇒ The **Nurses' Health Study**, a prospective observational study of over 100,000 women, found the relative risk (RR) of major coronary artery disease (CAD)-related events among current users of estrogen to be 0.56 versus RR among former users of estrogen 0.83. This translates to an estimated 37% to 44% risk reduction for CAD events in ever-users of estrogen (Stampfer et al., 1991).
  ⇒ Addition of progestin did not offset estrogen's cardiovascular benefits (Grodstein et al., 1996).
- Recent randomized clinical trials (RCTs) have challenged the observational trial data.
  ⇒ The **Heart and Estrogen/Progestin Replacement Study (HERS)** was an RCT of HRT for secondary prevention of cardiac events in postmenopausal women. No difference was seen in terms of coronary events; an increased incidence of cardiac events in women taking HRT was seen during first year despite improved lipid profiles (Hulley et al., 1998).
  ⇒ The **Estrogen Replacement and Atherosclerosis Trial (ERA)** found no difference between treatment and placebo groups in progression of atherosclerotic lesions or in development of new lesions. While this is not a clinical endpoint, its findings are consistent with those of HERS trial (Herrington et al., 2000).
- Potential explanations for discrepancy between observational data and RCTs include:
  ⇒ Women who choose HRT tend to be healthier and better educated.
  ⇒ Type of progestin used with estrogen may have reduced potential benefit of estrogen alone.
  ⇒ Benefits of HRT may be limited to younger women closer to menopause.
  ⇒ HRT may be beneficial only in primary prevention.
- American Heart Association recommends that HRT should not be initiated for purpose of primary or secondary prevention of cardiovascular disease (Mosca et al., 2001).
- In absence of definitive conclusion regarding cardiovascular benefits of HRT, must emphasize strategies proven to reduce cardiac events including smoking cessation, hepatic hydroxymethyl glutaryl coenzyme A (HMG CoA) reductase inhibitors, and β-blockers.

Osteoporotic Fracture Reduction (also see Chapter 25, Osteoporosis)

- Estrogen reduces rate of bone loss and improves bone density. Maximum benefit is seen among current, long-term users (more than 5 years) and if HRT is started near menopause (Felson et al., 1993).
- Estimated 73% reduction in risk in women ages 75 to 85 if taking estrogen continuously since menopause; 57% to 69% in women who begin therapy at age 65 (Ettinger and Grady, 1994).
- Dose required to prevent osteoporosis: 0.625 mg daily of Premarin (0.3 g with 1500 mg calcium daily may be as effective); transdermal estrogens have similar effect on bone density. Progestins do not diminish estrogen effect and may promote new bone formation.

- Bone loss resumes at accelerated rate after cessation; risk for hip fracture returns to near baseline 6 or more years after stopping therapy.
- Nonhormonal therapies exist for bone loss with equivalent or better efficacy.

Alzheimer's Disease

- Biological mechanisms by which estrogen may improve cognitive function have been elucidated.
- However, in the Alzheimer's Disease Cooperative Study, there was no difference in rates of disease progression in treatment groups versus placebo (Shaywitz and Shaywitz, 2000, Mulnard et al., 2000).
- Ongoing clinical trials will address whether HRT has role in primary prevention of Alzheimer's disease.

Endometrial Cancer

- Incidence of endometrial hyperplasia is approximately 40% after 2 years of *unopposed* estrogen (PEPI, 1995).
- Concurrent use of continuous or cyclic regimens of progestins prevents estrogen-induced endometrial hyperplasia; risk of hyperplasia with progestins becomes comparable to that in nonusers (PEPI, 1995).
- Minimum 10 to 12 days per month of progestin is necessary to prevent hyperplasia.

Breast Cancer

- Observational studies including the Nurses' Health Study have suggested an increased risk of breast cancer among users of HRT (Colditz et al., 1995).
- A metaanalysis of 51 different studies by the Collaborative Group on Hormonal Factors in Breast Cancer showed an increased risk in long-term users (greater than 5 years) with RR of 1.35. There was little difference in short-term users (1 to 4 years). The risk declined after discontinuation of HRT (Collaborative Group on Hormonal Factors in Breast Cancer, 1997).
- Controversial evidence exists that breast cancers that develop while on HRT are less aggressive.
- Recent studies have shown that adding progestins to estrogen does not protect against breast cancer (unlike the case of endometrial cancer).
- **Breast Cancer Detection Demonstration Project:** Higher incidence of breast cancer in women on combination regimens compared to estrogen alone (Schairer, 2000; Ross et al., 2000). Despite numerous limitations, this study indicates that progestins do not eliminate risk incurred with estrogen.
- While there may be an added risk of breast cancer with progestins, estrogen monotherapy confers too high a risk of endometrial hyperplasia to be safe in women with a uterus.
- Overall the evidence suggests that short-term use of HRT does not elevate risk of breast cancer, whereas long-term, current use modestly increases the risk.

Other Effects

- Two- to three-fold increased risk of gallstones confirmed in HERS trial (Hulley et al., 1998).
- Observational trials show three-fold increase in thromboembolic events in HRT users (also demonstrated in the HERS trial) (Daly et al., 1996; Grady et al., 2000). Given the low incidence of these events in healthy postmenopausal women (1 in 3,000 per year), the absolute increase in risk is actually small.
- No increase in obesity has been observed.
- Observational studies have shown reduction in risk of colorectal cancer (Nanda et al., 1999).

Prescribing HRT (Table 26.2)

- Combination therapy is necessary for women with a uterus receiving HRT to prevent endometrial hyperplasia. Women without a uterus need only estrogen.
- Either continuous or cyclic regimens of progestin are possible, depending on patient preference. Early in menopause, cyclic regimens are often better tolerated because of lower rate of spotting.

TABLE 26.2 SELECTED COMMONLY PRESCRIBED HORMONE REPLACEMENT THERAPIES

Preparations	Dosing	Comments
Estrogens		
Conjugated equine estrogen (CEE) (Premarin)	0.625 mg qd	Most commonly prescribed in United States
Oral estradiol (Estrace, Estradiol)	1 mg qd	Synthetic version of human estrogen
Transdermal estradiol (Estraderm, Climara)	0.05 mg/qd	Decreased first-pass liver effect
Oral esterified estrogen (Estratab)	0.625 mg/qd	
Progestins		
Medroxyprogesterone acetate (MPA) (Provera)	2.5 mg qd 5 mg qd cyclic	Available in combined pill
Micronized progesterone (Prometrium)	100 mg qd 200 mg qd cyclic	Less adverse effect on lipid profile
Intravaginal progesterone (Crinone)	45–90 mg qod cyclic	Minimizes blood levels and side effects

qd, every day; qod, every other day.

- Women on cyclic regimens usually experience monthly withdrawal bleeding. Endometrial biopsy is only necessary if bleeding is early or prolonged. Changes in bleeding pattern also warrant further investigation.
- On continuous therapy, spotting is frequent. If spotting persists for more than 6 months, an endometrial evaluation is recommended.

Selective estrogen receptor modulators (SERMs)

- The ideal HRT would confer the potential benefits of estrogen on the heart and bone without adversely affecting the uterus and breast; the development of SERMs is a step toward this goal.
- The first available SERM, raloxifene, favorably alters the lipid profile [decreases low density lipoproteins (LDLs)], although there are no long-term data about how this translates into cardiovascular risk reduction (Walsh et al., 1998).
- Raloxifene does not have proliferative effects on the endometrium and therefore can be used without a progestin in women with a uterus.
- Raloxifene beneficially modulates bone density and prevents fractures (Khovidhunkit and Shoback, 1999).
- Raloxifene does not treat vasomotor symptoms, and hot flashes are a common side effect.

SELECTED REFERENCES

1. Colditz GA, Hankinson SE, Hunter DJ, et al. The use of estrogens and the risk of breast cancer in postmenopausal women. *N Engl J Med* 1995;332:1589–1593.
2. Collaborative Group on Hormonal Factors in Breast Cancer. Breast cancer and hormone replacement therapy: collaborative reanalysis of data from 51 epidemiological studies of 52,705 women with breast cancer and 108,411 women without breast cancer. *Lancet* 1997;350:1047–1059.
3. Daly E, Vessey MP, Hawkins MM, et al. Risk of venous thromboembolism in users of hormone replacement therapy. *Lancet* 1996;348:977–980.
4. Effects of estrogen or estrogen/progestin regimens on heart disease risk factors in postmenopausal women. *JAMA* 1995;273:199–208.
5. Ettinger B, Grady D. Maximizing the benefit of estrogen therapy for the prevention of osteoporosis. *Menopause* 1994;1:19–24.
6. Felson DT, Zhang Y, Hannan MT, et al. The effect of postmenopausal estrogen therapy on bone density in elderly women. *N Engl J Med* 1993;329:1141–1146.
7. Gerhard-Herman M, Hamburg NM, Ganz P. Hormone replacement therapy and cardiovascular risk. *Cur Cardiol Rep* 2000;2:288–292.
8. Grady D, Wenger NK, Herrington D, et al. Postmenopausal hormone therapy increases risk for venous thromboembolic disease: the Heart and Estrogen/Progestin Replacement Study. *Ann Intern Med* 2000;132:689–696.
9. Greendale GA, Lee NP, Arriola ER. The menopause. *Lancet* 1999;353:571–580.
10. Grodstein F, Stampfer MJ, Manson JE, et al. Postmenopausal estrogen and progestin use and the risk of cardiovascular disease. *N Engl J Med* 1996;335:453–461.

11. Grodstein F, Stampfer MJ, Colditz GA, et al. Postmenopausal hormone therapy and mortality. *N Engl J Med* 1997;336:1769–1775.
12. Herrington DM, Reboussin DM, Brosnihan BK, et al. Effects of estrogen replacement on the progression of coronary-artery atherosclerosis. *N Engl J Med* 2000;343:522–529.
13. Hulley S, Grady D, Bush T, et al. Randomized trial of estrogen plus progestin for secondary prevention of coronary heart disease in postmenopausal women (HERS study). *JAMA* 1998;280:605–613.
14. Khovidhunkit W, Shoback DM. Clinical effects of raloxifene hydrochloride in women. *Ann Intern Med* 1999: 120:431–439.
15. Manson JE, Martin KA. Postmenopausal hormone-replacement therapy. *N Engl J Med* 2001;345:34–40.
16. McNagny SE. Prescribing hormone replacement therapy for menopausal symptoms. *Ann Intern Med* 1999; 131:605–616.
17. Mosca L, Collins P, Herrington DM, et al. Hormone replacement therapy and cardiovascular disease: a statement for healthcare professionals from the American Heart Association. *Circulation* 2001;104:499–503.
18. Mulnard RA, Cotman CW, Kawas C, et al. Estrogen replacement therapy for treatment of mild to moderate Alzheimer disease: a randomized controlled trial. *JAMA* 2000;283:1007–1015.
19. Nabel EG. Coronary heart disease in women—an ounce of prevention. *N Engl J Med* 2000;343:572–574.
20. Nanda K, Bastian LA, Hasselblad D, et al. Hormone replacement therapy and the risk of colorectal cancer: a meta-analysis. *Obstet Gynecol* 1999;93:880–888.
21. Ross RK, Paganini A, Wan PC, et al. Effect of hormone replacement therapy on breast cancer risk: estrogen versus estrogen plus progestin. *J Natl Cancer Inst* 2000;92:328–332.
22. Schairer C, Lubin J, Troisi R, et al. Menopausal estrogen and estrogen-progestin replacement therapy and breast cancer risk. *JAMA* 2000;283:485–491.
23. Shaywitz BA, Shaywitz SE. Estrogen and Alzheimer disease: plausible theory, negative clinical trial. *JAMA* 2000;283:1055–1056.
24. Stampfer MJ, Colditz GA, Willet WC, et al. Postmenopausal estrogen therapy and cardiovascular disease. Ten-year follow-up from the nurses' health study. *N Engl J Med* 1991;325:756–762.
25. Walsh BW, Kuller LH, Wild RA, et al. Effects of raloxifene on serum lipids and coagulation factors in healthy postmenopausal women. *JAMA.* 1998;279:1445—1451.
26. Willett WC, Colditz G, Stampfer M. Postmenopausal estrogens—opposed, unopposed, or none of the above. *JAMA* 2000;283:534–535.

AMENORRHEA

INTRODUCTION

- Primary amenorrhea: Absence of menarche in a female 16 or older with normal secondary sexual development or in a female 14 or older who lacks secondary sexual characteristics. Found in 0.3% of population (Kiningham and Schwenk, 1996).
- Secondary amenorrhea: Absence of menses for 3 or more cycles or 6 months or more in previously menstruating woman; 12-month absence with prior oligomenorrhea (Hobart and Smucker, 2000). Found in 1% to 3% of general population, 3% to 5% of college students, and 5% to 20% of competitive athletes (Kiningham and Schwenk, 1996).

PATHOPHYSIOLOGY

Normal Menstrual Cycle

- Normal menstruation requires an intact hypothalamic-pituitary-ovarian axis, a hormonally responsive uterus, and an anatomically unobstructed outflow tract.
- Follicular (proliferative) phase (menses through ovulation):
  ⇒ Hypothalamus secretes gonadotropin-releasing hormone (GnRH) in a pulsatile manner, causing pituitary release of follicle-stimulating hormone (FSH), which stimulates ovarian follicles to mature and secrete estradiol. Via positive feedback, high estradiol causes luteinizing hormone (LH) surge, resulting in ovulation.
  ⇒ Endometrium sloughs during menses, then proliferates rapidly under the influence of estrogen.
- Luteal (secretory) phase:
  ⇒ Progesterone predominates, produced by the ruptured follicle which has become a corpus luteum. If fertilization does not occur, the corpus luteum involutes and estrogen and progesterone levels rapidly decrease.
  ⇒ Endometrium responds to progesterone with secretory changes, then becomes ischemic and prepares to slough as progesterone levels drop.
  ⇒ Low estrogen and progesterone stimulate hypothalamic secretion of GnRH, restarting the cycle.
- Chronic amenorrhea is associated with osteoporosis, endometrial cancer, and infertility.

DIFFERENTIAL DIAGNOSIS

- Primary amenorrhea: gonadal dysgenesis (Turner's syndrome, 45%), physiologic delay of puberty (20%), Müllerian agenesis (15%), transverse vaginal septum or imperforate hymen (5%), absent production of GnRH (hypogonadotropic hypogonadism, 5%), anorexia nervosa (2%), hypopituitarism (2%) (Reindollar et al., 1981).
- Secondary amenorrhea (see Table 27.1): ovarian disease (40%), hypothalamic dysfunction (35%), pituitary disease (19%), uterine disease (5%) (Reindollar et al., 1986).

TABLE 27.1 DIFFERENTIAL DIAGNOSIS OF SECONDARY AMENORRHEA

Physiologic	Prepuberty, pregnancy, lactation, postmenopause
Hypothalamic dysfunction	Functional hypogonadotropic amenorrhea: decrease in GnRH pulse frequency/amplitude, with loss of LH surge/ovulation; due to emotional stress, psychopathology, weight loss (>10% below ideal body weight), nutritional deficiencies, concurrent illness, increased exercise, competitive athletics (Taylor, 2001).
Pituitary disease	Prolactinoma: 33% of secondary amenorrhea (Kiningham and Schwenk, 1996).
	Empty sella syndrome: 4%–16% of patients with amenorrhea and galactorrhea; generally benign (Kiningham and Schwenk, 1996).
	Pituitary infarction (Sheehan's syndrome) and granulomatous disease (sarcoidosis).
Ovarian problems	Polycystic ovary syndrome.
	Premature ovarian failure (POF): ovarian failure before age 35; associated with autoimmune disorders (thyroid, rheumatoid arthritis, ITP, myasthenia gravis), radiation, chemotherapy, endometriosis, oophoritis (Fogel, 1997).
Uterine and outflow tract abnormalities	Asherman's syndrome (obliteration of uterus by intrauterine scarring and synechiae formation due to curettage, infection, or uterine surgery).
	Cervical scarring with os closure.

GnRH, gonadotropin-releasing hormone; LH, luteinizing hormone; ITP, idiopathic thrombocytopenic purpura.

EVALUATION

History

- Age at menarche, development of secondary sexual characteristics
- Previous menstrual pattern, timing of missed periods, presence of symptoms associated with ovulation
- Duration of amenorrhea
- Previous pregnancies and gynecologic procedures
- Risk factors (weight loss, athletic training, stress, depression/anxiety, comorbid illness)
- Weight, nutritional assessment, exercise patterns
- Use of oral contraceptive pills (OCPs):
    ⇒ Progesterone only pills
    ⇒ Discontinuation of OCPs can cause temporary amenorrhea, but not for more than 6 months.
- Medication use:
    ⇒ Increased prolactin [antipsychotics, tricyclics, monoamine oxidase inhibitors (MAOIs), and antihypertensives]
    ⇒ Estrogenic activity (digitalis, marijuana, OCPs, flavonoids)
    ⇒ Ovarian toxicity [chemotherapeutics (Kiningham and Schwenk, 1996)]
- Endometriosis or radiation
- Family history of early menopause, infertility, or congenital abnormalities
- Review of systems: hirsutism, headache, visual changes, thyroid or adrenal disease, galactorrhea, body habitus

Physical Exam

- Goals: assess for abnormal anatomy and physical signs of estrogen deficiency/excess or androgen excess
- General: stature, secondary sexual characteristics
- Skin: hair distribution (alopecia/hirsutism), striae, acne
- Thyroid: nodules, goiter, enlargement
- Breasts: development, galactorrhea
- Pelvic: normal external genitalia, vagina, cervix, uterus; adequacy of estrogenization (vaginal moisture). Evaluate for clitoromegaly, scarring of the cervical os, and uterine or ovarian masses.
- Neurologic: visual fields, sense of smell
- Signs of estrogen deficiency: dry, atrophic vaginal mucosa; scarce cervical mucus (Kiningham and Schwenk, 1996)

- Signs of androgen excess: truncal obesity, hirsutism, acne, male pattern baldness, clitoromegaly (Kiningham and Schwenk, 1996)

Laboratory and Diagnostic Testing (Figure 27.1)

- Check beta human chorionic gonadotropin (βhCG) to rule out pregnancy.
    ⇒ If negative and there is evidence of hypothalamic stress in an otherwise healthy woman, wait 2 to 3 months to see if menstrual cycles return spontaneously.
- Check thyroid-stimulating hormone (TSH) and prolactin levels.
- Check FSH and LH if menopause is likely.
- If hyperprolactinemia found [prolactin (PRL) over 80 ng/ml or PRL under 80 with symptoms), verify that patient not on medication that increases PRL (see above), then image the pituitary (MRI) to evaluate for prolactinoma.
- Perform progesterone challenge test to assess adequacy of endometrial estrogenization and patency of outflow tract.
    ⇒ Medroxyprogesterone (Provera) 100 mg intramuscularly or 10 mg by mouth daily for 5 to 10 days.
    ⇒ If no bleeding occurs, repeat in 1 month at double dose.
    ⇒ Positive test is any bleeding 2 to 7 days after progesterone course.
- Positive progesterone challenge test: adequate estrogen, likely cause of amenorrhea is anovulation.
    ⇒ Measure LH, FSH, and androgen levels: serum and free testosterone, serum dehydroepiandrosterone sulfate (DHEA-S), serum 17-hydroxyprogesterone (17-HP).
    ⇒ Hyperandrogenic chronic anovulation [polycystic ovary syndrome (PCOS)]: menstrual irregularities and evidence of virilization; high androgen levels, elevated LH with LH/FSH ratio of 2:1; strong association with obesity
    ⇒ Mild hypothalamic dysfunction: normal LH and androgen levels
- Negative progesterone challenge test (no bleeding): suggests inadequate estrogen stimulation, nonreactive endometrium, or outflow tract abnormality.
    ⇒ Evaluate for uterine disease: trial of estrogen (1.25 mg on days 1 to 21) and progesterone (5 to 10 mg Provera on days 17 to 21)
    ⇒ Absence of bleeding during days 21 to 28 confirms a uterine or outflow tract abnormality; need hysteroscopy for further evaluation and possible treatment.
    ⇒ Presence of withdrawal bleeding confirms inadequate estrogen stimulation: check FSH and LH to evaluate etiology of hypoestrogenic amenorrhea.
- Elevated FSH and LH: primary ovarian failure
    ⇒ If patient is under age 30, check karyotype to rule out presence of Y chromosome (testicular feminization or Turner's mosaic). If Y chromosome present, intraabdominal gonads must be removed due to risk of malignancy.
    ⇒ If patient is age 30 to 40, diagnosis is premature menopause, associated with autoimmune disorders. Check antinuclear antibodies (ANA), RF, erythrocyte sedimentation rate (ESR), TSH, free thyroxine (T4), antithyroid antibodies, morning cortisol (Kiningham and Schwenk, 1996).
    ⇒ If over age 40, diagnosis is menopause.
- If FSH and LH are normal or low, disorder is in the pituitary or hypothalamus.
    ⇒ Check brain MRI to rule out pituitary tumor, hemorrhage, and empty sella.
    ⇒ Check testosterone or cortisol levels if physical exam suggests androgen excess or Cushing's syndrome.
- If MRI negative, diagnosis is severe hypothalamic dysfunction.

TREATMENT

- Women with adequate estrogen but anovulatory cycles (positive progesterone challenge): cyclic progestin (e.g., Provera 10 mg for 7 to 10 days a month) to prevent endometrial hyperplasia and cancer. An OCP can be used if contraception is desired.
- Hypoestrogenic women (negative progesterone challenge): high risk for osteoporosis; calcium supplements and hormone replacement therapy should be offered to all young women who are hypoestrogenic.

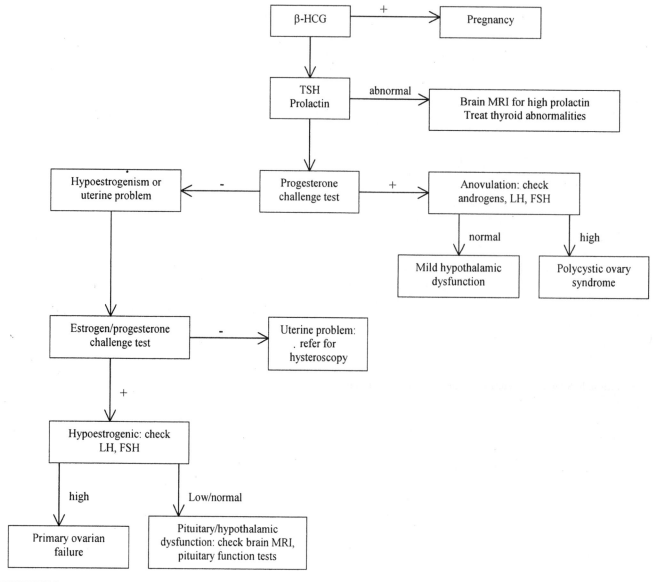

FIGURE 27.1.

- Mild hypothalamic dysfunction (positive progesterone challenge): usually resolves when the precipitating factor (situational stress, weight loss, excessive exercise) resolves.
  ⇒ If amenorrhea persists, use monthly progesterone or OCPs to regulate cycles.
  ⇒ For polycystic ovary syndrome (PCOS), OCPs, GnRH analogs, and clomiphene can be used.
- Severe hypothalamic dysfunction:
  ⇒ Anorexia nervosa: Menstrual cycle will not be restored until adequate weight gain is achieved.
  ⇒ If there is estrogen deficiency (negative progesterone challenge), hormone replacement therapy is necessary.
- Pituitary dysfunction:
  ⇒ Hyperprolactinemia: if PRL is below 80 and MRI shows a normal sella, observe and check PRL yearly. Repeat MRI every 2 to 3 years; treat with bromocriptine for bothersome galactorrhea or desired fertility. If PRL is above 80 or MRI is abnormal, treatment options include bromocriptine and surgery.
  ⇒ Destructive pituitary lesion: Patient will need replacement therapy tailored to her specific hormone deficiencies.

- Premature ovarian failure: Treat with hormone replacement therapy.
- Uterine scarring or outflow obstruction: hysteroscopy and lysis of synechiae.

RESOURCES

- http://www.advancedfertility.com/amenor.htm
- http://www.medem.com/default.cfm, search "amenorrhea"
- http://www.healthlinkusa.com, search "amenorrhea"
- National Women's Health Resource Center: http://www.womens-health.com
- American College of Obstetricians and Gynecologists: http://www.acog.com
- Other good internet sites for women's health: http://www.womenshealth.org and http://www.estronaut.com

SELECTED REFERENCES

1. Baird DT. Amenorrhea. *Lancet* 1997;350:275–279.
2. Couzinet B, Young J, Brailly S, et al. Functional hypothalamic amenorrhea: a partial and reversible gonadotrophin deficiency of nutritional origin. *Clin Endocrinol (Oxf)* 1999;50:229–235.
3. Fogel CI. Endocrine causes of amenorrhea. *Lippincotts Prim Care Pract* 1997; 1(5):507–518.
4. Franks S. Polycystic ovary syndrome. *N Engl J Med* 1995;333:853–861.
5. Goldenberg RL, Grodin JM, Rodbard D, et al. Gonadotropins in women with amenorrhea: the use of serum follicle-stimulating hormone to differentiate women with and without ovarian follicles. *Am J Obstet Gynecol* 1973;116:1003–1012.
6. Hobart JA, Smucker DR. The female athlete triad. *Am Fam Physician* 2000;61:3357–3364,3367.
7. Kiningham R, Schwenk T. Evaluation of amenorrhea. *Am Fam Physician* 1996;53:1185–1194.
8. Laughlin GA, Dominguez CE, Yen SS. Nutritional and endocrine-metabolic aberrations in women with functional hypothalamic amenorrhea. *J Clin Endocrinol Metab* 1998;83:25.
9. Reindollar RH, Novak M, Tho SP, et al. Adult-onset amenorrhea: a study of 262 patients. *Am J Obstet Gynecol* 1986;155:531.
10. Reindollar RH, Byrd JR, McDonough PG. Delayed sexual development: a study of 252 patients. *Am J Obstet Gynecol* 1981;140:371.
11. Santoro N, Filicori M, Crowley WF. Hypogonadotropic disorders in men and women: diagnosis and therapy with pulsatile gonadotropin-releasing hormone. *Endocr Rev* 1986; 7:11.
12. Warren MP. Clinical review 40: amenorrhea in endurance runners. *J Clin Endocrinol Metab* 1992;75:1393.

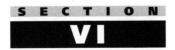

GYNECOLOGY/GENITOURINARY

CONTRACEPTION

INTRODUCTION

- Approximately 50% of pregnancies are unplanned (3.2 million per year).
- Women over age 40 have unintended pregnancy rate of 77%; those between ages 40 and 50 have second-highest rate of abortion (after those under age 15).
- Sterilization is most common form of birth control worldwide; oral contraceptive pills (OCPs) are second. In 1990, nearly 60% of all women of reproductive age were using contraception (see Table 28.1).

TABLE 28.1 OVERVIEW OF THE TYPES OF CONTRACEPTION AND THEIR EFFICACY

Method	Percent Accidental Pregnancy in First Year of Use		Percent Continuing Use at 1 Year
	Typical Use	Perfect Use	
No contraception	85	85	
Spermicides	21	6	43
Periodic abstinence	20		67
• Calendar		9	
• Ovulation method		3	
• Symptom-thermal		2	
• Postovulation		1	
Withdrawal	19	4	
Cervical cap:			
• Parous	36	26	45
• Nulliparous	18	9	58
Diaphragm	18	6	58
Condom			
• Female	21	5	56
• Male	12	3	63
Pill	3		72
• Progestin only		0.5	
• Combined		0.1	
IUD			
• Progesterone T	2	1.5	81
• Copper T 380A	0.8	0.6	78
• Lng20	0.1	0.1	81
Depo-Provera	0.3	0.3	70
Norplant	0.09	0.09	85
Female sterilization	0.4	0.4	100
Male sterilization	0.15	0.1	100

TREATMENT

Hormonal Methods

- Combined Oral Contraceptives
    - ⇒ OCPs inhibit follicle-stimulating hormone (FSH) and luteinizing hormone (LH) production, thereby decreasing follicle development and limiting ovulation. Progestin atrophies

endometrium, thickens cervical mucus, and inhibits fallopian tube function. Estrogen prevents implantation and stabilizes the endometrium, decreasing breakthrough bleeding and heavy menstruation.

⇒ Noncontraceptive benefits:

○ Increased regularity of menstrual cycle; decreased menstrual blood loss, iron deficiency anemia

○ Decreased incidence of ovarian cancer (30% with any use, 50% with use for more than 5 years), endometrial cancer (38% after 2 years, 51% after 4 years, 64% after 8 years), benign breast disease, functional ovarian cysts, acute pelvic inflammatory disease, endometriosis, acne and hirsutism

○ Increased bone density in women over 35

⇒ Multiple mild and a few more serious side effects may occur. Screen for contraindications, including family history of thromboembolism (see Tables 28.2 and 28.3); check blood pressure, breast exam, Pap smear.

⇒ Have patient begin pills either the first Sunday after menses start (Sunday start requires backup contraception for the first month) or the first day of menses (immediate protection). Take at the same time every day.

⇒ Start with a basic, generic pill. Follow-up in 2 to 3 months to check blood pressure and screen for side effects (40% of women; most resolve within 3 months); change pill formulation as needed (see Table 28.4).

⇒ OCPs do not protect from sexually transmitted diseases (STDs); a barrier method should be added for at-risk women.

⇒ Missed pills:

○ One or two pills: take forgotten pills immediately, resume normal pill-taking. Use backup method if two consecutive pills missed.

○ More than three pills: skip those pills, use backup for the month. Alternatively, stop pills entirely for that cycle and start next pill pack on usual schedule (bleeding will occur).

TABLE 28.2 ORAL CONTRACEPTIVE PILLS SIDE EFFECTS AND CONTRAINDICATIONS

Mild side effects/lab abnormalities	**More serious adverse effects**
Breakthrough bleeding, amenorrhea, or late spotting	Thromboembolic/cardiovascular disease: estrogen causes dose-dependent increase in clotting factors, potentiated by nicotine. Risk highest in smokers, pills ≥ 50 mg. No CV risk with low dose pills. ?increased DVT risk with third gen. progestins; minimal in absolute terms.
Weight gain, bloating, breast swelling, tenderness	
Acne and hirsutism	
Decreased libido	
Alopecia	Hypertension: 4%–5% incidence, with BP increase in 9%–16% of normotensive women
Fatigue/depression	Glucose intolerance: rarely clinically significant
Nausea and vomiting	Breast cancer: no clear evidence of increased risk, although question of slightly increased risk with more than 8 years of use
Lipid alteration	
Increased amylase, coagulation factors, magnesium, platelets, renin, thyroid binding globulin, cortisol, aldosterone, prolactin.	
Decreased albumin, haptoglobin, alkaline phosphatase, Vitamin B_6, B_{12}	Cervical cancer: increased incidence, ? lifestyle-related
Absolute contraindications	Cholelithiasis
Smoker over age 35	Hepatocellular adenoma
Abnormal vaginal bleeding of unknown cause	**Relative contraindications**
Known or suspected estrogen-dependent cancers (breast)	Migraines without aura/focal symptoms
	Active renal, hepatic, or gallbladder disease
Thromboembolic disorder	Hypertension (uncontrolled)/hyperlipidemia/diabetes mellitus
Cardiovascular disorders: CAD, CVA, structural heart disease, pulmonary hypertension, AF, history of SBE	High risk for CAD
	Smoker under age 35
	Known prolonged immobility
Liver disease: benign hepatic adenoma, history of liver cancer, active viral hepatitis, cirrhosis	Medications which may interfere with absorption/ metabolism
Pregnancy or lactation (< 6 weeks postpartum)	Sickle cell disease
Migraine with focal neurological symptoms or prolonged aura	Malabsorption
	Postpartum (3–4 weeks)

CV, cardiovascular; DVT, deep venous thrombosis; BP, blood pressure; CAD, coronary artery disease; CVA, cerebrovascular accident; AF, atrial fibrillation; SBE, subacute bacterial endocarditis.

TABLE 28.3 CHANGING ORAL CONTRACEPTIVE PILLS BASED ON SIDE EFFECTS

Headache, nausea, breast tenderness, and swelling	Excess estrogen. Try low estrogen pill or nighttime dosing.
Hirsutism, acne, noncyclic weight gain	Progestin and/or androgen excess. Try third generation progestin pill.
Mood changes and decreased libido	Progestin excess. Try third generation or less androgenic progestins.
Breakthrough bleeding	Multifactorial. Late cycle bleeding: Increase progestin content. Early cycle bleeding: Increase estrogen content. Switching progestin category or increasing estrogen content may be effective. Consider missed pills.
Amenorrhea	Multifactorial. Rule out pregnancy, then consider change to a third generation progestin, triphasic oral contraceptive pills, lower dose progestin, or higher dose estrogen.

- Progestin-only oral contraceptives
  ⇒ "Mini-pill" does not consistently suppress ovulation (40% of women on the mini-pill still ovulate); mechanism is partial ovulation suppression, alteration of cervical mucus, and atrophy of the endometrium.
  ⇒ Indications: intolerable estrogen side effects; lactation (no effect on milk production, minimally secreted into breast milk.). Must be taken at same time every day.
  ⇒ Side effects: irregular vaginal bleeding, amenorrhea; minimal effect on lipids, carbohydrate metabolism or blood coagulation
- Long-acting progestin contraceptives
  ⇒ Mechanism: Long-acting progestin suppresses LH surge (and thus ovulation) in 30% to 50% of women and alters cervical mucus and endometrium.
  ⇒ Side effects: irregular bleeding/amenorrhea (50% within 1 year for Depo-Provera), weight gain, nausea, acne, ovarian cysts, depression. Safe in women with contraindications/intolerable side effects to estrogen
  ⇒ **Norplant:** five 5-year implants containing levo-norgestrel inserted under the skin
    ○ Decreased efficacy in very obese women due to lower serum progestin levels
    ○ Difficult removal stimulated development of Norplant 2, a two-implant version not available in the United States.
  ⇒ **Depo-Provera:** injection of 150 mg of medroxyprogesterone acetate (Provera) every 3 months
    ○ Check pregnancy test prior to first injection, during week 1 of cycle; send reminders for follow-up injections.
    ○ Can be used during lactation, although milk production will decrease slightly.
    ○ Fertility returns 4 to 9 months after the last injection.

TABLE 28.4 COMMONLY USED ORAL CONTRACEPTIVE PILL FORMULATIONS

Name	Estrogen (mcg)	Progestin (mg)	Approximate price	
Monophasic				**Estrogens:**
Loestrin 1/20	EE 20	NEA I	$$$	EE, ethinyl estradiol (potent estrogen)
Microgestin			$ generic	ME, mistranol (low potency estrogen)
Alesse	EE 20	LN 0.1	$$	
Levlite			$$	
Aviane			$ generic	
Orthocept	EE 30	DG 0.15 (low potency)	$$	**Progestins:**
Desogen			$$	NG, norgestrel (potent androgen)
Apri			$ generic	ED, ethylnodiol diacetate (estrogenic)
Nordette	EE 30	LN 0.15	$$$	NEA, norethindrone acetate (potent androgen)
Levlen			$$	
Levora			$ generic	
Lo-Ovral	EE 30	NG 0.3 (potent)	$$$	
Low-Ogestrol			$ generic	
Loestrin 1.5/30	EE 30	NEA 1.5	$$$	

(continued)

TABLE 28.4 *(continued)*

Name	Estrogen (mcg)	Progestin (mg)	Approximate price	
Ovcon 35	EE 35	NE 0.4	$$$	*Second generation:*
Brevicon	EE 35	NE 0.5	$$	LN, levonorgestrel (intermediate
Modicon			$	androgenic potency, higher than NE)
NeCon .5/35			$ generic	NE, norethindrone (intermediate
Ortho-Novum 1/35	EE 35	NE 1	$$$	androgenic potency, lower than LN)
Genora 1/35			$	
NeLova 1/35			$ generic	
NeCon 1/35			$	
Demulen 1/35	EE 35	ED 1 (estrogenic)	$$$	*Third generation:*
Zovia 1/35			$ generic	NGT, norgestimate (low potency
Orthocyclen	EE 35	NGT 0.25	$$$	androgen)
Biphasic				DG, desogestrel (lowest potency
Mircette	EE 20/10 days 23–28	DG 0.15	$$$	androgen)
Ortho 10/11	EE 35	NE 0.5/1		
Triphasic				
Ortho 7/7/7	EE 35	NE 0.5/0.75/0.5	$$$	
TriNorinyl	EE 35	NE 0.5/1/0.5		
Triphasil,	EE 30/40/30	LN.05/.075/.125	$$$	
Trilevlen			$$$	
Trivora			$ generic	
Orthotricyclen	EE 35	NGT 0.18/0.215/0.25		
Estrostep	EE 20/30/35	NEA 1	$$	
Progestin				
Micronor		NE 0.35	$$$	
Nor-Q.D.				
Ovrette		NG 0.075	$$$	

Intrauterine Devices (IUDs)

- Mechanism: *Copper* IUDs (replace after 8 to 10 years) induce foreign body response with inflammation; *progesterone-releasing* IUDs (Progestasert, replaced annually) and *levonorgestrel* IUDs (Marena, replaced every 5 years) affect cervical mucus and endometrium.
- Inserted by trained practitioner during first 3 days of menses; immediate return of fertility on removal.
- Mild side effects: Cramping after insertion; increased vaginal discharge or bleeding; 5% to 20% expulsion rate; perforation very rare. No increased risk of infertility with long-term use
- Serious adverse effects: Increased risk of pelvic inflammatory disease in those at risk for STDs; increased incidence of ectopic pregnancy with Progestasert (decreased with copper and levonorgestrel).

TABLE 28.5 CONTRAINDICATIONS TO INTRAUTERINE DEVICE (IUD) USE

Absolute	Relative
Active, recent, or recurrent pelvic inflammatory disease	Nulligravidity
	Immunosuppression or valvular heart disease (? risk of endocarditis)
Pregnancy	Uterine abnormalities (large fibroids, bicornuate uterus)
Known or suspected pelvic malignancy	Abnormal Pap smears
Undiagnosed vaginal bleeding	History of infertility in a woman desiring pregnancy
Behavior placing individual at high risk for STD	History of ectopic pregnancy
Wilson's disease	

STD, sexually transmitted diseases;

Barrier Methods

- Diaphragm or cervical cup
  - ⇒ Fitted by trained clinician (reassess fit after childbirth or 10% body weight change); use with spermicide for full efficacy; patient must be capable of correct insertion.
  - ⇒ Diaphragm should remain in place for 6 to 8 hours after intercourse and then be removed; cervical cap may be left in for a maximum of 24 hours.
  - ⇒ Significant protection against STDs; decreased risk of cervical dysplasia.

TABLE 28.6 CONTRAINDICATIONS TO AND ADVERSE EFFECTS OF DIAPHRAGM USE

Contraindication	Adverse Effects
Allergy to latex or spermicide	Toxic shock syndrome (TSS) (very rare)
Recurrent urinary tract infections	Allergy
Active sexually transmitted disease	Irritation
History of toxic shock syndrome (TSS)	Recurrent candidiasis
Difficulty learning insertion technique	Pelvic discomfort
Anatomic abnormalities influencing fit (prolapse, prior OB laceration)	Recurrent cystitis from spermicide
Within 6 weeks postpartum	

OB, obstetric.

- Condoms
  - ⇒ Latex condoms: excellent protection against STDs; opportunity for men to participate in contraception
  - ⇒ Contraindication: latex allergy
  - ⇒ Use with spermicide more effective than either alone; lubricants must be water-based, as oil-based lubricants (petroleum) weaken the condom. A new condom must be used for each act of intercourse.
  - ⇒ Average breakage rate is 1% to 2%; counsel regarding morning-after pill for emergencies.
- Female condoms
  - ⇒ Disposable, prelubricated polyurethane sheath between two rings; one fits inside the vagina, the other sits exteriorly on the vulva. Failure rate similar to male condom, although less clinical experience.
  - ⇒ Protects against STDs, including HIV.

Sterilization

- Describe as being irreversible when counseling patients.
- Contraindications: ambivalence, poor surgical or anesthesia candidate
- Vasectomy
  - ⇒ Office procedure involving ligation of the vas deferens through a small incision in the scrotum; reversible about 60% of time depending on timing and type of vasectomy.
  - ⇒ Check sperm counts after procedure; backup contraception necessary until semen sperm count is zero.
  - ⇒ Side effects rare: hematoma, granuloma, epididymitis, infection
  - ⇒ Cost is 3 times less than tubal ligation; 20 times fewer complications.
- Tubal ligation
  - ⇒ Fallopian tube may be ligated, coagulated, or mechanically occluded; performed immediately postpartum or electively at any point.
  - ⇒ Clip ligation reversible less than 50% of the time if tube remains healthy and intact.
  - ⇒ Side effects: complications from anesthesia; damage to ovaries or laparoscopic complications occur rarely.

- Hysterectomy
  ⇒ Never used solely for contraception; consider if other indications exist.
  ⇒ Mortality is 10 to 100 times more than tubal ligation; morbidity and cost is also higher.

Postcoital "emergency" contraception: "morning-after pill"

- Risk of pregnancy after unprotected sex is 8%; reduced to 2% with emergency contraception.
- Initiate within 72 hours of unprotected sex, most effective within 48 hours; associated with 1% failure rate.
- Mechanism: inhibits ovulation, fertilization, or endometrial development
- Standard regimen: Ovral, 2 pills [100 mcg ethinyl estradiol (EE) and 1 mg norgestrel (NG) total], repeat once 12 hours later. High dose conjugated estrogens (5 mg by mouth for 5 days, causes severe nausea) or progesterone-only regimens (levonorgestrel 0.75 mg by mouth every 12 hours for 2 days) are also effective.
- Side effects: Nausea, vomiting; consider prescribing an antiemetic with estrogen containing pills.
- Emergency contraception hotline: 1-888-NOT-2-LATE.

Medical Abortion

- RU 486, an antiprogesterone and contragestive agent, used to terminate pregnancies under 8 weeks; most effective within 63 days of last menstrual period.
  ⇒ Only available to registered, qualified physicians with surgical backup.
  ⇒ Mifepristone 600 mg by mouth in office. Return to office 48 hours later for 400 mg misoprostol by mouth and 4 hours of observation. Follow-up visit in 2 weeks to confirm successful abortion.
  ⇒ 92% successful termination, 5% incomplete abortion, 2% require dilatation and curettage, 1% continued pregnancy.
- Methotrexate and misoprostol also used to induce abortion in pregnancies under 8 weeks, although not Food and Drug Administration (FDA) approved.

Surgical Abortion

- 1.6 million performed in the United States each year, more than 90% within the first trimester.
- Risks of abortion lowest at approximately 7 to 8 weeks gestation; risks double every 2 weeks thereafter.
- Birth control information and supplies are important after abortion; patient acceptance is high.

Pregnancy/Preconception Counseling

- Prenatal vitamin with 400 mcg of folic acid daily for at least 3 months prior to conception
- Review medication list for drugs contraindicated during pregnancy, including coumadin, nonsteroidal antiinflammatory drugs (NSAIDs), angiotensin-converting enzyme inhibitors (ACEIs), antiseizure medications, and isotretinoin.
- Check varicella and rubella immunoglobulin G (IgG) titers. If negative and patient not yet pregnant, vaccinate 3 months prior to conception (live attenuated vaccines). If the patient is already pregnant, counsel to avoid exposure to these viruses, and vaccinate after delivery.
- Pregnant women should abstain from alcohol and drugs, excessive caffeine, soft unpasteurized cheeses, shellfish, fish with high mercury levels (shark, swordfish, tilefish, king mackerel), and hot tubs. Women who smoke should be strongly urged to quit.
- Patients with abnormal bleeding, abdominal cramping, or pain should report to the local emergency room.
- Refer to obstetrics during first trimester; high-risk patients (hypertension, diabetes) should be seen for preconception counseling. Refer to infertility specialist after 1 year of unsuccessful attempts at conception.

FUTURE DIRECTIONS

- Lunelle: Estrogen-progesterone monthly injectable recently FDA-approved; very effective (less than 1 pregnancy per 100 women-years); monthly withdrawal bleed with rapid return of fertility.
- Nuvaring: Silicone vaginal ring releases low-dose estrogen/progestin; worn for 3 weeks then removed for the fourth to allow menstruation; effective; minimal side effects; one size fits all. Approved by FDA in 2001.
- Other new hormonal contraceptives pending FDA approval: transdermal estrogen/progesterone patch (Evra), applied every week for 3 out of 4 weeks; single rod etonorgestrel implant (Implanon) effective for 3 years; 8 to 12 week OCP (Seasonale), which reduces bleeding to four episodes annually.
- New barrier methods under development: Lea's contraceptive, worn for 48 hours in the upper vagina; FemCap, a silicone cervical cap designed for over-the-counter use; spermicides with bactericidal and virucidal activity.

SELECTED REFERENCES

1. Archer D. New contraceptive options. *Clin Obstet Gynecol* 2001;44(1):122–126.
2. Audet MC, Moreau M, Koltun WD, et al. Evaluation of contraceptive efficacy and cycle control of a transdermal contraceptive patch vs an oral contraceptive: a randomized controlled trial. *JAMA* 2001;285:2347.
3. Cardiovascular disease and use of oral and injectable progestogen-only contraceptives and combined injectable contraceptives. Results of an international, multicenter, case-control study. World Health Organization Collaborative Study of Cardiovascular Disease and Steroid Hormone Contraception. *Contraception* 1998;57:315.
4. Dardano KL, Burkman RT. The intrauterine contraceptive device: an often-forgotten and maligned method of contraception. *Am J Obstet Gynecol* 1999;181:1.
5. Fu H, Darroch JE, Haas T, et al. Contraceptive failure rates: new estimates from the 1995 National Survey of Family Growth. *Fam Plann Perspect* 1999;31:56.
6. Glasier A. Emergency postcoital contraception. *N Engl J Med* 1997;337:1058–1064.
7. Hendrix NW, Chauhan SP, Morrison JC. Sterilization and its consequences. *Obstet Gynecol Surv* 1999;54: 766–782.
8. Hubacher D, Lara-Ricalde R, Taylor DJ, et al. Use of copper intrauterine devices and the risk of tubal infertility among nulligravid women. *N Engl J Med* 2001;345(8):561–567.
9. Leblanc ES, Laws A. Benefits and risks of third-generation oral contraceptives. *J Gen Intern Med* 1999;14: 625–632.
10. Mulders TM, Dieben TO. Use of the novel combined contraceptive vaginal ring NuvaRing for ovulation inhibition. *Fertil Steril* 2001;75:865—870.
11. Rivera R, Yacobson I, Grimes D. The mechanism of action of hormonal contraceptives and intrauterine contraceptive devices. *Am J Obstet Gynecol* 1999;181:1263–1269.
12. Sherif K. Benefits and risks of oral contraceptives. *Am J Obstet Gynecol* 1999;180:S343–S348.
13. Spitzer WO, Lewis MA, Heinemann LA, et al. Third generation oral contraceptives and risk of venous thromboembolic disorders: an international case-control study. *BMJ* 1995;312:83–88.
14. Vasilakis C, Jick H, del Mar, Melero-Montes M. Risk of idiopathic venous thromboembolism in users of progestagens alone. *Lancet* 1999;354:1610.
15. Williams RS. Benefits and risks of oral contraceptive use. *Postgrad Med* 1992;92:155–171.

ABNORMAL PAP SMEAR

INTRODUCTION

- The Papanicolaou (Pap) smear is a primary screening tool which has dramatically improved early detection of cervical cancer and decreased death rates.
- Cervical cancer is the second leading cause of worldwide cancer deaths in women and accounts for nearly 400,000 new cases annually.
- The American Cancer Society estimates 12,900 new U.S. cases and 4,400 deaths in 2001 (American Cancer Society, 2001).

PATHOPHYSIOLOGY (TABLE 29.1)

- Human papilloma virus (HPV) is a common sexually transmitted infection. It is strongly associated with cervical intraepithelial neoplasia (CIN), the precursor to cervical cancer; HPV DNA is detected in 70% to 78% of CIN I patients and 83% to 89% CIN II/III patients (Wright et al., 2000; Manos et al., 1999).
- Over 70 HPV subtypes have been identified, 30 of which infect the cervix.
  ⇒ Types 6, 11, and 42: low-grade lesions and anogenital warts (condyloma acuminata, noncervical warts)
  ⇒ Types 16, 18, 33, 35, and 39: high-grade lesions and invasive cancer
- Exact prevalence unknown, ranging from 6% to 84% on polymerase chain reaction (PCR) of normal cervices (Wright and Richart, 1990). Over a 3-year period, cumulative risk of any HPV infection was 44% in one study of adolescent women (Woodman et al., 2001).
- Transmission may occur via labial-scrotal contact; condoms not protective. Incubation ranges from 3 weeks to 8 months (average 3 months); carriers are usually asymptomatic.
- Infection generally transient (under 2 years); median duration was only 8 months in one group of college women followed for 3 years (Ho et al., 1998). Persistence of HPV for over 6 months was associated with older age, cancerous types of HPV, and infection with multiple HPV types.
- A DNA test, the Hybrid Capture II test by Digene, is the only available HPV subtyping test. Its use remains unclear; it may be helpful in triaging atypical squamous cell of undetermined significance (ASCUS) Pap smears for repeat Pap versus colposcopy (Manos et al., 1999).

TABLE 29.1 RISK FACTORS FOR CERVICAL CANCER

High-risk HPV subtypes (types 16, 18)	Lower socioeconomic status
Cigarette smoking (7-fold risk)	Radiation exposure
Multiple partners (>2)	HIV infection
Early age at first intercourse (< age 17)	Immunosuppression

HPV, human papilloma virus.

EVALUATION

Conventional Pap Smear

- Endocervical brushings and scrapings of cervical area evaluates cells sloughed during previous 6 weeks; sampling artifacts such as clumping, mucus, blood, pus, or bacteria can prevent adequate evaluation (Bethesda, 1989).
- Metaanalysis of 94 studies found moderate accuracy for conventional Pap testing; sensitivity was 30% to 87% and specificity was 86% to 100% in the 12 least biased studies (Nanda et al., 2000).

Thin Smear (Thin Prep)

- Thin prep solution passes through filter that removes blood and mucous, leaving pure population of epithelial cells in a monolayer and increasing the yield of adequate Pap smears.
- High-quality data lacking (Nanda et al., 2000); generally accepted as equally effective in diagnosing intraepithelial lesions and better at detecting low-grade lesions.

Adequacy of Specimen (Table 29.2)

- *Satisfactory for evaluation*
- *Satisfactory for evaluation but limited by . . . :* 50% to 75% of the cellular material is obscured but some can still be interpreted.
- *Unsatisfactory for evaluation:* > 75% of cells are uninterpretable due to inflammation, blood, or debris.

Categorization of Abnormalities (Bethesda Classification)

- Atypical squamous or glandular cells of undetermined significance
- Intraepithelial neoplasia (low-grade also known as CIN I, or high-grade known as CIN II and III)
- Reactive changes or infection
- Other malignancies

Colposcopy

- Office procedure performed during pelvic examination that allows visualization of the cervix under magnification. Abnormal epithelial areas turn white upon application of acetic acid and may be biopsied under guidance of the colposcope.

TREATMENT

- The following management strategies are for immunocompetent patients; immunocompromised patients require aggressive follow-up of any abnormality given significantly increased risk of invasive disease.

Atypical Squamous Cells of Undetermined Significance (ASCUS)

- ASCUS is not a precancerous or cancerous condition, but may be first indication of intraepithelial neoplasia. Also seen in benign atrophic, inflammatory, or reactive changes.
- Majority of ASCUS reflects transient, benign abnormalities. However, the incidence of squamous intraepithelial neoplasia on subsequent colposcopy is 36%, with 5% to 10% high-grade disease (Lachman and Cavallo-Calvanese, 1998). Early reports using HPV subtyping to select women with ASCUS and a high-risk HPV subtype for colposcopy found a high-grade lesion in 5.1% of 56.1% of women referred (Solomon et al., 2001).
- Repeat Pap after treatment of reversible process decreases overdiagnosis of trivial abnormalities.

Atypical Glandular Cells of Undetermined Significance (AGCUS)

- AGCUS may represent a precursor to endometrial or endocervical malignancy, also seen with squamous lesions.
- Retrospective study of 1381 patients with AGCUS revealed that more than a third had a histologic abnormality: squamous intraepithelial lesions (28%), adenocarcinoma in situ (4%), adenocarcinoma of the cervix (2%), and adenocarcinoma of the endometrium (2%) (Geier et al., 2001).

Low-Grade Squamous Intraepithelial Lesions (LGSIL, CIN I, Mild Dysplasia)

- LGSIL spontaneously regresses in approximately 60% of patients (Hunter and Holschneider, 2001); there is now a trend toward less aggressive intervention.
- Possible role for HPV subtype testing in LGSIL: low-risk women (HPV oncogenic DNA negative) with biopsy-proven mild dysplasia in a visible lesion may opt for ablation/excisional procedure or close monitoring with colposcopy and Pap smears every 3 months. High-risk patients (HPV oncogenic DNA positive) should have ablation/excision.
- Current practice (no HPV testing): Patient preference dictates treatment with ablation/excision versus serial smears if the entire lesion is visualized.

High-Grade Squamous Intraepithelial Lesions (HGSIL, CIN II and III, Moderate and Severe Dysplasia)

- Approximately 20% of women with HGSIL will develop invasive cancer (McIndoe et al., 1984); all such patients should undergo colposcopy, endocervical curettage, and biopsy.
- Treatment options to remove the abnormal area: excision (conization) via scalpel or laser, or loop electrosurgical excision procedure (LEEP), also called large loop excision of the transformation zone (LLETZ); ablation via cryotherapy or laser.

Abnormal Cervical Examination (Table 29.2)

- False negative Pap smears occur in the setting of obscuring blood or inflammatory cells; a normal Pap smear is not reassuring if there is a visible lesion suspicious for dysplasia. Any cervical lesion that is raised, friable, or appears to be a condyloma should be referred for biopsy.
- A history of postcoital bleeding or irregular vaginal bleeding unexplained by hormonal imbalance should prompt referral for colposcopy and biopsy.

TABLE 29.2 MANAGEMENT OF ABNORMAL PAP SMEAR

Pap Smear Result	Management
No abnormality, but no endocervical cells, or limited evaluation	Repeat in 3 months (high risk patient) or 1 year (low risk patient).
Benign cellular changes	May be caused by infection (i.e., fungal, Trichomonas, coccobacillus c/w Actinomyces, cellular changes associated with HSV):
Squamous metaplasia	
Inflammatory cellular changes	Treat identified infections if symptomatic (may not need to treat if asymptomatic), repeat Pap after therapy.
Hyperkeratosis	
Parakeratosis	Otherwise, routine follow-up.
	Associated with infections, radiation, inflammation, or atrophy:
	If postmenopausal and signs of atrophy, treat with topical conjugated estrogen 1 gram per vagina twice weekly for 2–3 months, and repeat Pap after therapy.
Reactive cellular changes	If identified symptomatic infection, treat.
	If inflammation in low-risk patient, repeat Pap in 1 year.
	Premenopausal woman, cycle day 1–14: Routine follow-up.
Endometrial cells, normal appearing	Postmenopausal woman during withdrawal phase of HRT: Routine follow-up.
	Any other postmenopausal woman or premenopausal woman out of phase: Endometrial biopsy.

(continued)

TABLE 29.2 *(continued)*

Pap Smear Result	Management
Atypical glandular cells of undetermined significance (AGUS)	Colposcopy and possible endometrial biopsy in older women. Treat reversible processes. Treat any identified infections.
Atypical squamous cells of undetermined significance (ASCUS)	Postmenopausal woman: Treat for atrophic vaginitis with topical conjugated estrogen cream 1 gram per vagina twice weekly for 2–3 months. Repeat Pap smear after above treatments: If normal, repeat every 3 to 6 months until three normal smears. If any repeat Paps are abnormal, refer to gynecology; colposcopy recommended. If other risk factors, may refer to colposcopy without repeating Pap. Consider HPV DNA testing and triage of high-risk subtypes to colposcopy.
Low grade squamous intraepithelial neoplasia (LGSIL), CIN I	Refer for colposcopy and probable biopsy. Treatment, if selected, with ablation or excision. Growing evidence for conservative management with reliable patient.
High grade squamous intraepithelial neoplasia (HGSIL), CIN II/III, or CIS	Refer for immediate colposcopy, endocervical curettage, and biopsy.
Squamous cell carcinoma	Refer for immediate colposcopy and further management.

HSV, herpes simplex virus; HRT, hormone replacement therapy; HPV, human papilloma virus; CIN, cervical intraepithelial neoplasia; CIS, carcinoma in situ.
Source: Adapted from Goodman AK. Management of the abnormal Papanicolaou smear. UpToDate, Inc., 2001.

Follow-Up for Dysplasia

- Low-risk women: 12% chance of recurrence after complete treatment. Higher-risk women, especially HIV positive or HPV types 16 or 18: 50% risk of recurrence (Maiman et al., 1990)
- Pap smear every 3 months for the first year after treatment of dysplasia, accompanied by follow-up colposcopy with endocervical curettage every 6 months for 1 year.
- After the first year, routine follow-up if no recurrence (annual Pap for low-risk patients; twice per year if higher risk).

Prevention

- Smoking cessation (smoking increases risk of cervical cancer sevenfold)
- Folate and beta-carotene deficiencies may enhance development of dysplasia (Kwasniewska et al., 1997). Folic acid (1 mg daily) and beta-carotene (15 mg daily) suggested for all women with dysplasia.
- Avoidance of high-risk sexual practices that increase risk of HPV exposure and reinfection

SELECTED REFERENCES

1. ACOG committee opinion. Recommendations on frequency of Pap test screening Number 152—March 1995. Committee on Gynecologic Practice. American College of Obstetricians and Gynecologists. *Int J Gynaecol Obstet* 1995;49:210–211.
2. American Cancer Society. *Cancer Facts and Figures 2001.* American Cancer Society, 2001.
3. 1988 Bethesda Classification System for reporting cervical/vaginal cytologic diagnoses. *JAMA* 1989;262:931–934.
4. Geier CS, Wilson M, Creasman W. Clinical evaluation of atypical glandular cells of undetermined significance. *Am J Obstet Gynecol* 2001;184:64.
5. Ho G, Bierman R, Beardsley L, et al. Natural history of cervicovaginal papillomavirus infection in young women. *N Engl J Med* 1998;338:423–428.
6. Hunter M, Holschneider C. Cervical intraepithelial neoplasia: management. UpToDate, 2001.
7. Kwasniewska A, Tukendorf A, Semczuk M, et al. Folate deficiency and cervical intraepithelial neoplasia. *Eur J Gynaecol Oncol* 1997;6:526.
8. Lachman MF, Cavallo-Calvanese C. Qualification of atypical squamous cells of undetermined significance in an independent laboratory: is it useful or significant? *Am J Obstet Gynecol* 1998;179(2):421–429.

9. Maiman M, Fruchter RG, Serur E, et al. Human immunodeficiency virus infection and cervical neoplasia. *Gynecol Oncol* 1990;38:377–382.

10. Manos MM, Kinney WK, Hurley LB, et al. Identifying women with cervical neoplasia using human papillomavirus DNA testing for equivocal Papanicolaou results. *JAMA* 1999;281:1605–1610.

11. McIndoe WA, McLean MR, Jones RW, et al. The invasive potential of carcinoma in situ of the cervix. *Obstet Gynecol* 1984;64:451–458.

12. Moscicki A, Hills N, Shiboski S, et al. Risks for incident human papillomavirus infection and low grade intraepithelial lesion development in young females. *JAMA* 2001;285:2995–3002.

13. Nanda K, McCrory DC, Myers ER, et al. Accuracy of the Papinicolaou test in screening for and follow-up of cervical cytologic abnormalities: a systematic review. *Ann Intern Med* 2000;132:810–819.

14. Solomon D, Schiffman M, Tarone R. Comparison of three management strategies for patients with atypical squamous cells of undetermined significance: baseline results from a randomized trial. *J Natl Cancer Inst* 2001;93:293–299.

15. Woodman CBJ, Collins S, Winter H, et al. Natural history of cervical human papillomavirus infection in young women: longitudinal cohort study. *Lancet* 2001;357:1831–1836.

16. Wright TC, Richart RM. Role of human papillomavirus in the pathogenesis of genital tract warts and cancer. *Gynecol Oncol* 1990;37:151–164.

17. Wright TC, Denny L, Kuhn L, et al. HPV DNA testing of self-collected vaginal samples compared with cytologic screening to detect cervical cancer. *JAMA* 2000;283:81–86.

ABNORMAL VAGINAL BLEEDING

INTRODUCTION

- Defined as bleeding that occurs at an inappropriate time (cycle length <21 days or >36 days) or in an excessive amount (abundant bleeding or bleeding that lasts >7 days)
- Between menarche and menopause, nearly every woman has at least one episode; most common around the extremes of reproductive life

PATHOPHYSIOLOGY

- Estrogen primes the endometrium, cyclic withdrawal of progesterone stimulates sloughing of endometrium and menses.
- Normal menstrual cycle regulated by pituitary gonadotropins, luteinizing hormone (LH), and follicle-stimulating hormone (FSH), which stimulate follicular development and ovarian secretion of estradiol and progesterone (see Chapter 27)
- Ovulatory bleeding: Regular, cyclic, predictable bleeding associated with ovulatory cycles and normal function of the hypothalamic–pituitary–ovarian axis; dysmenorrhea is common.
- Anovulatory bleeding (dysfunctional uterine bleeding): unpredictable bleeding (onset, duration, frequency, amount) associated with anovulation (the absence of cyclic progesterone); usually painless; frequently seen at menarche, menopause, and with physical or emotional stress

DIFFERENTIAL DIAGNOSIS (TABLE 30.1)

- Vaginal bleeding is not necessarily uterine: Rectal, urethral, vulvar, vaginal, and cervical sources must be evaluated.
- Premenarchal: Vaginal bleeding before menarche is always abnormal. Etiologies: foreign body, sexual abuse, urologic abnormalities, vulvovaginitis, and malignancy (rare).
- Adolescents: Anovulation in >90% of cases, but pregnancy must be ruled out. Other etiologies: hematologic abnormalities, medical illness, infection, and rarely malignancy
- Premenopausal: Pregnancy and malignancy must be ruled out. Other common etiologies: polyps, fibroids, adenomyosis, infection, anovulation, and hematologic abnormalities
- Perimenopausal: Intermittent anovulation most common; prolonged periods of unopposed estrogen put perimenopausal women at increased risk for endometrial hyperplasia.
- Postmenopausal: Endometrial cancer most serious. More common causes: endometrial polyps, endometrial hyperplasia, and vaginal and endometrial atrophy

TABLE 30.1 CAUSES OF VAGINAL BLEEDING BY LOCATION AND ETIOLOGY

Vulva	Benign growths (skin tags, condylomata, angiokeratoma, sebaceous cyst), cancer, infection (STDs)
Vagina	Benign growths (polyps, Gartner duct cysts, adenosis), cancer, vaginitis (STDs, bacterial vaginosis, atrophic vaginitis).

(continued)

TABLE 30.1 *(continued)*

Cervix	Benign growths (polyps, ectropion, endometriosis), cancer (invasive or metastatic from uterus, choriocarcinoma), infection
Uterus	Anovulatory cycles (polycystic ovarian syndrome), benign growths (polyps, endometrial hyperplasia, adenomyosis, fibroids), cancer, infection, pregnancy
Upper tract disease	Fallopian tube cancer, ovarian cancer
Trauma	Sexual abuse, intercourse, foreign bodies, pelvic trauma, straddle injuries, fractures
Drugs	Contraception, hormone replacement therapy, anticoagulants, steroids, chemotherapy, antipsychotics, antibiotics (toxic epidermal necrolysis or Stevens-Johnson syndrome)
Systemic disease	Coagulation disorders, thyroid disease, chronic liver disease, Cushing syndrome, diseases that involve the vulva (Behçet, Crohn, lymphoma, pemphigoid)
Diseses not affecting the genital tract	Bladder cancer, urinary tract infection, inflammatory bowel disease, hemorrhoids, urethritis

Note: STD, sexually transmitted disease;
Source: Adapted from Goodman AK. Terminology and differential diagnosis of genital tract bleeding in women. UpToDate, Inc, 2001.

EVALUATION

History

- Amount, timing and precipitating factors of the bleeding; any associated symptoms
- Detailed menstrual history (duration, frequency, intensity)
- Prior medical problems
- Sexual history
- Weight loss or gain
- Emotional stress
- Medications, including type of contraception
- Personal or family history of coagulopathy
- Risk factors for gynecologic malignancy (see Table 30.2)

TABLE 30.2 RISK FACTORS FOR GYNECOLOGIC MALIGNANCIES

Vulva	Age, HPV infection, poverty, diabetes, hypertension, obesity, vulvar dystrophies, granulomatous pelvic infection, smoking
Vagina	Condylomata, HPV infection, diethylstilbestrol exposure
Cervix	Sexual activity at an early age, multiple sexual partners, HPV infection, cigarette smoking, history of sexually transmitted disease, human immunodeficiency virus
Uterus	Obesity, nulliparity or low parity, chronic anovulation, polycystic ovarian syndrome, early menarche, late menopause, unopposed estrogen, history of breast or ovarian cancer, family, history of endometrial cancer
Fallopian tube	Unknown
Ovarian	Uninterrupted ovulation (nulliparity or low parity, delayed childbearing, late menopause), history of breast cancer, high-fat diet, family history of breast or ovarian cancer

Note: HPV, human papillomavirus.

Physical Examination

- **Pelvic examination:** careful assessment of the external and internal anatomy of the genital tract looking for suspicious lesions, uterine or adnexal masses, focal tenderness, or abnormal discharge
- **General medical examination:** signs of systemic illness, evidence of coagulopathy (bruising, petechiae) or endocrinopathies (thyroid disease, Cushing disease, virilization)

Laboratory And Diagnostic Testing (Table 30.3)

- Pregnancy test, Papanicolaou (Pap) smear, and biopsy of any visible lesion
- **Transvaginal ultrasound:** Evaluate for endometrial hyperplasia (with endometrial biopsy as the gold standard). An endometrial stripe ≥4 mm yielded 96% sensitivity, 68% specificity for hyperplasia (Karlsson et al., 1995).
- **Endometrial biopsy:** Rule out endometrial hyperplasia or dysplasia. Sensitivity 91%, specificity >98% in premenopausal women; and >99% and >98%, respectively, in postmenopausal women (Dijkhuizen et al., 2000).
- **Pelvic ultrasound:** Assess uterine size, adnexal abnormalities; often unable to differentiate subtle intrauterine abnormalities.
- **Hysteroscopy:** Flexible fiberoptic hysteroscope is inserted into the endometrial cavity for direct intrauterine visualization; excellent for lesions such as polyps, fibroids, and neoplastic change.

TABLE 30.3 LABORATORY AND DIAGNOSTIC TESTING

Blood tests: Complete blood cell count, β-human chorionic gonodotropin workup as indicated by history
Cytology: Papanicolaou smear
Pathology: Biopsy of visible lesion, endometrial biopsy
Radiology: Transvaginal and pelvic ultrasound, sonohysterogram
Operative techniques: Dilation and curettage, hysteroscopy, laparoscopy

Approach To Premenopausal Bleeding

- **Assess ovulatory status:** Menstrual charting (regular, cyclic bleeding every 21 to 36 days); basal body temperature charting (temperature rises after ovulation 0.5°); serum progesterone measurement in mid-luteal phase, 18 to 24 days after onset of menses (progesterone >2 ng/mL suggests normal ovulation; 6 to 25 ng/mL confirms ovulation).
- **Ovulatory cycles:**
  ⇒ Menorrhagia: Heavy or prolonged menstrual bleeding, usually due to fibroids, adenomyosis, endometrial hyperplasia or polyps, endometrial or cervical cancer, coagulopathy, or pregnancy complication. Check complete blood cell count, prothrombin time/partial thromboplastin time, β-human chorionic gonadotropin, and thyroid-stimulating hormone (TSH). Patients older than 35 years or with risk factors for endometrial cancer need endometrial biopsy plus/minus pelvic ultrasound.
  ⇒ Intermenstrual bleeding: Bleeding that occurs between regular menstrual periods, often due to oral contraceptives (OCs), infections, cervical polyps, cervical cancer, or trauma. Frequently occurs during first 3 months on OCs or with missed pills. If persistent after pill change and no explanation found on initial workup, refer to gynecology for endometrial biopsy with possible ultrasound or hysteroscopy.
- **Anovulatory cycles:** Manifestation of a disturbance in the hypothalamic–pituitary–ovarian axis, due to stress, weight loss, chronic illness, thyroid disease, hyperprolactinemia, and excess androgens/cortisol. The triad of obesity, hirsutism, and chronic anovulation with irregular menstrual cycles suggests polycystic ovarian syndrome (PCOS). Workup with TSH, prolactin level, pregnancy test, and Pap smear (dexamethasone suppression test and 24-hour urine free of cortisol if Cushing syndrome suspected). Women with risk factors for endometrial cancer or whose cycles do not stabilize on therapy should undergo endometrial biopsy or transvaginal ultrasound.

Approach to Perimenopausal Bleeding

- Irregular menses common; ovulation is possible, so consider pregnancy. Estrogen excess from chronic anovulation increases risk of hyperplasia and cancer; women with six or more irregular cycles or heavy bleeding should undergo endometrial biopsy or transvaginal ultrasound. Hormonal therapy is appropriate for most other women without further workup (see below).

Approach to Postmenopausal Bleeding

- All bleeding after menopause should be evaluated with an endometrial biopsy or transvaginal ultrasound.

TREATMENT

General Principles

- Institute appropriate treatment when a specific etiology is discovered (thyroid disease, hyperprolactinemia, pregnancy, cervical or endometrial cancer).
- Patients with menorrhagia or intermenstrual bleeding and concerning features on history or physical or in whom the below treatment fails should be referred to a gynecologist for further evaluation.

Premenopausal Women with Menorrhagia and No Anatomic Abnormality

- OCs: First line. Induce normal menstrual cycles with decreased blood flow (see Chapter 28 for details on OC use).
- Nonsteroidal antiinflammatory drugs: Cause vasoconstriction and platelet activation, thereby reducing blood loss. Naproxen sodium and mefenamic acid decreased blood flow by about 50% in one double-blind study (Hall et al., 1987). First line.
- Danazol: Synthetic steroid disrupts the hypothalamic–pituitary axis and decreases menstrual flow; androgenic side effects (hirsutism, acne, fluid retention) make it a less desirable option.
- Gonadotropin-releasing hormone analogues: induce a menopausal state. Generally used as a bridge to more definitive therapy (hysterectomy or myomectomy), because they are expensive, require parenteral administration, and need estrogen replacement if used for >3 months.

Intermenstrual Bleeding in A Woman on Oral Contraceptives

- Change to a pill with more estrogenic progesterone (see Chapter 28 for specific hormonal makeup of OCs).
- Include additional estrogen such as conjugated estrogen (Premarin), 0.625 mg orally every day (q.d.) for the first 21 days of one to two successive menstrual cycles, to stabilize the endometrium.

Anovulatory Bleeding With A Negative Workup and No Concerning Features

- Hormonal therapy including OCs or cyclic progesterone
- If no menstrual flow for >6 weeks, induce withdrawal bleeding (medroxyprogesterone acetate [Provera], 5 to 10 mg q.d. for 10 to 12 days) before OCs, to minimize breakthrough bleeding.
- If OCs are contraindicated or not desired, medroxyprogesterone acetate (5 to 10 mg q.d. for 10 to 12 days of every month) is a reasonable alternative to prevent endometrial hyperplasia.
- PCOS: OCs or cyclic medroxyprogesterone acetate for women not desiring fertility. Weight reduction in obese patients may break the cycle of excess androgens. If fertility desired, refer to gynecology for ovulation induction and discussion of surgical options.

Perimenopausal Women With No Evidence of Endometrial Hyperplasia

- OCs, cyclic progesterone, or hormone replacement therapy (HRT)
- Women with intermittent ovulatory cycles do better with OCs or cyclic medroxyprogesterone acetate as above; OCs have the additional benefit of providing contraception.
- Transition to HRT if desired once the woman is menopausal; assess by looking for a high FSH level when the patient is off the pill for 6 days (right before starting a new pill package).

SELECTED REFERENCES

1. American College of Obstetricians and Gynecologists. *Management of anovulatory bleeding.* Washington, DC: American College of Obstetricians and Gynecologists, 2000. ACOG practice bulletin 14.
2. Bayer SR, DeCherney AH. Clinical manifestations and treatment of dysfunctional uterine bleeding. *JAMA* 1993;269:1823.
3. Dijkhuizen FP, Mol BW, Brolmann HA, et al. The accuracy of endometrial sampling in the diagnosis of patients with endometrial carcinoma and hyperplasia. *Cancer* 2000;89(8):1765–1772.
4. Goldfarb JM, Little AB. Abnormal vaginal bleeding. *N Engl J Med* 1980;302:666.
5. Gull B, Carlsson S, Karlsson B, et al. Transvaginal ultrasonography of the endometrium in women with postmenopausal bleeding: is it always necessary to perform an endometrial biopsy? *Am J Obstet Gynecol* 2000;182:509.
6. Hall P, Maclachlan N, Thorn N, et al. Control of menorrhagia by the cyclo-oxygenase inhibitors naproxen sodium and mefenamic acid. *Br J Obstet Gynaecol* 1987;94(6):554–558.
7. Karlsson B, Granberg S, Wikland M, et al. Transvaginal ultrasonography of the endometrium in women with postmenopausal bleeding—a Nordic multicenter study. *Am J Obstet Gynecol* 1995;172:1488–1494.
8. Kilbourn CL, Richards CS. Abnormal uterine bleeding. Diagnostic considerations, management options. *Postgrad Med* 2001:109(1):137–138, 141–144, 147–150.
9. Munro MG. Medical management of abnormal uterine bleeding. *Obstet Gynecol Clin North Am* 2000;27(2): 287–304.
10. Rosenberg MJ, Waugh MS, Higgins JE. The effect of desogestrel, gestodene and other factors on spotting and bleeding. *Contraception* 1996;53:85.
11. Thorneycroft IH, Gibbons WE. Vaginal bleeding patterns in women receiving hormone replacement therapy. Impact of various progestogen regimens. *J Reprod Med* 1999;44[Suppl 2]:209–214.

BREAST CANCER AND BENIGN BREAST DISEASE

INTRODUCTION

- Over a 10-year period, 16% of women present with a breast complaint (22 episodes per 1,000 person-years), with a 4% incidence of cancer (Barton et al., 1999).
- Fibrocystic breast disease: Prevalence 8% to 30%; autopsy studies report microcysts, macrocysts, or epithelial hyperplasia in 50% to 60% of women (Goehring and Morabia, 1997).
- About 190,000 new cases of breast cancer are reported each year in the United States; most common malignancy in women; second most common cause of cancer death in women; main cause of death in women ages 45 to 55 years.

PATHOPHYSIOLOGY

- Cyclic hormonal changes associated with mild tenderness, lumpiness, swelling, and pain in up to 60% of women (estrogen stimulates ductal proliferation; progestins stimulate lobular differentiation and proliferation) (Ader and Browne, 1997).
- Eight percent to 10% of premenopausal women experience moderate to severe perimenstrual pain (Ader et al., 1999).
- Most benign breast conditions (fibrocystic disease, fibroadenomas, papillomas, duct ectasia) are likely triggered by changes in progesterone and estrogen levels during menstrual cycle.
- Exposure to estrogen remains chief risk factor for breast cancer (see Table 31.1).

TABLE 31.1 RISK FACTORS FOR DEVELOPMENT OF BREAST CANCER

Female gender	<1% breast cancer cases in men
Age	77% new cancers, 84% deaths in women older than 50 yr
Reproductive factors	Early menarche, late menopause, nulliparity, late first pregnancy (age >30)—markers for increased estrogen exposure
Susceptibility genes	BRCA1 and BRCA2 (high prevalence in Ashkenazi Jews), Li-Fraumeni cancer syndrome, Cowden syndrome
Family history	First- degree relative yields relative risk of 2.5
Benign breast disease	Number of total biopsies, risk highest with atypical hyperplasia
Lifestyle factors	Two to three drinks alcohol/d raises risk; no good evidence for diet effect

DIFFERENTIAL DIAGNOSIS

- Palpable breast mass: fibrocystic disease, benign tumor (fibroadenoma), mastitis, fat necrosis, hematoma, ductal ectasia, malignancy
- Breast pain: physiologic, fibrocystic disease, mastitis, stretched Cooper ligaments (seen with large breasts), fat necrosis (usually from trauma); chest wall pain, costochondritis, ischemic heart disease, gallbladder disease

- Nipple discharge: galactorrhea (hyperprolactinemia, hypothyroidism, medications, breast stimulation, chest wall irritation, physiologic), blood (benign papilloma, intraductal carcinoma, Paget's disease), yellow or brown (fibrocystic disease, cysts communicating with ducts, ductal ectasia), purulent (infection, either mastitis or breast abscess)

EVALUATION

History

- Timing and nature of symptoms, including relationship to menses
- Risk factors for breast cancer (see Table 31.1), including prior breast biopsies
- Lactation status
- Medication history, including psychiatric drugs and hormones
- Nipple discharge, fever, chills, systemic symptoms

Physical Examination

- Breasts are best examined early in the follicular phase (1 week after onset of menses), when estrogen stimulation is minimal.
- Systematically palpate breast and axillary nodes with patient both lying flat and sitting with hands on hips. Goals are to document and localize nodules or skin changes, reproduce areas of pain, elicit any nipple discharge, and feel for lymphadenopathy.
- **Fibrocystic changes:** common in younger women; prominent plaques of glandular tissue, poorly defined, often in upper outer quadrant, associated with cyclical pain
- **Fibroadenoma:** Painless, freely mobile, well circumscribed, with a firm round or rubbery feel; median age at diagnosis is 30 years.
- **Cyst:** Round or oval, well demarcated, smooth, and mobile; may vary with the menstrual cycle; frequent in women in their 30s and the perimenopause.
- **Mastitis:** Pain, tenderness and erythema, particularly during lactation (usually *Staphylococcus aureus*). Nonlactating women may develop chronic relapsing and remitting periductal mastitis, with inflammatory changes causing nipple inversion, subareolar masses, and recurrent periareolar abscesses (Edmiston et al., 1990).
- **Nipple discharge:** Bilateral discharge is almost never malignant (usually galactorrhea); unilateral discharge is rarely malignant (13% in one series [Leis et al., 1988]); send cytology on bloody discharge (increased risk of malignancy, although usually due to intraductal papilloma). Sticky, colored, nonbloody discharge often from duct ectasia; pus from infection.
- **Suspicious mass:** Solitary, hard, irregular, usually nonpainful, often fixed. Malignancy cannot be distinguished from a benign finding by clinical features; any questionable lesion needs evaluation.

Laboratory

- Routine laboratory workup is not indicated except for galactorrhea, when β-human chorionic gonadotropin, prolactin, and thyroid-stimulating hormone levels should be sent.

Diagnostic Studies

- Mammography:
  ⇒ Diagnostic mammogram with radiologist present for any palpable breast mass in women older than 35 years (high breast density decreases sensitivity in younger patients); evaluates the rest of the breast along with the lesion in question.
  ⇒ Includes ultrasound and compression or magnification views as needed.
  ⇒ May fail to detect 10% to 15% of palpable breast lesions, so cannot be used to exclude malignancy.
- Ultrasound:
  ⇒ Helpful in younger women, differentiating between solid and cystic masses, or when a palpable mass is partially or poorly seen on mammogram (Zylstra, 1999).
  ⇒ Used to guide some interventional procedures.

- **Biopsy and tissue diagnosis** may be accomplished in one of three ways:
  - ⇒ *Fine needle aspiration (FNA):* Office procedure using a small needle to aspirate fluid or cells from a palpable mass; distinguishes solid from cystic lesions, and yields tissue for cytology for solid lesions. Fluid may be discarded if nonbloody but should be sent for pathology if bloody (cancer in 1% cases). False-negative rate is 6%, with no false-positive results in one study, but institution dependent (Pruthi, 2001).
  - ⇒ *Core needle biopsy:* 14- to 18-gauge needle, under ultrasound or stereotactic mammographic guidance, yields a core of tissue for histology. Often used for nonpalpable lesions, slightly less sensitive than FNA.
  - ⇒ *Excision biopsy:* local surgical excision of a mass, often using needle localization (mammographically placed needle helps the surgeon locate the lesion)
- **"Triple diagnosis"** uses clinical breast examination, mammogram, and FNA to evaluate a palpable mass; decreases excision biopsies for benign disease; allows women with definitive malignancy to have a one-stage operative procedure, bypassing excision biopsy:
  - ⇒ Benign disease suggested by all three tests: follow clinically every 3 to 6 months. There is an approximately 1% false-negative risk, which the patient should understand (Layfield, 1989).
  - ⇒ Malignant disease suggested by all three tests: refer for definitive therapy; 99.4% cancer rate (Layfield, 1989).
  - ⇒ Any discordant test: excision biopsy
- Management of suspected cyst (see Fig. 31.1) or solid mass:
  - ⇒ No fluid on aspiration suggests solid mass, which may be managed by triple diagnosis or by excision biopsy directly (with preceding diagnostic mammogram), depending on institutional and patient preference.

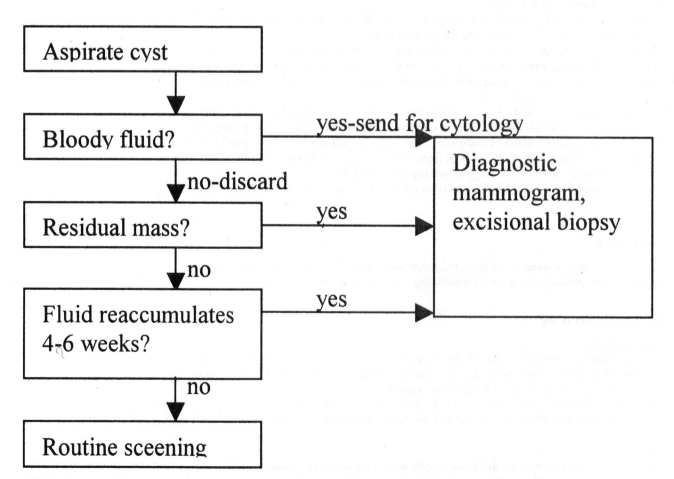

FIGURE 31.1. Management of suspected cyst. (From Pruthi S. Detection and evaluation of a palpable breast mass. Mayo Clin Proc 2001;76:641–648, with permission.)

TREATMENT

Fibrocystic Disease

- Pain may be relieved by reassurance, a supportive bra, and acetaminophen or antiinflammatory agents.
- Further options include caffeine avoidance; vitamin E (400 IU twice daily); evening primrose oil (1,500 to 3,000 mg every day [q.d.]); the androgen danazol (100 to 200 mg q.d.); the antiestrogen tamoxifen; androgenic oral contraceptive agents (Belieu, 1994). The first three are preferred, given absence of side effects.

Galactorrhea

- Prolactin adenomas may be treated with dopamine agonists such as bromocriptine or cabergoline if symptoms are troubling or for amenorrhea and/or infertility; also effective in idiopathic hyperprolactinemia.
- Macroadenomas require surgical excision if mass effects are not responsive to medical therapy.

Mastitis

- Hot packs to affected area to help with drainage; antibiotics with efficacy against *S. aureus*
- Chronic subareolar abscess may require surgical excision.

Breast Cancer

- *Lobular carcinoma in situ:*
  ⇒ Marker for increased risk of invasive disease in either breast; options include close monitoring, tamoxifen, or bilateral prophylactic mastectomies.
- *Ductal carcinoma in situ:*
  ⇒ Twenty percent may progress to invasive disease.
  ⇒ Treated as early stage invasive cancer with local therapy plus/minus tamoxifen
- *Locally invasive disease:*
  ⇒ Local therapy including sentinel lymph node biopsy or axillary node dissection: equal survival with mastectomy and lumpectomy/radiation; more local recurrence with breast-conserving therapy, but salvageable
  ⇒ Adjuvant therapy: tamoxifen, 20 mg q.d. for 5 years for women with estrogen-receptor–positive tumors
  ⇒ Polychemotherapy: women with poor prognostic indicators, including lymph node positivity, tumors larger than 1 cm, lymphatic or vascular invasion
- *Metastatic disease:*
  ⇒ Median survival, 2 to 3 years; 5-year survival, 10% to 15%. Goals of therapy are palliation (improve quality of life) and prolongation of life.
  ⇒ Hormonal therapy: tamoxifen, ovarian ablation, aromatase inhibitors
  ⇒ Polychemotherapy: cyclophosphamide (Cytoxan), doxorubicin (Adriamycin), taxane, capecitabine, gemcitabine, among others
  ⇒ Biological agents: trastuzumab (Herceptin), a recently approved anti-HER2/neu agent
  ⇒ Symptomatic therapy: bisphosphonates for bone metastases or hypercalcemia, radiation for painful bone metastases

FUTURE DIRECTIONS

- *Prevention:* Tamoxifen was recently approved by the Food and Drug Administration for high-risk women based on a trial showing a 50% reduction in cancer (increased risk of endometrial cancer and deep venous thrombosis). Other selective estrogen-receptor modulators may have similar benefit; Study of Tamoxifen and Raloxifene trial comparing tamoxifen with raloxifene for prevention is ongoing.
- The development of computer models of breast cancer susceptibility as a screening tool allows identification of women at high risk who may benefit from prevention trials or close monitoring.

- Future imaging modalities: digital mammography; computer-aided diagnosis; power Doppler ultrasound; magnetic resonance imaging; isotope imaging (methoxyisobutyl-isonitrile and positron emission tomography). Their role in management is not yet defined (Jochelson, 2001).

RESOURCES

- American Cancer Society: http://www.cancer.org
- The Breast Cancer Awareness and Solutions Network: http://www.bce.army
- The National Cancer Institute: 301-496-6641; http://rex.nci.nih.gov
- Women's Cancer Network: http://www.wcn.org

SELECTED REFERENCES

1. Ader DN, Browne MW. Prevalence and impact of cyclic mastalgia in a United States clinic-based sample. *Am J Obstet Gynecol* 1997;177(1):126–132.
2. Ader DN, Shriver CD, Browne MW. Cyclical mastalgia: premenstrual syndrome or recurrent pain disorder? *J Psychosom Obstet Gynecol* 1999;20(4):198–202.
3. Barton MB, Elmore JG, Fletcher SW. Breast symptoms among women enrolled in a health maintenance organization: frequency, evaluation and outcome. *Ann Intern Med* 1999;130:651–659.
4. Bergh J, Jonsson PE, Glimelius B, et al. (SBU-group). Swedish Council of Technology Assessment in Health Care. A systematic overview of chemotherapy effects in breast cancer. *Acta Oncologica* 2001;40(2-3):253–281.
5. Bodian CA. Benign breast diseases, carcinoma in situ, and breast cancer risk. *Epidemiol Rev* 1993;15:177–187.
6. Brinton LA, Schairer C. Estrogen replacement therapy and breast cancer risk. *Epidemiol Rev* 1993;15:66–79.
7. Bywaters JL. The incidence and management of female breast disease in a general practice. *J R Coll Gen Pract* 1977;27:35.
8. Edmiston CE, Walker AP, Krepel CJ, et al. The nonpuerperal breast infection: aerobic and anaerobic microbial recovery from acute and chronic disease. *J Infect Dis* 1990;162(3):695–699.
9. Fornage BD. Sonographically guided needle biopsy of nonpalpable breast lesions. *J Clin Ultrasound* 1999;27(7):385–398.
10. Goehring C, Morabia A. Epidemiology of benign breast disease, with special attention to histologic types. *Epidemiol Rev* 1997;19(2):510–527.
11. Jochelson M. Breast cancer imaging: the future. *Semin Oncol* July 2001;28(3):221–228.
12. Leis HP. Concepts regarding breast biopsies. *Breast Dis* 1991;4:223.
13. Leis HP, Green FL, Cammarata A, et al. Nipple discharge: surgical significance. *South Med J* 1988:81:20.
14. Leris C, Mokbel K. The prevention of breast cancer: an overview. *Curr Med Res Opin* 2001;16(4):252–257.
15. Layfield LJ, Glasgow BJ, Cramer H. Fine needle aspiration in the management of breast masses. *Pathol Annu* 1989;24pt2:23–62.
16. National Center for Health Statistics. *Seer cancer statistics review, 1973–1995.* Bethesda, MD: US National Cancer Center Institute; 1998.
17. Pena KS. Evaluation and treatment of galactorrhea. *Am Fam Physician* 2001;63(9):1763–1770.
18. Pruthi S. Detection and evaluation of a palpable breast mass. *Mayo Clin Proc* 2001;76(6):641–648.
19. Zylstra S. Office management of benign breast disease. *Clin Obstet Gynecol* 1999;42(2):234–248.

URINARY INCONTINENCE

INTRODUCTION

- Urinary incontinence (UI) affects 15% to 30% of adults older than 65 years living in the community and >50% of patients in long-term care facilities. The incidence in women is twice that in men.
- Morbidity: psychological distress; local and systemic infections; skin breakdown from moisture and irritation; may influence decisions on when to institutionalize incontinent elders
- Providers should include continence in the adult review of symptoms, because patients rarely volunteer symptoms of incontinence.

PATHOPHYSIOLOGY

- Risk factors: chronic obstructive pulmonary disease, chronic cough, diabetes, transient ischemic attack and stroke, depression, constipation, multiple pregnancies, vaginal delivery, episiotomy, estrogen depletion, genitourinary (GU) surgery, radiation
- Physical changes of the aging body that predispose to, but do not cause, UI:
  ⇒ Decreased bladder capacity limits ability to postpone voiding.
  ⇒ Decreased detrusor contractility decreases urinary flow rate.
  ⇒ Increased involuntary bladder muscle contractions, decreased physical mobility may impair continence.
  ⇒ In men, the prostate enlarges; in women, the urethra shortens.
- Tonic inhibition of bladder wall detrusor muscle and tonic contraction of urethral smooth muscle (via T11-L2) maintain continence; sphincter closure augmented by urethral support from pelvic musculature and S2-4 cholinergic stimulation of striated sphincter muscle.
- With voluntary micturition, cholinergic activity initiates detrusor contraction and urethral smooth muscle relaxation.

DIFFERENTIAL DIAGNOSIS

Transient Urinary Incontinence (Table 32.1)

- Multiple precipitants (**DIAPERS**); often reversible with identification and treatment of the acute etiology.
  ⇒ Delirium/dementia: lack of central nervous system (CNS) tonic inhibition detrusor hyperreflexia
  ⇒ Infection: local irritation detrusor hyperreflexia
  ⇒ Atrophic vaginitis: pelvic floor atrophy → bladder outlet incompetence
  ⇒ Pharmaceuticals: detrusor hyporeflexia, bladder outlet obstruction, altered mental status (see Table 32.1)
  ⇒ Excess urine output: volume overload, glycosuria, diuretics
  ⇒ Restricted mobility: rheumatologic disease, Parkinson disease, severe dyspnea, catatonic depression
  ⇒ Stool: impaction bladder outlet obstruction

TABLE 32.1 PHARMACOLOGIC CAUSES OF TRANSIENT URINARY TRACT INFECTION

Drug Class	Mechanism
Antidepressants (tricyclic antidepressants, selective serotonin reuptake inhibitors)	Detrusor hyporeflexia
Antipsychotics (anticholinergic)	Detrusor hyporeflexia
α-adrenergic blockers	Urethral relaxation; stress incontinence in women
α-adrenergic agonists (cold and diet preparations)	Bladder outlet obstruction, urinary retention
Alcohol	Polyuria, sedation, immobility, delirium
Calcium channel blockers	Urinary retention, due to smooth muscle relaxation
Diuretics	Polyuria, frequency, urgency
Narcotics/sedatives	Fecal impaction, muscle relaxation, immobility, delirium

Long-term Urinary Incontinence

- *Detrusor hyperreflexia* (urge incontinence: frequent, sudden, imminent need to void); most common cause of intrinsic UI in elderly population; seen equally in men and women
  ⇒ Etiologies: loss of CNS tonic inhibition (stroke, cervical stenosis); bladder irritation (infections, neoplasms, bladder stones; early bladder outlet obstruction; urethral hypermobility (due to pelvic floor laxity)
- *Detrusor hyporeflexia* (overflow incontinence: dribbling small amounts, high postvoid residual [PVR]); least common etiology of UI
  ⇒ Etiologies: lower motor neuron disease (diabetes, alcohol, vitamin B_{12} deficiency, syphilis); damage to the lumbar afferents (disc herniation, spinal stenosis, tumor); prolonged or chronic obstruction; drugs
- *Bladder outlet obstruction* (overflow incontinence: dribbling small amounts, high PVR); affects men far more frequently than women
  ⇒ Etiologies: benign prostatic hyperplasia (BPH), prostate cancer, urethral stricture, stones, acute spinal cord lesion
- *Bladder outlet incompetence* (stress incontinence: losing urine with coughing, lifting, usually not nocturnal); generally seen only in women
  ⇒ Etiologies: laxity of urethral support from pelvic floor (after childbirth/surgery, estrogen deficiency); drugs

EVALUATION

History

- Identify physiologic reasons behind incontinence and any remediable factors:
  ⇒ Onset of incontinence, precipitants, frequency, volume, timing, type of incontinence based on symptoms (urge, stress, overflow)
  ⇒ Bowel and sexual function
  ⇒ Medical history, including medications
  ⇒ Presence of transient, exacerbating factors (see above)

Physical Examination

- General alertness and functional status
- Orthostatic hypotension, evidence of dehydration
- *Neck:* cervical spine mobility; evidence for cervical stenosis including interosseous muscle wasting
- *Back:* evidence of previous back surgery; tuft of hair or dimple at the spinal cord base (suggests spina bifida occulta)
- *Abdomen:* distended or tender bladder
- *Pelvic (women):* atrophy; prolapse/pelvic-floor laxity or weakness; urine loss with cough; bulging of the anterior wall (cystocele) or posterior wall (rectocele) with cough; masses
- *GU (men):* phimosis or paraphimosis in uncircumcised men

- *Rectal:* fecal impaction; prostatic hypertrophy or mass
- *Neurologic:* perianal sensation; weakness in lower extremities or toes; abnormal lower extremity reflexes

Initial Diagnostic Tests

- Blood urea nitrogen/creatinine, glucose, calcium, vitamin B_{12}, rapid plasma reagin
- Urinalysis, with culture if suspected infection
- Suspected overflow incontinence: If PVR is high (>100 mL), obtain immediate renal ultrasound to assess for hydronephrosis and potential obstructive renal failure.
- 48- to 72-hour voiding diary (timed entry of each void and episode of incontinence): may clarify mechanism of incontinence by highlighting symptoms, frequency, and possible precipitants; monitors effectiveness of interventions

Urodynamic Testing

- Routine testing not recommended: invasive, expensive, rarely needed for diagnosis after careful history and physical examination
- May offer precise diagnosis necessary when surgical correction is being considered

TREATMENT

- *Detrusor hyperreflexia (urge incontinence)*
  - ⇒ *Bladder training* (timed voiding with use of relaxation techniques to suppress any intervening urgency, prompted voiding for demented patients). Biofeedback may help patients identify and use volitional pelvic muscles to maintain continence.
  - ⇒ Antispasmodic and anticholinergic agents: *oxybutynin (Ditropan)* and *tolterodine (Detrol)*. Side effects: dry mouth and constipation (can exacerbate incontinence); may precipitate urinary obstruction in patients with component of urethral obstruction (consider α-adrenergic blocker in men with BPH); tolterodine interacts with warfarin to raise international normalized ratio.
- *Detrusor hyporeflexia (overflow incontinence)*
  - ⇒ *Decompression* with indwelling catheter for 14 days, followed by voiding trial. If unsuccessful, intermittent straight catheterization may be necessary.
  - ⇒ Bethanechol (cholinergic) is occasionally helpful in stimulating detrusor function.
- *Bladder outlet obstruction (overflow incontinence)*
  - ⇒ *Surgical relief* of the obstruction
  - ⇒ α-Blockers (*terazosin [Hytrin]* may require 6 weeks for response; *tamsulosin [Flomax]*, increase dose after 2 to 4 weeks if inadequate response); 5α-reductase inhibitor (*finasteride [Proscar]* less effective than α-blockers, may take 1 year for full response) (see Chapter 33).
- *Bladder outlet incompetence (stress incontinence)*
  - ⇒ *Kegel exercises;* pessaries for bladder or uterine prolapse; weight loss for morbidly obese
  - ⇒ Surgery (bladder neck suspension): best cure rate (>75%), but associated surgical morbidity
  - ⇒ *Estrogen* (topical cream or intravaginal rings, transdermal, or oral); α-adrenergic agonists (propanolamine) stimulate urethral muscle contraction but are contraindicated in patients with hypertension or heart disease; imipramine is helpful in mixed stress and urge UI given both α-agonist and anticholinergic properties.
- *Reasons to refer*
  - ⇒ Unsatisfactory response to adequate therapeutic trial
  - ⇒ Need for specialized treatment including pessary or surgical correction
  - ⇒ Suspicion for urinary tract malignancy, including hematuria without infection
  - ⇒ Suspicion for prostate cancer, including nodule or asymmetry on examination
  - ⇒ Suspicion for gynecologic cancer, including pelvic abnormality or urinary obstruction
  - ⇒ Neurologic findings of CNS compromise, such as multiple sclerosis or cord compression

SELECTED REFERENCES

1. Brown JS, Sawaya G, Thom DH, et al. Hysterectomy and urinary incontinence: a systematic review. *Lancet* 2000;356:535.
2. Burgio KL, Locher JL, Goode PS, et al. Behavioral vs drug treatment for urge urinary incontinence in older women: a randomized controlled trial. *JAMA* 1998;280:1995.
3. *Clinical practice guideline: urinary incontinence in adults.* Rockville, MD: US Dept of Health and Human Services, Agency for Health Care Policy and Research; 1992. AHCPR publication 92-0038.
4. DuBeau CE, Resnick NM. Evaluation of the causes and severity of geriatric incontinence: a critical appraisal. *Urol Clin North Am* 1991;18:243.
5. Fantl JA, Newman DK, Colling J, et al. *Clinical practice guideline number 2: urinary incontinence in adults: acute and chronic management.* Rockville, MD: US Dept of Health and Human Services, Agency for Health Care Policy and Research; 1996. AHCPR publication 96-0682.
6. Fantl JA, Wyman JF, McClish DK, et al. Efficacy of bladder training in older women with urinary incontinence. *JAMA* 1991;265:609.
7. Jackson S, Shepherd A, Brookes S, et al. The effect of oestrogen supplementation on post-menopausal urinary stress incontinence: a double-blind placebo-controlled trial. *Br J Obstet Gynaecol* 1999;106:711.
8. Millard R, Tuttle J, Moore K, et al. Clinical efficacy and safety of tolterodine compared to placebo in detrusor overactivity. *J Urol* 1999;161:1551.
9. Resnick NM. Noninvasive diagnosis of the patient with complex incontinence. *Gerontology* 1990;36[Suppl 2]:8.
10. Skelly J, Flint AJ. Urinary incontinence associated with dementia. *J Am Geriatr Soc* 1995;43:286.
11. Weidner AC, Myers ER, Visco AG, et al. Which women with stress incontinence require urodynamic evaluation? *Am J Obstet Gynecol* 2001;184:20.

BENIGN PROSTATIC HYPERPLASIA

INTRODUCTION

- Defined as benign glandular and stromal nodules arising in the periurethral prostatic tissue.
- Prevalence increases with age (Roylance et al., 1995):
  ⇒ Age 30: <10% prevalence
  ⇒ Age 50: 50% prevalence
  ⇒ Age 85: 90% prevalence
- 25% of U.S. men will be treated for benign prostatic hyperplasia (BPH) by age 80 (McConnell et al., 1994).
- Morbidity related to lower urinary tract symptoms, acute retention, infection, and rarely, renal failure secondary to unrelieved outflow obstruction

PATHOPHYSIOLOGY

- Three components of lower urinary tract symptoms:
  ⇒ *Mechanical obstruction:* In the prostate cell, testosterone is converted by 5α-reductase to dihydrotestosterone, causing cell proliferation. Prostatic hyperplasia leads to mechanical bladder outlet obstruction.
  ⇒ *Dynamic obstruction:* α-Adrenergic receptors control smooth muscle tone in the bladder neck and prostate; stimulation increases bladder outlet obstruction.
  ⇒ *Detrusor hypertrophy:* Bladder (detrusor) muscle response to obstruction, leads to uninhibited muscular contraction and further obstruction.
- Risk factors: increasing age, normal testicular function. Family history of early prostatectomy (before age 64) is controversial (Barry et al., 1997).
- Natural history: Slowly progressive in most men, but waxing and waning symptoms are common. One third of patients with mild BPH have spontaneous regression of symptoms without treatment (Barry, 1990), whereas those with severe symptoms at baseline tend toward persistent symptoms or opt for surgery.

DIFFERENTIAL DIAGNOSIS

- Most commonly due to BPH, but other etiologies are in the differential (see Table 33.1).

TABLE 33.1 DIFFERENTIAL DIAGNOSIS OF LOWER URINARY TRACT INFECTION SYMPTOMS

Medication side effects
Urethral stricture
Bladder calculi
GU infection: urinary tract infection, prostatitis
GU cancer
Neurogenic bladder
Metabolic disturbances: hyperglycemia, hypercalcemia

Note: GU, genitourinary.

EVALUATION

History (Table 33.2)

- Obstructive symptoms ("voiding"): hesitancy, terminal dribbling, overflow incontinence, straining, prolonged voiding, retention, weak stream
- Irritative symptoms ("filling"): frequency, urge incontinence, nocturia, urgency, small voided volume
- Review medications: diuretics, sympathomimetics (increase outflow resistance), anticholinergics (impair bladder function), calcium channel blockers
- Evaluate for other etiologies of voiding dysfunction: primary bladder disease, urethral stricture, genitourinary cancer or infection, diabetes mellitus, congestive heart failure, hypercalcemia. If rapid symptom onset or age younger than 50 years, other cause is more likely.

Physical Examination

- Digital rectal examination (enlarged, symmetrically firm prostate; feels like "tip of nose")
- Focused neurologic examination (evidence of peripheral/autonomic neuropathy, bladder dysfunction)

Laboratory Studies

- Urinalysis (rule out pyuria, hematuria)
- Serum creatinine clearance, other chemistries as indicated
- Prostate-specific antigen (PSA) (optional): Controversial test requiring discussion with patient; does not definitively reduce mortality; may generate morbidity from acting on results. Discuss testing if life expectancy is >10 years and diagnosis of prostate cancer would change treatment plan (Barry et al., 1997). DRE does not change PSA; ejaculation may cause mild elevation; prostatitis, prostate biopsy, acute retention may increase level for weeks. PSA predicts preventive benefit of finasteride.

Further Diagnostic Studies (Fig. 33.1)

- Noninvasive urinary flow rate recording: electronic recording of urinary flow rate throughout micturition. Peak flow rate <15 mL/sec supports diagnosis of BPH.
- *Postvoid residual:* measurement of urine remaining in the bladder immediately after micturition. Poorly reproducible; generally not helpful.
- *Formal urodynamics (pressure–flow studies):* measures pressure in bladder during voiding. Differentiates between low peak flow rate secondary to obstruction and neurogenic bladder; "gold standard" for diagnosis of bladder outlet obstruction but may not improve outcome
- *Upper urinary tract (ultrasound or intravenous pyelogram) imaging:* patients with hematuria, urinary tract infection (UTI), renal insufficiency, history of urolithiasis or urinary tract surgery
- *Urethrocystoscopy:* helps plan invasive therapy in patients with hematuria, urethral strictures, bladder cancer, or prior surgery of lower tract

TABLE 33.2 AMERICAN UROLOGICAL ASSOCIATION SYMPTOM INDEX FOR BENIGN PROSTATIC HYPERPLASIA (BARRY ET AL., 1992)

Question to be answered:

1. Over the past month, how often have you had a sensation of not emptying your bladder completely after you finished urinating?
2. Over the past month, how often have you had to urinate again less than 2 hours after you finished urinating?
3. Over the past month, how often have you found you stopped and started again several times when you urinated?
4. Over the past month, how often have you found it difficult to postpone urination?
5. Over the past month, how often have you had a weak urinary stream?
6. Over the past month, how often have you had to push or strain to begin urination?

Not at all	Less than one time in five	Less than half the time	About half the time	More than half the time	Almost always
0	1	2	3	4	5

7. Over the past month, how many times did you most typically get up to urinate from the time you went to bed at night untill the time you got up in the am?

None	One time	Two times	Three times	Four times	Five or more times
0	1	2	3	4	5

Sum of 7 circled number (AUA Symptom Score):____

MILD	0–7
MODERATE	8–19
SEVERE	20–35

Note: AUA, American Urological Association.

TREATMENT

Goals

- Primary goal is to improve quality of life by decreasing symptoms and preventing complications; age-related conditions and patient preferences should be considered, along with symptom severity (see Fig. 33.1).

Watchful Waiting

- For *mild symptoms* of BPH (American Urological Association [AUA] score <7), risks of interventions usually outweigh benefits. Reassure patient and review condition each year.
- Potential complications: chronic or acute (1.0% to 2.5% per year) urinary retention; recurrent UTIs; renal failure from obstructive uropathy; bladder stones; irreversible bladder decompensation

Pharmacologic Therapies

- Patients with *moderate-severe* symptoms (AUA score >8) should be informed about all treatment options.
- α-Blockers are more effective than 5α-reductase inhibitors in improving symptoms of BPH and peak urinary flow rate (Lepor, 1996; Debuyne et al., 1998). No evidence for combination therapy (although trials <12 months); no direct comparisons of these medications with surgical treatment.
- α-Blockers: decrease prostatic smooth muscle tone; improve urinary flow rates by approximately 50% (McConnell, et al. 1994). Symptomatic improvement is seen in 60% to 80%; no clear reduction in complications, need for future surgery.
  ⇒ Doxazosin and terazosin: benefit in concomitant hypertension, although α-blocker monotherapy inadvisable given ALLHAT study (see Chapter 3)
  ⇒ Tamsulosin: more selective antagonist of α_{1A}-receptor; doesn't lower blood pressure; possibly fewer systemic side effects; less need for titration
  ⇒ Adverse effects: orthostatic hypotension, nasal congestion, dizziness, fatigue
- *5α-Reductase inhibitors (finasteride)*: competitive inhibitor of 5α-reductase; blocks testosterone to dihydrotestosterone conversion, causing involution of hyperplastic prostatic tissue.
  ⇒ Reduces prostate volume (20%), PSA levels (50%), BPH symptoms (30% to 40%), particularly among men with large prostate glands (>40 g) (Boyle et al., 1996). May take up to 12 months for full effect. Reduces risk of acute retention and surgery for men with larger prostates (or higher PSA levels).
  ⇒ Adverse effects: decreased libido, impotence, ejaculatory dysfunction; sexual side effects in 5%
- *Saw palmetto:* plant extract obtained from *Serenoa repens* inhibits 5α-reductase in animals; systematic review of human data found self-reported symptom improvement similar to finasteride (Wilt et al., 2000).
- *β-Sitosterol plant extract:* significant reductions in symptom scores versus placebo in several small difficult-to-interpret studies using different preparations

Surgical Therapies

- Patients with *severe symptoms* (AUA score >20) benefit most from surgery, usually used after medical therapy fails.
- Definite indications for surgery: *acute retention* without a predisposing cause; *hydronephrosis;* repeated *UTIs;* recurrent or refractory gross *hematuria;* an *elevated creatinine clearance* clearly related to BPH; *bladder stones*
- Urology referral also indicated persistent symptoms, despite maximal medical therapy
- *Transurethral incision, transurethral resection (TURP), open prostatectomy:* "gold standard" in terms of outcome; symptomatic improvement in 75% to 96% of patients; best overall improvement of symptoms/objective voiding parameters (Guthrie, 1997)
  ⇒ 0.2% mortality
  ⇒ 20% complications (TURP < open procedure): retrograde ejaculation (70%); urinary incontinence (2% to 4%); impotence (5% to 10%); persistent urinary symptoms; dilutional hyponatremia; bleeding requiring transfusion; bladder neck contracture; infection

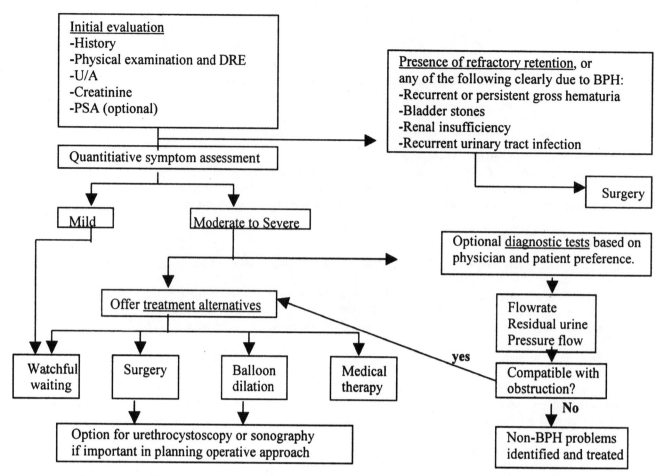

FIGURE 33.1. Possible treatment algorithm. (From McConnell JD. Why pressure flow studies should be optional and not mandatory studies for evaluating men with BPH. *Urology* 1994:44:156–158, with permission.)

- Newer surgical treatments:
  ⇒ *Laser prostatectomy:* less bleeding than standard TURP but relative effectiveness uncertain
  ⇒ *Transurethral microwave thermotherapy:* effectiveness versus TURP is controversial
  ⇒ *Transurethral needle ablation:* fewer side effects than TURP, but less effective
  ⇒ *Prostatic stents:* few or no data

SELECTED REFERENCES

1. Barry MJ. Epidemiology and natural history of BPH. *Urol Clin North Am* 1990;17:495–507.
2. Barry MJ, Fowler FJ, Bin L, et al. The natural history of PTS with BPH as DX by North American urologists. *J Urol* 1997;157:10–15.
3. Barry M, Fowler F, O'Leary M, et al. The American Urological Association Symptom Index for benign prostatic hyperplasia. *J Urol* 1992;148:1549.
4. Boyle P, Gould AL, Rochrborn CG. Prostate volume predicts outcome of treatment of BPH. *N Engl J Med* 1996;335:533–539.
5. Debuyne FMJ, Jardin A, Colloi D, et al. Sustained-release alfuzosin, finasteride and the combination of both in the treatment of benign prostatic hyperplasia. *Eur Urol* 1998;34:169–175.
6. Guthrie R. Benign prostatic hyperplasia in elderly men. *Postgrad Med* 1997;101(5):141–160.
7. Lepor H. A Department of VA cooperative randomized placebo controlled clinical trial of the safety and efficacy of terazosin and finasteride monotherapy and terazosin/finasteride combo therapy in men with clinical BPH. *J Urol* 1996;155:587A.
8. Lepor H, Williford WO, Barry MJ, et al. The efficacy of terazosin, finasteride, or both in benign prostatic hyperplasia. VA cooperative studies benign prostatic hyperplasia study group. *N Engl J Med* 1996;335:533–539.
9. McConnell JD. Why pressure flow studies should be optional and not mandatory studies for evaluating men with BPH. *Urology* 1994;44:156–158.

10. McConnell JD. The effect of finasteride on the risk of acute urinary retention and the need for surgical treatment among men with benign prostatic hyperplasia. *N Engl J Med* 1998;338(9):557–563.
11. McConnell JD, Barry MJ, Bruskewitz RC, et al. *Clinical practice guidelines number 8: BPH: diagnosis and treatment.* Rockville, MD: US Dept of Health and Human Services, Agency for Health Care Policy and Research; 1994. AHCPR publication 94-0582.
12. Roylance P, Gibelin B, Espie J. Current treatment of BPH. *Biomed Pharmacother* 1995;49:332–338.
13. Wilt T, Ishani A, Stark G, et al. Serenoa repens *for benign prostatic hyperplasia* [the Cochrane Library, issue 3]. Oxford: Update Software; 2000.

ERECTILE DYSFUNCTION

INTRODUCTION

- Defined as inability to acquire or maintain an erection sufficient for sexual intercourse in >75% of attempts; differs from loss of libido, premature ejaculation, or anorgasmia.
- 20 to 40 million men are estimated to suffer from erectile dysfunction (ED) (Nehra, 2000).
- Prevalence increases with age: Nearly 40% of men age 40 years and 70% of men age 70 years report occasional difficulty in obtaining or maintaining erection (Goldstein et al., 1998).

PATHOPHYSIOLOGY

- Normal erections require vascular, hormonal, neural, and psychogenic contribution to activate penile blood flow into the corpora cavernosa and stimulate intrapenile synthesis of the neurotransmitter nitric oxide. Problems at any point within the pathway may cause ED.
  ⇒ **Vascular:** Sexual excitement leads to relaxation of arteriolar smooth muscle via nitric oxide and parasympathetic nerves, causing engorgement of the sinusoids and compression of venous outflow.
  ⇒ **Nervous system:** Sacral autonomic nerves converge into penile cavernous nerves, which control blood flow through parasympathetic (erection) and sympathetic (ejaculation) activation; pudendal nerve controls penile sensation, activating reflex erection via S2-4; central nervous system processes psychogenic stimuli, which are relayed to the spinal cord at T1-L2.
  ⇒ **Hormonal mediators:** Sexual stimulation causes nitric oxide release by intrapenile nerves and endothelial cells (Lue, 2000), activating intracellular cyclic guanosine monophosphate, which relaxes arteriolar smooth muscle. Prostaglandin E, prostaglandin I_2, and vasoactive intestinal polypeptide (VIP) also contribute to penile smooth muscle relaxation via cyclic adenosine monophosphate formation.

DIFFERENTIAL DIAGNOSIS (TABLES 34.1 AND 34.2)

TABLE 34.1 DIFFERENTIAL OF ERECTILE DYSFUNCTION

Psychogenic	Performance anxiety, depression, mental stress; 90% of severely depressed patients
Diabetes mellitus	50% of diabetic men have erectile dysfunction (Melman and Gingell, 1999); etiology multifactorial: neuropathy, vascular disease, psychiatric conditions
Vascular disease	Inadequate arteriolar flow or impaired venoocclusion in patients with hypertension, peripheral vascular disease, ischemic heart disease, smoking history, diabetes, trauma
Hormonal dysfunction	Testosterone deficiency depresses libido and erection; hyperprolactinemia; hypothyroidisum and hyperthyroidism; Addison disease

(continued)

TABLE 34.1 *(continued)*

Urologic/pelvic surgery	Radical prostatectomy, radical cystectomy for bladder cancer, colorectal surgery can disrupt autonomic nerves
	All treatment modalities for prostate cancer (surgical, brachytherapy seed placement, external beam therapy); occurs after simple prostatectomy (transurethral erection or open suprapubic prostatectomy) but much more rare
Spinal cord injury	No erection or sensation if S2-4 destroyed; ejaculation impaired with damage to sympathetic nerves to 1-3, although reflex erection via penile stimulation possible
Medications/drugs	See Table 34.2

TABLE 34.2 DRUGS THAT CAUSE ERECTILE DYSFUNCTION

Drug Class	Specific Categories/Drugs	Comments
Antihypertensives	thiazides, centrally acting sympatholytics (clonidine, methyldopa), β-blockers	Fewer sexual side effects for ACE inhibitors, calcium channel blockers
Antiandrogens	spironolactone, H_2-blockers (especially cimetidine), finasteride, ketoconazole	
Antidepressants	tricyclics, SSRIs, monoamine oxidase inhibitors	Impaired orgasm with SSRI—erectile function often maintained
Antipsychotics	phenothiazines, butyrophenones	Due to anticholinergic actions
Central nervous system depressants	alcohol, benzodiazepines, barbiturates, opiates	Chronic alcohol use causes penile neuropathy, hypogonadism
Other drugs of abuse	cocaine, amphetamines, marijauna	May increase libido but impair performance

Note: SSRI, selective serotonin reuptake inhibitor.

EVALUATION

History

- Goal is to distinguish between problems of libido, erection, ejaculation, and orgasm.
- *Medical history:* diabetes mellitus, smoking, hypertension, depression, medications, alcohol or drug use
- *Psychosocial factors:* relationship conflicts, anxiety, depression
- *Rapidity of onset:* Acute etiologies include psychogenic (suggested by inability to complete intercourse in a man with no history of sexual dysfunction, pelvic trauma, or surgery), radical prostatectomy, or pelvic trauma.
- *Morning erections:* Presence of any spontaneous erection, often during rapid eye movement sleep, confirms intact neurologic reflexes and adequate penile blood flow. Loss of nocturnal erections implies vascular or neurologic ED, although severely depressed men may have transient loss of morning erections.
- *Degree of libido:* Decreased sexual desire suggests psychogenic or endocrinologic etiology (thyroid disease, hyperprolactinemia, hypogonadism, Addison disease).
- *Degree of erection:* nonsustained erection after penetration due to either anxiety (sympathetic release leading to detumescence) or vascular steal syndrome (high oxygen requirement of the thrusting pelvis diverts blood from the vasodilated corpora cavernosa [Michal et al., 1978])

Physical Examination

- *Cardiovascular:* blood pressure, femoral and peripheral pulses, femoral bruits
- *Endocrine:* thyroid goiter, visual field cuts (assessing for pituitary tumor)
- *Breasts:* gynecomastia (Klinefelter syndrome, liver disease, antiandrogenic drugs)
- *Genitalia:* anatomic abnormalities, Peyronie disease (plaques along dorsolateral shaft causing penile curvature), testicular atrophy or asymmetry, prostate (nodules)

- *Neurologic:* genital/perineal sensation, cremasteric reflex (inner thigh touch elicits scrotal contraction, suggesting intact thoracolumbar erection center)

Laboratory Studies and Further Diagnostic Testing

- *Distinguish organic from psychogenic cause:* Extensive workup should only be undertaken if organic etiologies are strongly suspected; empiric treatment is often indicated regardless of exact etiology.
- *Nocturnal tumescence testing:* Formal study of nocturnal erectile ability is performed in a sleep laboratory to monitor REM, electroencephalogram, and erections; less expensive alternative is the RigiScan monitor, which monitors similar information at home. Absence of nocturnal erections implies organic etiology of ED.
- *Screening labs* if clinically warranted: fasting blood glucose level, fasting lipid levels, thyroid-stimulating hormone (TSH) level. Yield is low for serum total testosterone concentration, but occasionally indicated:
  ⇒ If low, measure *serum free testosterone, luteinizing hormone,* and *prolactin.*
  ⇒ If high, check *TSH* to rule out hyperthyroidism.
- Medical therapy attempted before further testing in most situations. Potentially useful tests in some situations (usually in consultation with a specialist):
  ⇒ *Duplex ultrasonography* is a minimally invasive method to study the arterial supply and venoocclusive mechanism; also assesses for plaques in Peyronie disease.
  ⇒ *Direct injection of VIP* helps to assess penile vascular function; may also be used as a therapeutic test in men who desire intracavernosal injections.
  ⇒ *Pelvic arteriography* or *cavernosography* is performed in young men with traumatic arterial insufficiency or congenital/traumatic venous leakage, respectively.

TREATMENT (TABLE 34.3)

General Principles

- Eliminate offending drugs when possible.
- Correct any reversible causes (endocrine abnormalities, tobacco, depression); testosterone patches should only be used in men with demonstrated hypogonadism.
- Psychosexual therapy is first-line therapy for men with psychogenic ED and a helpful adjunct in all cases.
- Referral to urology is indicated if patients choose vacuum constriction devices, intraurethral therapy, penile self-injections, or penile prostheses; or with evidence of Peyronie disease or other anatomic problem.

TABLE 34.3 TREATMENT OPTIONS FOR MEN WITH ERECTILE DYSFUNCTION

Treatment	Cost	Effect	Advantages	Disadvantages	Dose	Recommendation
Psychosexual therapy	$50–150 per session		Noninvasive; partner involved; curative;	Time consuming; patient resistance		First-line treatment; may be combined with other treatments
Oral sildenafil (Viagra)	$10 per dose	Blocks cyclic guanosine mono-phosphate breakdown, prolonging the vasodilatory effect of nitric oxide; requires sexual stimulation	Oral dosage; 50–85% efficacy (Morgantaler, 1999)	Contraindicated with active cardiac disease; 1 hr wait; HA, flushing, dyspepsia, visual changes	25–50 mg, max 100; 1 dose/day	First-line treatment; **contraindicated with nitrates–may cause hypotension/ death**

(continued)

TABLE 34.3 *(continued)*

Treatment	Cost	Effect	Advantages	Disadvantages	Dose	Recommendation
Intraurethral suppository: alprostadil (Muse)	$18–24 per treatment	Prostaglandin E$_1$ gel placed into penile meatus, induces vasodilation	Up to two treatments/d; less penile fibrosis and priapism than with penile injections	Not recommended with pregnant partner; mild penile curethral pain	250–1,000 µg, 5–10 min before sex, lasts 1 hr	Second-line treatment
Penile self-injections: alprostadil or drug mixtures	$5–25 per dose	Prostaglandin E$_1$ injected into base of penis; causes smooth muscle relaxation in cavernosum	Effective in 50–85%; few systemic side effects	Requires injection; high dropout rate; can cause penile pain, priapism, fibrosis; not for daily use	2.5–20 µg titrated for effect; 10–20 min before sex	Second-line treatment if patient prefers not to use intraurethral alprostadil
Yohimbine	$24 for 100 tablets	Blocks central α$_2$ receptors; improves libido	May have placebo effect	Anxiety, insomnia, tremor, nausea; may increase labile hypertension	5.4 mg p.o. t.i.d.	Second-line treatment; for men with psychogenic component; continue treatment if good response.
Vacuum constriction device (pump)	$150–450 per device.	Vacuum draws blood into penile cavernosa Elastic band holds blood in penis	Least expensive, easy to use; no systemic side effects	Unnatural erection; causes petechiae, numbness (20%), trapped ejaculation		Second-line treatment, but high satisfaction rate
Penile prosthesis (all types)	$8,000–15,000	Semirigid or inflatable	Highly effective	Unnatural erection (semirigid device); infection; requires replacement in 5–10 yrs; requires anesthesia and surgery		For men not satisfied with medical treatment
Vascular surgery	$10,000–15,000	Arterial bypass	Curative	Poor results in older men with generalized vascular disease; requires anesthesia and surgery		For young men with traumatic erectile dysfunction

Note: p.o., per os; t.i.d three times a day.
Source: Adapted from Lue T. Erectile dysfunction. *N Engl J Med* 2000; 342(24): 1802–1813, and Spark RF. Treatment of male sexual dysfunction. UpToDate, 2001, with permission.

Future Therapies

- New oral medications are currently undergoing phase 1 and 2 trials. These drugs are "on demand," rather than taken in advance like sildenafil.

SELECTED REFERENCES

1. Cheitlin MD, Hutter AM, Brindis RG, et al. Use of sildenafil (Viagra) in patients with cardiovascular disease. *Circulation* 1999;99:168–177.
2. Diokno AC, Brown MB. Sexual function in the elderly. *Arch Intern Med* 1990;150:197–200.
3. Ernst E, Pittler MH. Yohimbine for erectile dysfunction: a systematic review and meta-analysis of randomized clinical trials. *J Urol* 1998;159:433–436.
4. Goldstein I, Lue TF, Padma-Nathan H, et al. Oral sildenafil in the treatment of erectile dysfunction. *N Engl J Med* 1998;338:1397–1404.
5. Herrmann HC, Chang G, Klugherz BD, et al. Hemodynamic effects of sildenafil in men with severe coronary artery disease. *N Engl J Med* 2000;342:1622–1626.
6. Korenman SG. New insights into erectile dysfunction: a practical approach. *Am J Med* 1998;105:135–144.
7. Levy A, et al. Non-surgical management of erectile dysfunction. *Clin Endocrinol* 2000;52:253–260.
8. Linet OI, Ogring FG, for the Alprostadil Study Group. Efficacy and safety of intracavernosal prostaglandin in men with erectile dysfunction. *N Engl J Med* 1996;334:873–877.
9. Lue T. Erectile dysfunction. *N Engl J Med* 2000;342(24):1802–1813.

10. Melman A, Gingell JC. The epidemiology and pathophysiology of erectile dysfunction. *J Urol* 1999;161:5–11.
11. Michal V, Kramar R, Pospichal J. External iliac "steal syndrome." *J Cardiovasc Surg* 1978;19:55–57.
12. Morgentaler A. Male impotence. *Lancet* 1999;345:1713–1718.
13. Nehra A, et al. Pharmacotherapeutic advances in the treatment of erectile dysfunction. *Mayo Clin Proc* 1999;74:709–721.
14. Nehra A. Treatment of endocrinologic male sexual dysfunction. *Mayo Clin Proc* 2000; 75:40–45.
15. Padma-Nathan H, Hellstrom WJG, Kaiser FE, et al. Treatment of men with erectile dysfunction with transurethral alprostadil. *N Engl J Med* 1997;336:1–7.
16. Rendell MS, Rajfer J, Wicker PA, et al., for the Sildenafil Diabetes Study Group. Sildenafil for treatment of erectile dysfunction in men with diabetes. A randomized controlled trial. *JAMA* 1999;281:421–426.

ABNORMAL URINALYSIS: PROTEINURIA, HEMATURIA, LEUKOCYTURIA

PROTEINURIA

Introduction

- Proteinuria: daily urinary protein excretion >150 mg
- Nephrotic syndrome: urinary protein concentration >3.5 per day
- Proteinuria may be isolated or associated with renal disease or systemic illness.

Pathophysiology

- Four basic mechanisms:
  ⇒ Increased glomerular permeability (nephrotic syndrome)
  ⇒ Increased production of proteins small enough to pass freely through glomerulus (multiple myeloma)
  ⇒ Decreased tubular reabsorption of small amounts of filtered proteins (Fanconi's syndrome)
  ⇒ Increased secretion of tissue proteins associated with inflammatory conditions (pyelonephritis)

Differential Diagnosis

- **Nonnephrotic, normal urine sediment and glomerular filtration rate (GFR)**
  ⇒ *Transient proteinuria* generally occurs during a nonrenal illness and resolves with that illness (common etiologies: febrile illness, congestive heart failure [CHF], seizures, vigorous exercise, cold exposure).
  ⇒ *Orthostatic (postural) proteinuria:* asymptomatic, normal examination, normal GFR, normal urinalysis, proteinuria (usually <1.5 g per day) detected only when erect
  ⇒ *Isolated proteinuria:* same criteria as above without postural change in proteinuria
- **Nonnephrotic, abnormal urine sediment or GFR**
  ⇒ Generally secondary to a systemic illness (hypertension, diabetes mellitus, CHF, peripheral vascular disease) or early/mild glomerular disease or early/mild tubulointerstitial disease
- **Nephrotic-range proteinuria**
  ⇒ 75% associated with *systemic disease:* diabetes mellitus, amyloidosis, light-chain disease, membranous lupus nephropathy, human immunodeficiency virus (HIV) nephropathy, infective endocarditis, hepatitis B virus, malignancy
  ⇒ *Toxins:* heroin, angiotensin-converting (ACE) enzyme inhibitors, nonsteroidal antiinflammatory drugs (NSAIDs)
  ⇒ *Primary renal disease:* minimal-change disease, membranous glomerulonephritis, focal segmental glomerulosclerosis (FSGS), immunoglobulin A (IgA) nephropathy

- Nephritic syndrome
  ⇒ *Immune complex–mediated glomerulonephritis:* lupus, bacterial endocarditis, postinfectious glomerulonephritis, hepatitis B and C associated, cryoglobulinemia, IgA nephropathy, shunt nephritis
  ⇒ *Antineutrophil cytoplasmic antibodies (ANCA) associated:* Wegener glomerulonephritis, idiopathic rapidly progressive glomerulonephritis, polyarteritis nodosa
  ⇒ *Anti–glomerular basement membrane (anti-GBM) associated:* Goodpasture syndrome, anti-GBM disease
  ⇒ *Vascular thrombosis:* hemolytic–uremic syndrome/thrombotic thrombocytopenic purpura, preeclampsia
  ⇒ *Primary renal disease:* membranoproliferative glomerulonephritis, FSGS, IgA nephropathy

Evaluation

History

- Present condition: febrile illness, seizures, vigorous exercise, recent upper respiratory infection (URI), vasculitic rash, shortness of breath, cough, edema, nocturia, arthralgias
- Medication use: NSAIDs, ACE inhibitors, heroin
- Medical history: hypertension, diabetes, congestive heart failure, HIV, hepatitis B, malignancy
- Family history: renal disease or abnormal urinalysis

Laboratory and Diagnostic Testing

- Urine dipstick: Detects proteinuria in the range of 30 to 1,000 mg/dL; does not consistently detect microalbuminuria (range of 30 to 300 mg per 24 hour).
  ⇒ False-negative results: dilute urine or positively charged proteins (light chain).
  ⇒ False-positive result: concentrated urine, high pH level, 3+ hematuria (>50 to 100 red blood cells [RBCs] per high-power field [HPF]), radiocontrast, bacteruria
- Perform urinalysis to verify finding. If negative on subsequent measures, consider transient proteinuria.
- 24-hour collection of urine for protein, creatinine, and volume (the gold standard):
  ⇒ Men excrete 15 to 25 mg of creatinine per kilogram per day; women, 12 to 18 mg/kg per day; use to verify adequacy of collection.
- Spot tests (allow compensation for urinary dilution; units in milligrams per deciliter):
  ⇒ Spot urine protein/creatinine ratio: approximately equal to grams of protein excreted in 24 hours.
  ⇒ Spot urine protein/osmolality ratio: >2.5 corresponds to >3 g of protein excreted in 24 hours.
- Suspected orthostatic proteinuria: Split 24-hour urine into overnight and daytime samples; check dipstick on early morning sample (should be negative) and evening sample (should be positive).
- Evaluate renal function:
  ⇒ Cockroft-Gault formula estimates GFR: $(140 - \text{age}) \times \text{lean body weight} \div P_{Cr} \times 72$ ($\times 0.85$ for women)
  ⇒ 24-hour urine creatinine clearance gives exact GFR; inulin or iothalamate clearance are used occasionally.
- Check urine sediment:
  ⇒ *Dysmorphic RBCs* or *RBC casts* suggest glomerulonephritis.
  ⇒ *RBCs* suggest glomerular disease or urinary tract lesion.
  ⇒ *White blood cells (WBCs)* or *WBC casts* suggest tubulointerstitial disease or urinary tract infection (UTI).
  ⇒ *Oval fat bodies* or *fatty casts* suggest nephrotic syndrome.
  ⇒ *Maltese cross* (refractile lipid contained in macrophages) suggests nephrotic syndrome.
  ⇒ *Eosinophils* suggest allergic interstitial nephritis (AIN), pyelonephritis, renal transplant rejection, prostatitis, and cystitis.
- Look for evidence of other tubular dysfunction (RTA [Renal Tubular Acidosis], concentrating defect, renal wasting of sodium, potassium, magnesium, calcium, phosphaturia, uricosuria). Their presence may suggest Fanconi syndrome, analgesic nephropathy, pyelonephritis, or toxin-mediated nephropathy.
- Other labs: serum lipids, serum/urine electrophoresis, albumin (nephrotic syndrome); comple-

ment levels, antinuclear antibody, hepatitis B and C serologies, cryoglobulins, ANCA, anti-GBM antibody (nephritic syndrome)
- Renal biopsy for nephrotic-range proteinuria without obvious etiology

Treatment

- Primary goal of therapy is treatment of the underlying disorder. If no specific therapy exists, supportive care is important.
- General measures to decrease proteinuria and preserve renal function:
  ⇒ Dietary protein restriction (0.6 g/kg plus protein added to match urinary losses) may reduce proteinuria.
  ⇒ Control of hypertension (ACE inhibitors have a beneficial effect on proteinuria separate from their blood pressure–lowering effects, particularly in diabetic patients).

HEMATURIA

Introduction

- Gross hematuria is blood in the urine that is visible to the naked eye.
- Microscopic hematuria is >3 to 5 RBC/HPF (>1,000 RBC per minute).

Pathophysiology

- The pathogenesis of *glomerular hematuria* (glomerulonephritis) can be attributed to humoral and cell-mediated immune glomerular inflammation.
  ⇒ Antibodies can bind directly to components of the glomerulus (Goodpasture syndrome).
  ⇒ Antigen–antibody complexes can be deposited in the glomerulus (poststreptococcal gonococcus).
  ⇒ Hematuria resulting from glomerulonephritis typified by RBC casts and/or dysmorphic RBCs as red cells are damaged by passage through the inflamed glomerulus.
- *Extraglomerular hematuria* results from inflammation, infection, or irritation of any part of the genitourinary system outside the glomerulus: renal parenchyma, ureter, bladder, urethra. Use of certain medications, particularly anticoagulants, may also contribute.

Differential Diagnosis (Table 35.1)

- Gross hematuria: neoplasm 28% (bladder > prostate > kidney > ureter), infection 34% (bladder > prostate > kidney), unknown 34%
- Microscopic hematuria: neoplasm 10%, infection 12%, calculi 20%, unknown 44%

TABLE 35.1 DIFFERENTIAL DIAGNOSIS OF HEMATURIA

Glomerular	Familial	Extrarenal (most common)
Primary glomerulonephritis	Thin basement membrane disease	Tumors (pelvic, ureter, bladder, prostate)
Immunoglobulin A nephropathy	Hereditary nephritis (Alport disease)	Benign prostatic hypertrophy
Postinfectious glomerulonephritis	Fabry disease	Nephrolithiasis
Focal glomerulosclerosis	Nail-patella syndrome	Infectious (cystitis, prostatitis, *Schistosoma hematobium*, tuberculosis)
Rapidly progressive glomerulonephritis	**Nonglomerular**	Drugs (anticoagulants, cyclophosphamide)
Secondary glomerulonephritis	Renal tumors (Hypernephroma)	Systemic bleeding disorders
Systemic lupus nephritis	Vascular (malignant hypertension, etc)	Trauma
Vasculitis	Metabolic (hypercalcemia, hyperuricosemia)	
Essential mixed cryoglobulinemia	Familial (polycystic kidney disease, medullary sponge kidney)	
Hemolytic–uremic syndrome	Infection (pyelonephritis, tuberculosis)	
Thrombotic thrombocytopenic purpura		

Source: Adapted from Ahmed Z, Lee J. Asymptomatic urinary abnormalities: hematunia and proteinuria. *Med clin north am* 1997; 81: 6.41–6.52, with permission.

Evaluation

History

- Timing of hematuria: initiation of stream suggestive of urethral source; end of stream suggests neck or trigone of bladder or posterior urethra; throughout stream consistent with bladder, ureteral, renal, or diffuse bleeding. Hematuria after catheter introduction or manipulation of catheter suggests trauma.
- Renal colic: stone or papillary necrosis
- Presence of clots: If large, suggests bladder source; if long and stringy, suggests a ureteral source; essentially rules out a glomerular source of bleeding.
- Recent URI with gross hematuria: suggestive of IgA nephropathy or poststreptococcal glomerulonephritis
- Purpuric rash, neuropathy, abdominal pain, cough, history of hepatitis: consider vasculitis.
- Frequency and hesitancy in an older man: suspicious for prostate pathology
- Family history of hematuria: Consider polycystic kidney disease or hereditary nephritis.
- Medications: anticoagulants, NSAIDs, cyclophosphamide, salicylates, sulfonamides, methenamine

Laboratory Testing

- Urine dipstick and urinalysis (UA):
  - ⇒ Grossly red urine with negative dipstick: ingestion of certain foods (beets, rhubarb, dyes), drugs (phenazopyridine, phenindione, phenothiazine), and porphyrins
  - ⇒ Grossly red urine with a positive dipstick but no RBCs on UA: myoglobinuria
  - ⇒ Significant proteinuria: Consider nephritic and/or nephrotic etiologies
- Urine sediment:
  - ⇒ Dysmorphic RBCs or RBC casts pathognomonic for glomerular source; if present, may biopsy directly.
  - ⇒ Laboratory evaluation for glomerulonephritis, as indicated by history: erythrocyte sedimentation rate, complement levels, anti–GBM antibody, ANCA, ANA, antistreptolysin O titer, cryoglobulin assay, SPEP (serum protein electrophoresis), blood cultures, hepatitis B and C, HIV
- Urine culture
- Complete blood cell count, blood urea nitrogen/creatinine clearance, prothrombin time/partial thromboplastin time, 24-hour urine for protein and creatinine

Imaging and Further Workup

- Renal ultrasound: Evaluate for masses, cysts or obstruction in asymptomatic, non-glomerular hematuria (microscopic or gross): If normal, further workup varies with age:
  - ⇒ Younger than 40 years; malignancy rare
    1. 24-hour urine collection for hyperuricosuria and hypercalciuria; family history and UA of family members to rule out familial hematuria
    2. If normal: intravenous pyelogram (IVP) to rule out medullary sponge kidney and small tumor; consider urine cytology.
    3. If negative: consider biopsy versus observation.
  - ⇒ Older than 40 years: malignancy more common (transient hematuria 2% to 9% risk of urinary malignancy; persistent hematuria 5% to 20% incidence of malignancy)
    1. IVP to rule out tumor
    2. If negative: cystoscopy, urine cytology to evaluate bladder/prostate disease. Cytology 80% sensitive for tumors of the collecting system
    3. If negative: computed tomographic scan with contrast for further malignancy evaluation
    4. If negative: 24-hour urine collection for hypercalciuria, hyperuricosuria
    5. If negative: consider observation, renal biopsy, or renal angiogram.

Treatment

- *Glomerular hematuria (glomerulonephritis):* supportive management; immunosuppressive therapy depending on the underlying condition. A renal consultant should be involved.

- *Non-glomerular hematuria:* direct treatment at the specific cause (antibiotics for infections; lithotripsy for nephrolithiasis; surgical, immunotherapy, chemotherapy, or radiotherapy for tumors)

LEUKOCYTURIA

Introduction

- Urine contains >3 to 5 WBC/HPF.
- Usually seen in UTIs, but found in other conditions including tubulointerstitial disease

Differential Diagnosis

- UTI
- Prostatitis
- Infection with *Chlamydia trachomatis*
- Renal tuberculosis (TB)
- AIN: drug therapy (penicillins, NSAIDs, sulfonamides); infection; immunologic disease; idiopathic

Evaluation

History

- Symptoms of dysuria, urinary frequency, and urgency may point to UTI.
- Use of certain medications or prior history of rheumatologic disease: consider AIN.
- Risk factors for TB

Physical Findings

- CVA (cerebrovascular accident) tenderness, inflamed prostate, rash

Laboratory and Diagnostic Testing

- Urine dipstick:
  - ⇒ Threshold for detection 5 to 15 WBC/HPF.
  - ⇒ False-negative results: glycosuria, high specific gravity, excessive oxalate excretion
  - ⇒ False-positive results: presence of vaginal debris
- Urine sediment:
  - ⇒ *WBC casts:* classic for pyelonephritis (distinguishes upper tract infection); may also be found in tubulointerstitial diseases such as AIN.
  - ⇒ *Urine eosinophils:* suggestive of AIN
- Urine culture
- Other tests if indicated by history (acid-fast bacilli in urine, mycobacterial culture, and others)

Treatment

- UTI: antibiotics
- AIN: primarily supportive. Immunosuppressive agents may be tried, but their routine use is controversial.

SELECTED REFERENCES

1. Ahmed Z, Lee J. Asymptomatic urinary abnormalities: hematuria and proteinuria. *Med Clin North Am* 1997;81:641–652.
2. Greenberg A. Urinalysis. In: Greenberg A, et al., eds. *Primer on kidney disease,* 2nd ed. San Diego: Academic Press, 1998:27–35.
3. Grossfeld GD, Carroll PR. Evaluation of asymptomatic microscopic hematuria. *Urol Clin North Am* 1998;25:661–676.

4. Hricik DE, Chung-Park M, Sedor JR. Medical progress: glomerulonephritis. *N Engl J Med* 1998;339:888–899.
5. Lewis EJ, Hunsicker LG, Bait RP, et al. The effect of angiotensin converting enzyme inhibition on diabetic nephropathy. *N Engl J Med* 1993;329:1456.
6. Meyers CM. Acute interstitial nephritis. In: Greenberg A, et al., eds. *Primer on kidney disease,* 2nd ed. San Diego: Academic Press, 1998:277–282.
7. Nieuwhof C, Doorenbos C, Grave W, et al. A prospective study of the natural history of idiopathic non-proteinuric hematuria. *Kidney Int* 1996;49:222.
8. Orth SR, Ritz E. The nephrotic syndrome. *N Engl J Med* 1998;338:1202–1211.
9. Springberg PD, Garrett LE Jr, Thompson AL, et al. Fixed and reproducible orthostatic proteinuria: results of a 20-year follow-up study. *Ann Intern Med* 1982;97:516.
10. Sutton JM. Evaluation of hematuria in adults. *JAMA* 1990:2475–2480.
11. Wingo CS, Clapp WL. Proteinuria: potential causes and approach to evaluation. *Am J Med Sci* 2000;320:188–194.

CHRONIC RENAL FAILURE

INTRODUCTION

- End-stage renal disease (ESRD), meaning the need for renal replacement therapy: 280,000 patients on dialysis in the United States; 100,000 patients with functioning kidney transplants. Prevalence growing by about 8% per year; projections for 2010 suggest that the number of patients will double compared with 1997.
- Mortality is higher in patients with ESRD versus the general population; most common causes are cardiac (sudden death, myocardial infarction), infection, cerebrovascular, and malignancy.

PATHOPHYSIOLOGY/CLINICAL PRESENTATION

- Stages of chronic renal failure (CRF): loss of renal reserve, renal insufficiency, renal failure (inadequate compensatory mechanisms), uremia, ESRD requiring renal replacement therapy
- Progression to ESRD unpredictable
- Complications of CRF
  ⇒ *Fluid balance:* impaired urinary concentrating mechanism, increasing sensitivity to water deprivation or volume depletion; oliguric patients at risk of volume overload
  ⇒ *Metabolic acidosis:* inability to excrete acid as urinary ammonium (in early stages) and titratable acid (in later stages); loss of bicarbonate in the urine exacerbates the problem.
  ⇒ *Hyperkalemia:* renal potassium excretion conserved initially; volume depletion, oliguria, and certain drugs (angiotensin-converting enzyme [ACE] inhibitors, nonsteroidal antiinflammatory drugs [NSAIDs], and potassium-sparing diuretics) worsen hyperkalemia.
  ⇒ *Renal osteodystrophy:* decreased renal function → phosphate retention and hyperphosphatemia → hypocalcemia → secondary hyperparathyroidism and bone disease. Decreased renal hydroxylation of 25-(OH) vitamin D lowers 1,25-$(OH)_2$ vitamin D (calcitriol), which normally enhances intestinal calcium absorption and bone mobilization of calcium.
    1. *Osteitis fibrosa:* Accelerated rates of bone turnover due to high levels of parathyroid hormone (PTH).
    2. *Osteomalacia and adynamic lesions:* low bone turnover states due to aluminum toxicity or relatively low levels of PTH
  ⇒ *Anemia:* usually multifactorial, normocytic, and normochromic; diminished erythropoietin production by atrophic kidneys; chronic iron deficiency; mucosal blood losses due to dysfunctional platelets; blood losses associated with dialysis
  ⇒ *Hyperuricemia:* occurs as urate excretion falls; predisposes to gout
  ⇒ *Peripheral neuropathy:* occurs at a glomerular filtration rate (GFR) <10% normal; often irreversible; patients experience crawling or pricking sensation in their lower extremities.
  ⇒ *Adverse drug effects:* due to failure to adjust dosing in renally cleared medications as the GFR falls
  ⇒ *Cardiovascular disease:* major cause of death in ESRD, due to dyslipidemia, co-morbidities including diabetes mellitus and hypertension, and in some patients, accelerated atherosclerosis

⇒ *Uremic syndrome:* may include fatigue, anorexia, weight loss, pruritus, muscle cramps, pericarditis, thirst, sleep disorders (day/night sleep reversal, sleep apnea), sensory and memory deficits, stupor, coma, and even death

DIFFERENTIAL DIAGNOSIS

● May present as a primary renal entity (nephrotic syndrome, renal artery stenosis), or as a component of other diseases (diabetes, hypertension, systemic lupus, urinary obstruction) (see Table 36.1).

TABLE 36.1. CAUSES OF END-STAGE RENAL DISEASE IN HEMODIALYSIS (HD) PATIENTS

Diabetic nephropathy	39.5%
Primary hypertensive disease	25.2%
Glomerulonephritis	9.1%
Missing	8.9%
Interstitial nephritis/pyelonephritis	3.8%
Etiology uncertain	3.6%
Miscellaneous	3.2%
Cystic/hereditary/congenital	2.8%
Secondary glomerulonephritis/vasculities	2.2%
Neoplasms/tumors	1.7%

Source: From Renal Data System. *USRDS 2000 annual data report.* Bethoda, MD: National Institutes of Health, National Institute of Diabetes and Digestive and Kidney Diseases; 2000, with permission

EVALUATION

History

● Medical history: diabetes mellitus, hypertension, collagen vascular diseases, human immunodeficiency virus (HIV) risk factors
● Urinary tract symptoms: dysuria, hematuria, colic, hesitancy, incontinence
● Medication use: NSAIDs, ACE inhibitors, diuretics, other renal toxins including heroin
● Systemic symptoms: hemoptysis, Raynaud symptoms, claudication
● Uremic symptoms: pruritus, fatigue, anorexia, restless legs, nausea
● Family history: renal failure including polycystic kidney disease, Alport syndrome, medullary sponge kidneys

Physical Examination

● Weight and blood pressure
● Enlarged kidneys to palpation (polycystic kidney disease or hydronephrosis)
● Signs of associated systemic disease: retinopathy (hypertensive or diabetic), keratopathy (hypercalcemia), hyporeflexia (hypercalcemia), peripheral neuropathy, vascular bruits, vasculitic skin rashes, gouty tophi
● Signs of volume overload: lower extremity edema, crackles and rales, elevated jugular venous pressure
● Signs of uremia: pericardial rub, abnormalities in mental status, excoriations from scratching

Diagnostic Laboratory Workup (As Indicated by History) for Newly Developed or Discovered Renal Failure

● Serum complement levels (C3 and C4), antinuclear antibody
● Antibodies for antistreptolysin O/B-antideoxyribonuclease
● Hepatitis B (membranous glomerulopathy), hepatitis C (cryoglobulinemia, send serum cryoglobulins if positive), HIV test

- Antineutrophil cytoplasmic antibody and anti–glomerular basement membrane
- Serum electrophoresis and Bence Jones proteinuria
- Peripheral blood for schistocytes
- Urine sediment for white blood cell or red blood cell casts, dysmorphic red cells

Laboratory Workup for Assessment of Renal Function and Progression of Renal Insufficiency

- Electrolytes, blood urea nitrogen, creatinine, glucose; hematocrit and mean corpuscular volume; calcium, magnesium, phosphate; albumin; uric acid; PTH
- 24-hour urine for protein and creatinine to calculate GFR
- Iron studies, consider erythropoietin level

Imaging and Pathology

- Renal ultrasound: to assess kidney size; rule out obstruction or polycystic kidneys
- Renal biopsy: for specific diagnosis in most patients with glomerulonephritis

TREATMENT

- Goals of therapy: Slow progression to ESRD; treat complications of renal insufficiency; prepare for eventual renal replacement therapy.

Slowing Disease Progression

- Aggressive *blood pressure control* with any effective antihypertensive limits further renal damage. May be additional benefit to ACE inhibitors, particularly in diabetics and those with marked proteinuria (Maschio et al., 1996). Discontinue if creatinine clearance increases >1 mg/dL, GFR falls, or hyperkalemia develops (check creatinine clearance and potassium concentration within several days). Contraindicated with known bilateral renal artery stenosis.
- *Tight glycemic control* in diabetic patients is crucial in limiting worsening renal function.
- *Protein restriction* is controversial: Slows progression of renal disease in some studies (Ikrizler et al., 1996), but protein malnutrition correlated with poor outcome in other studies (Klahr et al., 1994). Low-protein diets (0.5 to 0.75 g/kg per day) may benefit otherwise well-nourished patients with GFR 25 to 60 mL per minute. Not recommended with very high levels of proteinuria (15 g per day), superimposed catabolic illness, or steroid use.

Managing Complications of Renal Insufficiency

- Volume overload: fluid restriction for severe hypertension, congestive heart failure (CHF), or oliguria; sodium restriction to 2 g daily for patients with hypertension or mild CHF; severe CHF or oliguria mandates more intense restriction.
- Hyperkalemia: Monitor frequently; treat above 5.5 mEq/L (admit for intravenous treatment if electrocardiogram changes) with exchange resins such as sodium polystyrene sulfonate (Kayexalate); avoid constipation, given the gastrointestinal (GI) tract's role in potassium elimination.
- Hyperphosphatemia
  ⇒ GFR <30 mL per minute: calcium citrate (PhosLo) (667 mg three times a day) or calcium carbonate (1,250 mg twice a day [b.i.d.]) with meals
  ⇒ If calcium–phosphorus product is >75, initial lowering with aluminum-containing phosphorus binders prevents soft tissue calcifications.
- Hypocalcemia
  ⇒ *Calcium supplements* between meals (calcium carbonate [600 mg b.i.d.]) for symptomatic or severe hypocalcemia despite normalization of serum phosphate
  ⇒ Add *vitamin D* (calcitriol [0.025 mg every day]) for high PTH levels (>200 to 400 pg/mL), if calcium phosphorus product is <75 mg^2/dL^2 (may require an increase in the dose of phosphorus binders, because calcitriol increases GI absorption of phosphorus).

- Acidosis
  - ⇒ If serum bicarbonate concentration is <15 mEq/L, treat with *sodium bicarbonate,* 600 mg b.i.d., initially and titrate bicarbonate to >20 mEq/L.
  - ⇒ Monitor serum potassium and calcium concentrations during treatment of acidosis, because both may fall.
- Anemia
  - ⇒ Initially, *oral ferrous sulfate* for iron deficiency to maintain hematocrit goal 30 to 36
  - ⇒ With progressive renal failure, addition of *erythropoietin* (2,000 to 5,000 units subcutaneously three times a week) may be necessary. Monitor serum ferritin and percent transferrin saturation (serum ferritin/total iron-binding capacity × 100) for adequate iron stores: Transferrin saturation >30% predicts sufficient iron stores for erythropoiesis. Most frequent adverse effect of erythropoietin is worsening hypertension.
  - ⇒ Transfuse for high-output failure or angina; leukopore filter in potential transplant recipients.
- Impaired platelet function: bleeding diathesis possible in patients with uremic coagulopathy despite normal prothrombin time/partial thromboplastin time; DDAVP and cryoprecipitate can be used for acute bleeding.
- Cardiovascular complications (see Chapters 5 and 6)
  - ⇒ CHF: *furosemide* if CHF persists after dietary modifications; add *metolazone* for refractory fluid overload; *ACE inhibitors* unless contraindicated; digoxin potentially helpful but watch for toxicity.
  - ⇒ Accelerated atherosclerosis (U.S. Renal Data Systems, 2000): low threshold for *antilipid agents;* aggressive *risk factor modification* (smoking cessation, low-fat diet, exercise)
- Uremic complications
  - ⇒ Nausea: *oral antiemetics* such as Compazine or Phenergan.
  - ⇒ Pruritus: *topical agents* such as menthol, phenol lotion, or a trial of capsaicin cream; cholestyramine and ultraviolet light have also been successful.

Renal Replacement Therapy: Dialysis and Transplantation

- As creatinine clearance drops to 10 mg/dL despite maximal medical management, mean survival drops to 100 to 150 days. Early referral to a nephrologist who treats ESRD allows patients and their families to learn about their options, make educated choices, and prepare for eventual dialysis or transplantation.
- *Indications* for dialysis or transplantation in CRF:
  - ⇒ Uremic symptoms (including encephalopathy, coagulopathy)
  - ⇒ Hyperkalemia resistant to medical management
  - ⇒ Acidosis resistant to medical management
  - ⇒ Fluid overload with cardiopulmonary symptoms (including refractory hypertension)
  - ⇒ Peripheral neuropathy with severe symptoms
  - ⇒ Pericarditis
- *Hemodialysis:* filtration of the blood through a semipermeable membrane to remove fluid and balance electrolytes; three times a week in 4- to 5-hour sessions; requires vascular access. Placement of an atrioventricular fistula (at creatinine clearance around 4 to 5) 3 to 6 months before expected use permits maturation of the fistula and any necessary revisions.
- *Peritoneal dialysis:* dialysate fluid instilled directly into the peritoneum, which acts as a biological filter; allows home exchange of fluid in ambulatory patients; risk of spontaneous bacterial peritonitis.
- *Transplant:* cadaveric, living related, and living unrelated donors all increasingly used; rates of graft loss in both cadaveric and living donor transplants decreased by half in the last decade (11% for cadaveric and 5.5% in living donor recipients in the first year); patients with living donors may proceed directly to transplantation without preceding dialysis (Hariharan et al., 2000).

SELECTED REFERENCES

1. Cockcroft DW, Gault MH. Prediction of creatinine clearance from serum creatinine. *Nephron* 1976;16:13.
2. Goodman WG, Godlin J, Kuizon BD, et al. Coronary artery calcification in young adults with end stage renal disease who are undergoing dialysis. *N Engl J Med* 2000;342:1478–1482.

3. Greenberg A, Cheung AK, Coffmann TM, et al., eds. *Primer on kidney diseases,* 2nd ed. San Diego: Academic Press, 1998:431–454.
4. Hariharan S, Johnson CP, Bresnahan BA, et al. Improved graft survival after renal transplantation in the United States, 1988 to 1996. *N Engl J Med* 2000;342:602–612.
5. Ikrizler TA, et al. Nutrition in end-stage kidney disease. *Kidney Int* 1996;50:343–357.
6. Klahr S, Levey AS, Beck GJ, et al. The effects of dietary protein restriction and blood-pressure control on the progression of chronic renal disease. *N Engl J Med* 1994;330:877–884.
7. Lazarus JM, Bourgoignie JJ, Buckalew VM, et al. Achievement and safety of a low blood pressure goal in chronic renal disease. The Modification of Diet in Renal Disease Study Group. *Hypertension* 1997;29:641.
8. Maschio G, et al. Effect of ACE inhibitor benazepril on progression of chronic renal insufficiency. *N Engl J Med* 1996;334:939–945.
9. Peterson JC, Adler S, Burkart JM, et al. Blood pressure control, proteinuria, and the progression of renal disease. The Modification of Diet in Renal Disease Study. *Ann Intern Med* 1995;123:754.
10. Renal Data Systems. *USRDS 2000 annual data report.* Bethesda, MD: The National Institutes of Health, National Institutes of Diabetes and Digestive and Kidney Diseases, 2000.
11. Slatopolsky EA, Burke SK, Dillon MA, and the Renagel study group. Renagel, a nonabsorbed calcium- and aluminum-free phosphate binder, lowers serum phosphorus and parathyroid hormone. *Kidney Int* 1999;55:299.
12. Slatopolsky E, et al. Pathogenesis of secondary hyperparathyroidism. *Am J Kidney Dis* 1994;23:229–236.
13. Suthhanthiram M, et al. Renal transplantation. *N Engl J Med* 1994;331:365–376.
14. Tonelli M, Bohm C, Pandeya S, et al. Cardiac risk factors and the use of cardioprotective medications in patients with chronic renal insufficiency. *Am J Kidney Dis* 2001;37:484.
15. Walker R. General management of end-stage renal disease. *Lancet* 1997;315:1429–1432.

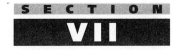

GASTROINTESTINAL

GASTROINTESTINAL COMPLAINTS: DYSPEPSIA, GERD, PEPTIC ULCER DISEASE

DYSPEPSIA

Introduction

- 20% to 40 % of people in United States experience recurrent pain in upper abdomen each year.

Differential Diagnosis

- Up to 60% of those who seek care have no definite diagnosis; classified as having functional or nonulcer dyspepsia (NUD).
- 30% diagnosed with peptic ulcer disease (PUD); remaining diagnosed with gastroesophageal reflux disease (GERD), biliary disease, irritable bowel syndrome, and other disorders

Evaluation

- Symptoms dominated by "heartburn" (retrosternal burning, particularly after meals and with recumbency) are likely to be **GERD**.
- Symptoms such as epigastric pain, early satiety, and bloating are likely to be **PUD**; cancer almost never seen in patients older than 45 years. Diagnose with endoscopy.
- Diagnosis is **NUD** if no abnormality is seen on endoscopy.
- **Chronic dyspepsia** is characterized by pain or discomfort in the upper abdomen for at least 3 months in previous year without metabolic or structural disease.

Treatment

- Management recommendations are geared toward minimizing risk of missed gastric cancer.
- "Alarm symptoms" (weight loss, bleeding, anemia, dysphagia, early satiety, strong family history of gastric cancer) warrant endoscopy, as do older patients with new-onset dyspepsia. Gastric cancer is seen in 1% to 2% of patients referred for endoscopy, primarily patients older than 45 years.
- If early endoscopy is not indicated, noninvasive *Helicobacter pylori* test by serology or urea breath testing may guide management. If *H. pylori* test result is negative, empiric trial of antisecretory agent is indicated.
- If symptoms persist after 8 weeks of therapy, endoscopy is recommended.
- Differentiate dyspeptic symptoms from biliary colic. Confusing diagnosis may lead to unnecessary cholecystectomy that does not relieve symptoms.

GASTROESOPHAGEAL REFLUX DISEASE

Introduction

- 44% of general population has heartburn at least once a month, 14% weekly, and 7% daily.
- More than one half of patients with pathologic GERD will not have visible esophagitis at esophagogastroduodenoscopy (EGD).

Pathophysiology/Clinical Presentation

- Classic presentations: pyrosis (heartburn), acid regurgitation, relief with antacids, chest pain (possibly from esophageal spasm), asymptomatic (33% of patients with Barrett esophagus have no symptoms)
- Esophageal damage proportional to amount and duration of acid–pepsin–bile exposure. Five mechanisms implicated in GERD development:
    ⇒ Lower esophageal sphincter (LES) abnormalities: Transient LES relaxations account for 60% to 83% of reflux episodes; hypotensive LES (mechanism by which most drugs and foods cause GERD); hiatal hernia.
    ⇒ Delayed esophageal acid clearance: esophageal motility aperistalsis (seen in patients with scleroderma); diminished saliva as in patients with Sjögren disease
    ⇒ Impaired epithelial resistance to acid
    ⇒ Gastric acid hypersecretion (Zollinger-Ellison syndrome)
    ⇒ Bile acid refluxate
- Complications
    ⇒ *Esophagitis:* most common
    ⇒ *Stricture:* 10% of patients with severe esophagitis
    ⇒ *Barrett esophagus:* replacement of esophageal squamous epithelium with metaplastic columnar epithelium; 10% of patients with GERD; 10% risk for development of adenocarcinoma
    ⇒ *Asthma*
    ⇒ *Ears, nose, throat:* laryngitis, tracheal stenosis, and possibly laryngeal cancer
- Little correlation between severity of symptoms and presence of mucosal disease (esophagitis)

Differential Diagnosis

- Given appropriate clinical scenario, consider infectious esophagitis (herpes simplex virus, cytomegalovirus, candida, human immunodeficiency virus), pill esophagitis (quinidine, potassium chloride, tetracyclines, alendronate), lye injury, alkaline reflux (postgastrectomy), and radiation injury.

Evaluation

- Most cases diagnosed clinically
- Patients who present atypically, fail to respond to conventional therapy, have GERD complications, or are considering antireflux surgery should undergo further evaluation.
- Five diagnostic approaches:
    ⇒ *Empiric aggressive acid suppression:* trial of omeprazole (40 mg orally [p.o.] every morning and 20 mg p.o. every night for 7 days; 75% decrease in symptoms is considered "positive" for GERD; 83% sensitive.
    ⇒ *Bernstein test:* Infusion of normal saline followed by 0.1 normal hydrochloric acid to evoke pain has a sensitivity of 50% and specificity of 55% for GERD; useful to evaluate noncardiac chest pain.
    ⇒ *Barium swallow:* sensitivity 25% to 62%; useful in patients with dysphagia to evaluate for strictures
    ⇒ *24-hour pH monitoring:* "gold standard" with sensitivity 80%, specificity 90%
    ⇒ *EGD:* sensitivity 62%, specificity 95%; one third of patients with GERD have recognizable mucosal changes; Barrett esophagus and strictures can be detected and strictures treated by EGD.

Treatment

- **Lifestyle change:** Elevate head of bed 2 to 6 inches or place wedge under pillow; avoid smoking, caffeine, NSAIDs, citrus juices, large meals, postprandial recumbency; encourage weight loss.
- **Pharmacologic therapy:**
    ⇒ *Antacids:* better than placebo; do not decrease complications; use in mild cases or for "breakthrough" symptoms when proton pump inhibitors (PPIs) or H_2-receptor antagonists (H2RAs) are used.

⇒ *H2RAs:* 60% clinical response, 50% esophagitis healing response overall; higher than standard doses often required to achieve efficacy

⇒ *PPIs:* most effective therapy; reduce acid production by 95% (vs. 65% for H2RAs); 80% healing and symptom response for esophagitis at 8 weeks (vs. 40% for H2RAs); first-line therapy for moderate to severe disease.

- **Antireflux surgery (fundoplication):**
  ⇒ Indications for surgery: young, healthy patients seeking to be free of chronic drug therapy; anatomically or mechanically defective LES; failure to heal with prolonged PPI therapy; esophageal bleeding or perforation; refractory extraesophageal complications
  ⇒ Contraindications: serious co-morbidities; esophageal dysmotility by manometry; lack of 24-hour pH test to prove GERD as etiology
  ⇒ Requires prior evaluation with 24-hour ambulatory pH monitoring, esophageal manometry, endoscopy, and gastric emptying scan
  ⇒ Not yet studied against aggressive acid suppression therapy with PPI
  ⇒ Main complication is dysphagia.
- **Refractory GERD:**
  ⇒ Step 1: PPI before meal
  ⇒ Step 2: PPI b.i.d. before meals
  ⇒ Step 3: Endoscopy; if manifestations of GERD → PPI b.i.d. before meals plus H2RA at bedtime (h.s.); if no manifestations of GERD → 24-hour pH monitoring. Two-drug regimen more effective than adding a third dose of PPI.
  ⇒ Step 4: PPI b.i.d. and H2RA h.s. inadequate; add prokinetic agent (metoclopramide) before meals and h.s.

Future Directions

- New endoscopic techniques to tighten the LES (simulation of fundoplication) by using radiofrequency probe to induce LES fibrosis; endoscopic placement of intraesophageal purse string sutures; endoscopic injection of collagen microspheres in the LES

PEPTIC ULCER DISEASE

Introduction

- Lifetime prevalence is 11% to 14% in men, 8% to 11% in women; overall prevalence of symptomatic PUD 1.8%.
- Incidence increases with age.

Pathophysiology

NSAID-related PUD

- After *H. pylori*, NSAIDs are most common cause of PUD (see Table 37.1).
- NSAIDs cause gastropathy (erosions, subepithelial hemorrhages) rather than gastritis (inflammatory response, like *H. pylori*).
- Mechanisms include reduction of prostaglandins and local, topical injury to epithelium.

H. pylori

- Spiral-shaped gram-negative bacteria that live in mucus overlying gastric and duodenal epithelial cells
- Associated with greatly increased risk of duodenal and gastric ulceration
- Infection rate correlates with age, socioeconomic status, and number of children living at home
- Level of antibody to *H. pylori* correlates with risk of duodenal or gastric ulcer; ulcers develop in 15% to 20%.
- Associated with gastric adenocarcinoma and low-grade mucosa-associated lymphoid tissue lymphoma

TABLE 37.1. DIFFERENTIAL DIAGNOSIS (OTHER THAN *HELICOBACTER PYLORI*, NONSTEROIDAL, ANTIINFLAMMATORY DRUGS)

5-Fluorouracil intrahepatic artery infusion	Zollinger-Ellison syndrome (suspect if multiple ulcers, early age, family history, diarrhea, hypercalcemia)	Stress ulcers
Cocaine via ischemic injury		Systemic mastocytosis
Crohn disease		Viral ulcers
Gastric malignancy (including lymphoma, adenocarcinoma)		(Cytomegalovirus, herpes simplex virus type 1)

Evaluation

Diagnostic Tests for H. pylori

- CLO (campylobacter-like organism) test: sensitivity and specificity 90% to 98%
- Urease breath test: sensitivity 90% to 95%, specificity 98% to 99%
- Serology (immunoglobulin G): sensitivity 95%, but does not distinguish current from past infection
- Histology: sensitivity and specificity 95% to 99%
- Endoscopic culture: 80% sensitivity, 100% specificity

Treatment

NSAID-related PUD

- Attempt to discontinue NSAIDs.
- Search for *H. pylori* and treat if positive.
- If continued use of NSAIDs, add PPI (more effective than H2RAs) or Misoprostol (though poorly tolerated due to diarrhea).
- COX-2 inhibitors less likely than nonselective NSAIDs to cause GI bleeding, but reports of significant GI bleeding even with use of these agents.

H. pylori

- 70% to 80% one-year relapse rate for DU (duodenal ulcer) after treatment with H2RAs only, rate decreases to <10% with eradication treatment (see Table 37.2).
- Confirmation of eradication is usually not necessary; only possible with urea breath test or biopsy.

TABLE 37.2. TREATMENT OF *HELICOBACTER PYLORI* INFECTION

Regimen	Dosing			Eradication	Cost
"OAC"[a]					
• **A**moxicillin	1,000 mg	b.i.d.	7	85–95%	$163
"OMC"					
• **M**etronidazole	As above	As above	7	85–95%	$161
"BMT"	*Dose*	*Interval*	*Days*		
• **B**ismuth	2 tabs	q.i.d.(meals + h.s.)	7	80–96%	$67
• **M**etronidazole	250 mg	b.i.d/q.i.d.(meals)	7		
• **T**etracycline	500 mg	q.i.d.(meals + h.s.)	7		
"BMT-O"					
• **O**meprazole	20 mg	b.i.d (meals)	7	Up to 98%	$75

Note: b.i.d, twice daily; q.i.d., four times a day;
[a] Preferred regimen in most cases on the basis of compliance and cost. Costs listed are Wholesale to pharmacy.
Sources: From The Sanford Guide (from JAMA 1996:275:622) and The Medical Letter 39(I).

SELECTED REFERENCES

1. Blum AL, Talley NJ, O'Morain C, et al. Lack of effect of treating *Helicobacter pylori* infection in patients with nonulcer dyspepsia. Omeprazole plus clarithromycin and amoxicillin effect one tear after treatment (OCAY) Study Group. *N Engl J Med* 1998;339:1875–1781.
2. The European *Helicobacter pylori* Study group. Current European concepts in the management of *Helicobacter pylori* infection. The Maastricht consensus report. *Gut* 1997;41:8–13.
3. Friedman LS. *Helicobacter pylori* and nonulcer dyspepsia. *N Engl J Med* 1998;339:1928–1930.
4. Graham DY, Lew GM, Klein PD, et al. *Ann Intern Med* 1992;116:705–708.
5. Lagergren J, Bergstrom R, Lindgren A, et al. Symptomatic gastroesophageal reflux as a risk factor for esophageal adenocarcinoma. *N Engl J Med* 1999;340:825–831.
6. Laine L, Harper S, Simon T, et al. A randomized trial comparing the effect of rofecoxib with that of ibuprofen on the gastroduodenal mucosa of patients with OA. *Gastroenterology* 1999;117:776–783.
7. McColl K, Murray L, El-Omar E, et al. Symptomatic benefit from eradicating *Helicobacter pylori* infection in patients with nonulcer dyspepsia. *N Engl J Med* 1998;339:1869–1874.
8. Parsonnett J, Friedman G, Vandersteen D, et al. *Helicobacter pylori* infection and the risk of gastric carcinoma. *N Engl J Med* 1991;325:1127–1131.
9. Parsonnett J, Hansen S, Rodriguez L, et al. *Helicobacter* infection and gastric lymphoma. *N Engl J Med* 1994;330:1267–1271.
10. Talley NJ, Vakil N, Ballard ED, et al. Absence of benefit of eradication Helicobacter pylori in patients with nonulcer dyspepsia. *N Engl J Med* 1999;341:1106–1111.
11. Vigneri S, Termini R, Leandro G, et al. *N Engl J Med* 1995;333:1106–1110.

EVALUATION OF ABNORMAL LIVER FUNCTION TESTS

INTRODUCTION

- When faced with abnormal liver function test results, first step is repetition and confirmation of results.
- History should focus on recent exposures, alcohol intake, medications (including herbs), family history, drug abuse history (intranasal and intravenous), history of blood transfusions.
- Physical examination may suggest chronicity of liver disease but usually does not reveal a specific etiology.
- Most patients in whom no etiology is clear after initial testing have alcoholic liver disease, steatosis (fatty liver), or steatohepatitis.

CLASSIFICATION

- **Enzyme tests** measure release of liver enzymes into bloodstream in response to hepatocyte inflammation, necrosis, and biliary obstruction.
    - ⇒ Hepatocellular damage: Serum aminotransferases (aspartate aminotransferase [AST] [serum glutamic-oxaloacetic transaminase], alanine aminotransferase [ALT] [serum glutamic-pyruvic transaminase])
    - ⇒ Cholestasis: Alkaline phosphatase (AP), 5′-nucleotidase, γ-glutamyl transpeptidase
- **Synthetic function** is measured by evaluating the liver's capacity to make serum proteins.
    - ⇒ Prothrombin time (not specific for hepatocellular injury; can be elevated with vitamin K deficiency)
    - ⇒ Albumin (low level suggests chronic process given its half-life of 21 days).
- **Serum bilirubin** is elevated in severe hepatocellular injury, obstruction, and nonhepatic conditions.

ELEVATED AMINOTRANSFERASE

- Aminotransferases normally circulate in the serum at low levels (<40 IU/L).
- Elevations of AST and/or ALT up to 250 IU/L are considered mild; elevation for >6 months is chronic.
- Both AST and ALT are elevated to some degree in most liver diseases. AST is found in many tissues (heart, skeletal muscle, kidney, brain, pancreas); ALT is more specific for liver.
- Absolute levels do not correlate well with severity of liver injury or prognosis; however, they may be useful to follow disease activity over time.
- See Tables 38.1 through 38.3 for differential and evaluation.

TABLE 38.1. MEDICATIONS AND HERBS

Amiodarone	
Antibiotics	Synthetic penicillins, ciprofloxacin, nitrofurantoin, ketoconazole, fluconazole, isoniazid
Antiepileptics	Phenytoin, valproate, carbamazepine
Herbal medications	Jin Bu Huan, mahuang, germander, valerian, mistletoe, skullcap, chaparral leaf, comfrey, atractylate, herbal teas with toxic alkaloids, pennyroyal oil
β-hydroxy-β-methylglutaryl-coenzyme A reductase inhibitors	
Hypoglycemics	Glipizide, "glitazone" class
Methyldopa	
Nonsteroidal antiinflammatory drugs	
Substances of abuse	Cocaine, anabolic steroids, MDMA ("ecstasy"), glues, solvents, phencyclidine ("angel dust")

TABLE 38.2. NONDRUG CAUSES OF ELEVATED AMINOTRANSFERASES

Alcoholic liver disease (ALD)	AST:ALT ratio of at least 2, with AST rarely >300 IU/L, ALT often normal.
	If GGTP 2x normal in patient with AST:ALT >2, sensitive and specific for ALD (too nonspecific as an independent marker).
Chronic hepatitis (hepatitis B, hepatitis C)	Hepatitis C most common cause of chronic liver disease and indication for liver transplant in United States; 400 million carriers of hepatitis B virus worldwide.
Nonalcoholic fatty liver diseases (NAFLD)	Usually asymptomatic and underdiagnosed; likely underlying condition in those who are diagnosed with "cryptogenic cirrhosis."
	AST: ALT usually <4x normal. Ratio of AST: ALT <1. Alkaline phosphatase may or may not be elevated (2x normal).
	Evaluate with right upper quadrant ultrasound.
	Liver biopsy for small subset (10%) patients who may go on to develop cirrhosis; those with diabetes mellitus and/or obesity if age >45 (Angulo et al., 1999), peripheral stigmata of chronic liver disease, abnormal iron studies, cytopenia, or splenomegaly.
	Therapy: modify risk factors.
Hereditary hemochromatosis	Initial tests serum iron and TIBC. If Fe/TIBC >45%, check serum ferritin. Ferritin >400 ng/mL in men and >300 ng/mL in women suggestive.
	Autosomal-recessive disorder of iron storage (overabsorption by intestines leads to iron deposition in various organs).
	If phenotypic screen positive, test for HFE gene.
	Perform liver biopsy if elevated LFTs, ferritin >1,000 ng/mL, or hepatomegaly.
	Therapy involves phlebotomy.
Autoimmune hepatitis (AIH)	Diagnosis based on elevation of aminotransferases, negative viral serologies, serologic and pathologic features consistent with AIH.
	Screening test is SPEP; >80% patients have hypergammaglobulinemia (two-fold polyclonal elevation specific for AIH). IgG elevation most common.
	If SPEP reveals polyclonal hypergammaglobulinemia, obtain ANA (28% sensitive), anti–smooth muscle antibody (40% sensitive), and possibly liver-kidney microsomal antibody (Pratt et al., 2000).
	Liver biopsy essential to confirm diagnosis, assess degree of fibrosis
	Therapy is trial of corticosteroids +/− azathioprine; usually steroid responsive.
Wilson disease	Autosomal-recessive disorder in cellular copper transport, results in copper deposition in liver (leading to cirrhosis), central nervous system, eyes (Kayser-Fleicher rings), and kidneys.
	Majority of patients age <40.
	Screening test is serum ceruloplasmin level (low <200 mg/L).
	More specific tests: 24-hr urine for copper (>100 μg/d), liver biopsy (>250 μg copper/g liver).
	Therapy: copper removal via chelation with penicillamine, trientine, or oral zinc.

(continued)

TABLE 38.2. *(continued)*

Celiac disease	Inflammatory enteropathy resulting from immune response to dietary gluten found in wheat, barley, and rye. Malabsorptive diarrhea and weight loss that improve with withdrawal of gluten from diet. Subclinical disease: mild fatigue, elevated aminotransferases (29–80 IU/L, ALT 60–130 IU/L [Bardella et al., 1999]) borderline iron deficiency, arthritis, osteopenia, vague abdominal pain (like IBS). Screen: serum antiendomysial IgA (97–100% sensitivity and nearly 100% specificity); virtually diagnostic. Antigliadin IgA, IgG, and antitissue transglutaminase IgA are other tests. Confirmed by biopsy of small intestine that reveals villous atrophy. Gluten-free diet results in resolution of mucosal changes, malabsorption, and LFTs.
α-antitrypsin deficiency	Autosomal-recessive disorder with low levels of α-antetrypsin, inhibitor of neutrophil elastase in lung. Most patients homozygous for ZZ alleles (PiZZ phenotype). Underrecognized, with one study finding a prevalence of 2–3% among 965 patients with COPD (Lieberman et al., 1986). Neonatal hepatitis, cirrhosis in children and adults, and hepatoma. Diagnosis made by low serum AAT levels (<80 mg/dL) and phenotype. Therapy options are intravenous AAT infusions, lung and liver transplant, gene therapy.

Note: AST:ALT ratio, the ratio of serum alanine aminotransferase to serum aspartate aminotransferase; GGTP, γ-glutamyl transpeptidase; TIBC, total iron-binding capacity; LFT, liver function test; SPEP, serum protein electrophoresis; IgG, immunogloubin G; ANA, antinuclear antibody; IBS, irritable bowel syndrome; COPD, chronic obstructive pulmonary disease; AAT, α-antitrypsin.

TABLE 38.3. ALOGRITHM TO EVALUATE ISOLATED ELEVATED AMINOTRANSFERASES

Step 1: Evaluate for the most common causes
- Consider medicines, herbs, and recreational drugs as etiologies
- Screen for alcohol abuse (AST:ALT ratio >2:1, elevated GGTP, elevated MCV)
- HCV antibody and HCV RNA (by PCR) (chronic hepatitis C)
- HBsAg, HBsAb, HBcAb (IgM and IgG) (chronic hepatitis B)
- Serum iron, total iron binding capacity (hemochromatosis suggestive if Fe/TIBC >45%)
- RUQ ultrasound (steatosis suggestive of NAFLD and liver morphology suggestive of cirrhosis)

Step 2: If the above is unrevealing, rule out nonhepatic causes
- Exclude muscle disorders (check CPK, aldolase)
- Thyroid disorders (hypothyroidism and hyperthyroidism can be evaluated with TFTs)

Step 3: Consider less common causes of liver disease
- Serum protein electrophoresis, ANA and anti–smooth muscle antibodies (autoimmune hepatitis)
- Ceruloplasmin (Wilson disease)
- Serum antiendomysial IgA or anti-TTG, +/− antigliadin IgA and IgG (celiac disease if history of diarrhea or unexplained iron deficiency)
- α-antitryspin level (AAT deficiency)

Step 4: Obtain a liver biopsy or observe
- If ALT and AST are < twofold elevated and patient is without evidence of hepatic decompensation
- Otherwise consider a liver biopsy. Although it may not provide a diagnosis or change management, a negative result may provide reassurance that there is no serious underlying liver disorder.

Note: AST:ALT ratio, ratio of serum alanine aminotransferase to serum aspartate aminotransferase; GGTP, γ-glutamyl transpeptidase; MCV, mean corpuscular volume; HCV, hepatitis C virus; PCR, polymerase chain reaction; HBsAg, hepatitis B surface antigen, HBsAb, hepatitis B surface antibody; HBcAb, hepatitis B core antibody; IgM, immunoglobulin, IgG, immunoglobulin G, Fe, ferritin; TIBC, total iron-binding capacity; RUQ, right upper quadrant; CPK, creatinine phosphokinase; NAFLD, nonalcoholic fatty liver disease; TFT, thyroid function test; ANA, antinuclear antibody; TTG, tissue transglutaminase.
Source: Adapted from Pratt, 2001, with permission.

ELEVATED ALKALINE PHOSPHATASE

- Enzyme bound to hepatic canalicular membrane. Elevation of hepatic AP due to increased liver synthesis; several other isoenzymes found in bone, intestine, kidney, and placenta
- Bone conditions associated with high AP include age older than 60 years, normal growth, Paget disease, osteoblastic bone metastases, and osteomalacia. Nonhepatic conditions associated with high AP include normal pregnancy and small-bowel obstruction.
- Degree of elevation of hepatobiliary AP may provide clue to etiology.
  ⇒ Mild elevations in AP (up to two to three times normal) are nonspecific; can occur in many forms of liver disease; often seen in hepatitis and cirrhosis.

⇒ Marked elevations of AP (more than ten times normal) generally indicate biliary obstruction in extrahepatic biliary obstruction (gallstone) or intrahepatic cholestasis (drugs or PBC [primary biliary cirrhosis]).
- Up to one third of patients with isolated AP of hepatobiliary origin have no identifiable source.
- See Tables 38.4 and 38.5 for differential and evaluation.

TABLE 38.4. DIFFERENTIAL DIAGNOSIS OF ELEVATED HEPATIC ALKALINE PHOSPHATASE

Cholestasis
- AIDS cholangiopathy
- Bile duct obstruction due to tumor (pancreas, gallbladder, cholangiocarcinoma, ampulla)
- Choledocholithiasis (most common cause of extrahepatic cholestasis)
- Chronic pancreatitis (leading to strictures of distal CBD)
- Drugs (cholestasis or cholestatic hepatitis seen with, e.g., amoxicillin/clavulanate, oral contraceptives, erythromycin, trimethoprim-sulfamethoxazole, penicillin derivatives, cimetidine, anabolic steroids, phenytoin, chlorpromazine)
- Infectious: EBV, CMV
- Primary biliary cirrhosis (progressive destruction of interlobular bile ducts)
- Primary sclerosing cholangitis (strictures of larger intrahepatic +/− extrahepatic bile ducts with proximal dilations)

Infiltration
- Amyloidosis
- Cancer (leukemia, Hodgkin's lymphoma, primary or metastatic cancer)
- Extrahepatic tumors (osteosarcoma, lung, gastric, head and neck, renal cell, ovarian, uterine)
- Granulomatous diseases (sarcoidosis, mycobacteria)
- Hepatic abscess

Note: AIDS, acquired immunodeficiency syndrome; CMV; cytomegalovirus; EBV, Epstein-Barr virus.

TABLE 38.5. ALGORITHM TO EVALUATE ELEVATED ALKALINE PHOSPHATASE (AP)

Step 1: Identify the source: bone vs. liver
- Initial test is 5'-nucleotidase or γ-glutamyl transpeptidase (GGTP).
  - ⇒ Parallel increase in AP and 5'-nucleotidase confirms hepatic etiology of AP elevation. Occasionally, there may be a dissociation between the rise of hepatic AP and 5'-nucleotidase.
  - ⇒ GGTP most useful in pregnancy, since GGTP is unaffected by pregnancy (unlike 5'-nucleotidase, which rises in pregnancy).
  - ⇒ Certain drugs such as phenytoin, barbiturates, and alcohol can increase GGTP. GGTP may be used to support suspicion of occult alcohol use in a patient with an AST:ALT>2.

Step 2: If the AP is of hepatobiliary origin: diagnostic evaluation
- Check a serum antimitochondrial antibody (AMA) and a right upper quadrant ultrasound.
  - ⇒ AMA is 95% sensitive and very specific for primary biliary cirrhosis.
  - ⇒ Ultrasound will allow assessment of liver parenchyma and bile ducts. If ultrasound reveals biliary obstruction or dilatation, endoscopic retrograde cholangiopancreatography (ERCP) should be performed to evaluate for choledocholithiasis and biliary duct strictures (as seen in primary sclerosing cholangitis).
  - ⇒ If ultrasound is negative but AMA is positive, or if ultrasound shows abnormal hepatic parenchyma but AMA is negative, liver biopsy should be performed.

Step 3: If both AMA and ultrasound are negative: assess degree of elevation of AP
- See above for differential.
- If AP >50% above normal, consider liver biopsy and ERCP. Magnetic resonance cholangiopancreatography is alternative as a noninvasive method to image biliary and pancreatic ducts.
- If AP <50% above normal, consider observation.

SELECTED REFERENCES

1. American Gastroenterological Association. *AGA guideline: Celiac sprue.* American Gastroenterological Association, 2000.
2. Angulo P, Keach JC, Batts KP, et al. Independent predictors of liver fibrosis in patients with nonalcoholic steatohepatitis. *Hepatology* 1999;30:1356.
3. Bardella MT, Vecchi M, Conte D, et al. Chronic unexplained hypertransaminasemia may be caused by occult celiac disease. *Hepatology* 1999;29:654.

4. Cohen JA, Kaplan MM. The SGOT/SGPT ratio: an indicator of alcoholic liver disease. *Dig Dis Sci* 1979;24:835.
5. Dienstag JL, Schiff ER, Wright TL, et al. Lamivudine as initial treatment for chronic hepatitis B in the United States. *N Engl J Med* 1999;341:1256.
6. Hultcrantz R, Glaumann H, Lindberg G, et al. Liver investigation in 149 asymptomatic patients with moderately elevated activities of serum aminotransferases. *Scand J Gastroenterol* 1986;21:109–113.
7. Lieberman J, Winter B, Sastre A. Alpha$_1$-antitrypsin PI-types in 965 COPD patients. *Chest* 1986;89:370.
8. McHutchinson JC, Gordon S, Schiff E, et al. Interferon alfa 2b alone or in combination with ribavirin as initial treatment for chronic hepatitis C. *N Engl J Med* 1998;339:1485–1492.
9. Pratt DS, et al. Evaluation of abnormal liver-enzyme results in asymptomatic patients. *N Engl J Med* 2000;342:1266.
10. Schuppan D, Jia JD, Brinkhaus B, et al. Herbal products for liver disease: a therapeutic challenge for the new millennium. *Hepatology* 1999;30:1099.
11. Silverman EK, Miletich JP, Pierce JA, et al. Alpha-1 antitrypsin deficiency: high prevalence in the St. Louis area determined by direct population screening. *Am Rev Respir Dis* 1989;140:961.

39

CHRONIC VIRAL HEPATITIS B AND C

CHRONIC HEPATITIS B

Introduction

- Affects 5% of world population; 5% to 10% of chronic liver disease and cirrhosis in United States (Lee, 1997).

Pathophysiology/Clinical Presentation (Tables 39.1 and 39.2; Fig. 39.1)

- Double-stranded DNA virus that belongs to the hepadnavirus family. Virus particle consists of outer envelope (with hepatitis B surface antigen [HBsAg]) and internal nucleocapsid (with hepatitis B core antigen [HBcAg]).
- Often asymptomatic at time of acute infection
- Routes of transmission: perinatal, percutaneous, and sexual

TABLE 39.1. SEROLOGY OF HEPATITIS B VIRUS (HBV)

Serologic test	Comments
HBV surface antigen (HBsAg)	Protein on outer surface of the virus.
	Presence in serum for >6 mo indicates chronic HBV infection
Antibody to HBV surface antigen (anti-HBs)	Appears on recovery from HBV infection or as a result of vaccination.
	Confers protective immunity.
Antibody to HBV core antigen (anti-HBc)	Detected in serum within 1 wk after HbsAg is detected.
	Lasts indefinitely in all patients who have been exposed to HBV.
	Unlike anti-HBs, anti-HBc does not confer protective immunity.
	Immunoglobulin M anti-HBc is marker of acute or recent HBV infection, whereas immunoglobulin G anti-HBc signifies recovery (in association with anti-HBs) or chronic infection (in association With HBsAg).
HBV e antigen (HBeAg)	Derived from the gene that codes for HBcAg.
	Marker of active viral replication and infectivity; correlates with high serum levels of HBV DNA.
	Predictor of perinatal transmission; 90% of mothers who have circulating HBeAg at the time of childbirth transmit the virus to their child.
	Infectivity of an HBeAg-positive needlestick is 20–30%.
Antibody to HBV e antigen (anti-HBe)	Indicates relative lack of infectivity (and lower serum levels of HBV DNA).
HBV DNA	A quantitative marker of HBV replication; used to assess infectivity and monitor response to antiviral therapy.

TABLE 39.2. INTERPRETATION OF HBV SEROLOGIC PROFILES

HBsAg	Anti-HBs	Anti-HBc	HBeAg	Anti-HBe	HBV DNA	Interpretation
+	−	IgM	+	−	+	Acute HBV
−	−	IgM	+/−	+/−	+/−	Acute HBV in "window period"
+	−	IgG	−	+	−	Late acute HBV or chronic carrier with low infectivity
+	−	IgG	+	−	+	Chronic HBV, high infectivity
+	−	IgG	−	−	+	Chronic HBV with "precore" mutant and, high infectivity
−	−	IgG	−	+/−	−	Infection in remote past or false-positive anti-HBc
−	+	IgG	−	+/−	−	Recovery from acute HBV
−	+	−	−	−	−	Immunization with HBV or infection in remote past

Note: HBV, hepatitis B virus; HbsAg, HBV surface antigen; anti-HBs, antibody to HBV surface antigen; anti-HBc, antibody to HBV core antigen; HBeAg, HBV e antigen; anti-HBe, antibody to HBV e antigen; IGM, immunoglobulin M, IgG, immunoglobulin G.

Evaluation

- Often asymptomatic or mild symptoms such as fatigue. Some patients have right upper quadrant pain and jaundice, reflecting active hepatitis.
- Screening: *HBsAg*, antibody to HBsAg (*anti-HBs*), and antibody to HBcAg (*anti-HBc*) (*total and immunoglobulin M*)
- Diagnosis: persistence of circulating HBsAg for >6 months. If patient is a candidate for antiviral therapy, hepatitis B e antigen (HBeAg) and serum hepatis B virus (HBV) DNA levels should be determined.

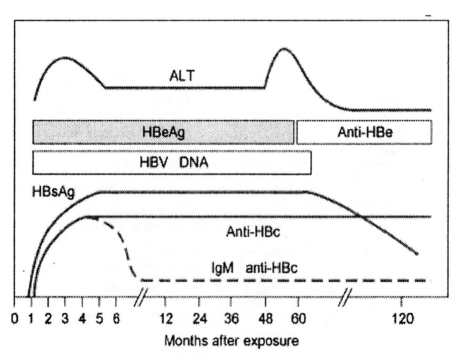

FIGURE 39.1. Serologic course of chronic hepatitis B. (From Dienstag JL, Isselbacher KJ. Acute viral hepatitis. In: Fauci AS, Braunwald E, Isselbacher KJ, et al., eds. *Harrison's principles of internal medicine*, 14th ed, vol 2. New York: McGraw-Hill, 1998;1677–1692, with permission.)

- Liver biopsy is useful to assess severity of disease (grade of inflammation and stage of fibrosis) and to exclude other causes.

Treatment

- Goal is suppression of HBV replication to prevent cirrhosis. Liver injury occurs mainly in patients with active viral replication. The serologic goal is clearance of HBV DNA and HBeAg from serum (sustained virologic response) and HBeAg to antibody to HBeAg (anti-HBe) seroconversion.
- **Interferon-α (IFN-α):** immunomodulatory, antiviral, and antiproliferative effects
  - ⇒ Efficacy: 16-week course of IFN-α (5 million units every day [q.d.] or 10 million units three times a week subcutaneously) leads to sustained loss of HBV DNA and HBeAg in 30% to 40% of patients and, in responders, delays progression of fibrosis (Niederau et al., 1996).
  - ⇒ Contraindications: decompensated cirrhosis, depression, history of suicidal tendency, severe leukopenia (white blood cell count <3,000) or thrombocytopenia (platelets <75,000), or other severe systemic disorders
  - ⇒ Side effects: initial flulike syndrome, fatigue, myalgias, anorexia and nausea, depression, irritability, insomnia, hair loss, thyroid abnormalities
- **Lamivudine (Epivir-HBV):** oral nucleoside analogue and inhibitor of HBV (and human immunodeficiency virus) DNA polymerase; alternative first-line therapy for chronic HBV with active viral replication.
  - ⇒ Efficacy: 100 mg q.d. as effective as a 16-week course of IFN-α monotherapy in inhibiting viral replication; loss of HBeAg in 30% to 40% and seroconversion to anti-HBe in 17% who receive lamivudine for 12 months. Therapy beyond 1 year is recommended if HBeAg to anti-HBe seroconversion fails to occur.
  - ⇒ Well tolerated; resistance may develop.
  - ⇒ For patients who do undergo HBeAg to anti-HBe seroconversion, lamivudine can be stopped after a minimum treatment period of 12 months; patients who do not develop anti-HBe should continue lamivudine indefinitely.
- Future therapy: New nucleoside analogues such as adefovir dipivoxil appear to be as effective without leading to resistance; under investigation.
- Universal precautions for handling all blood and body fluids minimize risk of HBV infection.

CHRONIC HEPATITIS C

Introduction

- About 170 million people worldwide are infected; 2.7 million people in the United States.
- Most common cause of chronic liver disease and indication for liver transplantation in the United States

Pathophysiology

- Transmission: parenteral contact via intravenous drug use and blood transfusions
- Mean incubation period after acute exposure: 8 weeks, with a range of 2 to 15 weeks
- Acute hepatitis C virus (HCV) infection is generally undiagnosed because it causes no or mild nonspecific symptoms.
- 20% to 30% progress to cirrhosis slowly over 20 to 30 years. Risk of hepatocellular carcinoma is 1% to 4% per year once cirrhosis is established.
- Prognosis: The best predictor is liver histology.
- Extrahepatic manifestations of HCV infection: essential mixed cryoglobulinemia, membranoproliferative glomerulonephritis, non-Hodgkin lymphoma, autoimmune thyroiditis, porphyria cutanea tarda, possibly diabetes mellitus

Evaluation (Fig. 39.2)

- Diagnosis: presence of antibody to HCV (anti-HCV) by serologic assays; HCV RNA by molecular assays

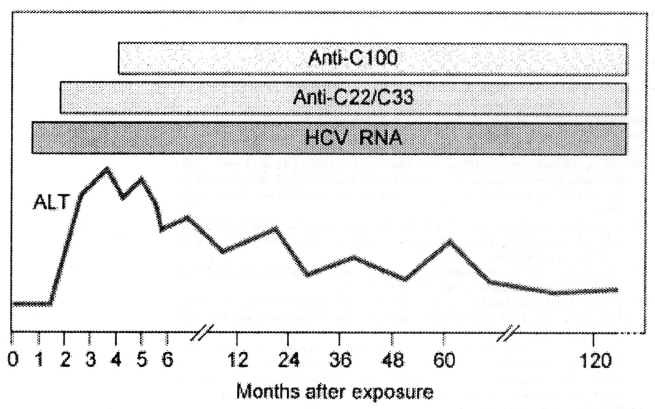

FIGURE 39.2. Serologic course of hepatitis C progression. (Adapted from Dienstag JL, Isselbacher KJ. Acute viral hepatitis. In: Fauci AS, Braunwald E, Isselbacher KJ, et al., eds. *Harrison's principles of internal medicine,* 14th ed, vol 2. New York: McGraw-Hill, 1998;1677–1692, with permission.)

- Screening: Anti-HCV appears in late acute and chronic infection. A third-generation enzyme immunoassay (EIA) can detect anti-HCV within 8 weeks of exposure with a sensitivity of 97%.
- Confirmation: Testing for HCV RNA follows a positive EIA result for anti-HCV.
- Genotype: Testing of HCV genotypes is used to help determine appropriate duration of therapy and to predict responsiveness to therapy.
- Liver biopsy: recommended before therapy to assess grade, stage, and prognosis, exclude other causes of liver disease, and aid in treatment decisions

Treatment

- Goal: Eradicate HCV; delay progression to cirrhosis, decompensated liver disease, and hepatocellular cancer.
- Sustained virologic response: absence of HCV RNA in serum (usually in combination with normalization of serum aminotransferase levels) 6 months after cessation of therapy; low likelihood of relapse
- Duration of treatment: 6 to 12 months depending on viral genotype, level of viremia, and presence or absence of cirrhosis
- **Pegylated IFN (PEG-IFN):** longer half-life and higher steady-state serum concentrations than standard IFN-α; requires only once-weekly subcutaneous injections, which improves compliance and quality of life.
  - ⇒ **PEG-IFN and ribavirin combination therapy is now standard of care.**
  - ⇒ Combination therapy with PEG-IFN and ribavirin for 48 weeks achieved a higher virologic response rate than with IFN-α and ribavirin (54% vs. 47%) (Manns et al., 2000).
- **Ribavirin** is synthetic guanosine analogue that appears to inhibit replication of HCV RNA; has a synergistic effect in decreasing RNA levels when used with IFN.
  - ⇒ IFN and ribavirin in combination induce a sustained response in 30% to 40% of patients, with approximately 60% experiencing histologic improvement (McHutchison et al., 1998).

⇒ Side effects: hemolytic anemia (hemoglobin <10 in 10% patients), nausea, pruritus, abnormal fetal development
- Patients with decompensated liver disease should not be treated with IFN-α and ribavirin.
- Check serum HCV RNA level at 3 months (for 6-month course of treatment), 6 months (for 12-month treatment), end of treatment, and 6 months after completion of therapy.
- **Liver transplantation:** only therapeutic option for patients with decompensated liver disease due to HCV. Antiviral therapy with IFN-α and ribavirin can limit impact of reinfection.
- Universal precautions should always be followed.
- Patients with HCV infection should be vaccinated against hepatitis A virus (HAV) and HBV if they do not already have antibody to HAV or anti-HBs.

SELECTED REFERENCES

1. Alter MJ, Kruszon-Moran D, Nainan OV, et al. The prevalence of hepatitis C virus infection in the United States, 1988 through 1994. *N Engl J Med* 1999;341:556–562.
2. Chang MH, Chen CJ, Lai MS, et al. Universal hepatitis B vaccination in Taiwan and the incidence of hepatocellular carcinoma in children. *N Engl J Med* 1997;336:1855–1859.
3. Cheng SJ, Bonis PAL, Lau J, et al. Interferon and ribavirin for patients with chronic hepatitis C who did not respond to previous interferon therapy: a meta-analysis of controlled and uncontrolled trials. *Hepatology* 2001;231–240.
4. Dienstag JL, Schiff E, Wright T, et al. Lamivudine as initial treatment for chronic hepatitis B in the United States. *N Engl J Med* 1999;341:1256–1263.
5. Lai C, Chien R, Leung N, et al. A one-year trial of lamivudine for chronic hepatitis B. *N Engl J Med* 1998;339:61–68.
6. Lauer GM, Walker BD. Hepatitis C virus infection. *N Engl J Med* 2001;345:41–52.
7. Lee WM. Hepatitis B virus infection. *N Engl J Med* 1997;337:1733–1745.
8. Liaw YF, Leung NW, Chang TT, et al. Effects of extended lamivudine therapy in Asian patients with chronic hepatitis B. Asia Hepatitis Lamivudine Study Group. *Gastroenterology* 2000;119:172–180.
9. Malik AH, Lee WM. Chronic hepatitis B virus infection: treatment strategies for the next millennium. *Ann Intern Med* 2000;132:723–731.
10. Manns MP, McHutchinson JG, Gordon S, et al. Peginterferon alfa-2b plus ribavirin compared to interferon alfa-2b plus ribavirin for the treatment of chronic hepatitis C 24 wk treatment analysis of a multicenter, multinational phase III randomized controlled trial [Abstract]. *Hepatology* 2000;32:297a.
11. McHutchison J, Gordon S, Schiff E, et al. Interferon alfa 2b alone or in combination with ribavirin in naïve chronic HCV patients: a US multicenter trial. *N Engl J Med* 1998;339:1485–1492.
12. Niederau C, Heintges T, Lange S, et al. Long-term follow-up of HBeAg-positive patients treated with interferon-alfa for chronic hepatitis B. *N Engl J Med* 1996;334:1422–1427.
13. Zuckerman AJ, Thomas HC, eds. *Viral hepatitis,* 2nd ed. London: Churchill Livingstone, 1998.

CHRONIC DIARRHEA

INTRODUCTION

- Defined as stools of loose consistency with or without increased frequency for >4 weeks or stool weight >200 g per day
- 90% of chronic diarrhea cases have identifiable causes; 80% of these can be diagnosed as outpatient. Of those with diagnoses, about 30% organic disease, 20% laxative or diuretic abuse, and remainder "functional" disease (Donowitz et al., 1995)
- Estimated prevalence 3% to 5% (Fine and Schiller, 1999); annual societal cost from lost work >$350,000,000 (Everhart, 1994)

PATHOPHYSIOLOGY

- Distinguish diarrhea from two mimics:
  - ⇒ Hyperdefecation: increased frequency of bowel movements without increase in stool weight above normal; occurs with proctitis, some cases of irritable bowel.
  - ⇒ Fecal incontinence: due to poor anal sphincter tone; often have liquid stools but normal volume
- Approximately 9 L of fluid pass through the normal gastrointestinal (GI) tract in 24-hour period: 2 L from direct ingestion, remaining from digestive fluids (1 L saliva, 2 L gastric fluid, 4 L biliary, pancreatic and small intestinal fluid).
- Absorption begins in lower small intestine, with 4 to 5 L absorbed from jejunum, 3 to 4 L from ileum. The colon reabsorbs 800 mL each day, leaving 200 mL to be excreted in stool.

DIFFERENTIAL DIAGNOSIS (TABLES 40.1 AND 40.2)

- **Chronic diarrhea of unknown etiology** after evaluation is likely due to laxative abuse, collagenous and lymphocytic colitis, irritable bowel syndrome (IBS) (abdominal pain with diarrhea), and fecal incontinence (not technically diarrhea).

TABLE 40.1. CLASSIFICATION OF CHRONIC DIARRHEA BY MECHANISM

Mechanism	Clinical Features	Examples
Inflammatory Damage to intestinal mucosa	Fever, abdominal pain, leukocytosis, blood and/or leukocytes in stool	Crohn's disease, ulcerative colitis, lymphocytic and collagenous colitis, radiation colitis, food allergy, human immunodeficiency virus.
Osmotic (malabsorptive) Nonabsorbed or nondigested intraluminal solute	Improves with fasting; nutrient deficiencies, weight loss; presence of fecal osmotic gap (>125 mOsm/kg of water)	Lactose or sorbitol intolerance, chronic pancreatitis, bacterial overgrowth, celiac disease, Whipple's disease, short-bowel syndrome

(continued)

TABLE 40.1. *(continued)*

Mechanism	Clinical Features	Examples

Secretory
  Excess electrolyte
  secretion
	Watery diarrhea, no change with
	  fasting, absence of fecal
	  osmotic gap
		Hormone-producing tumors,
		  limited terminal ileum
		  resection

Intestinal dysmotility
  Rapid transit time, some
  cases associated with
  bacterial stasis
	Alternating diarrhea and
	  constipation, neurologic
	  symptoms, bladder involvement
		Irritable bowel syndrome,
		  neurogenic bowel,
		  scleroderma, short bowel
		  syndrome

Factitious
  Self-induced
	Watery diarrhea with
	  hypokalemia, weakness, edema
		Laxative abuse

Miscellaneous		Amyloidosis, heavy metals, ischemic bowel, drugs, alcohol

Source: Adapted from Friedman et al. Diarrhea and constipation. Harrison's Principles of Internal Medicine, 14th edition. McGraw-Hill 1998, with permission.

TABLE 40.2. CAUSES OF CHRONIC DIARRHEA

Common causes
  Bacterial overgrowth of small intestine
  Carbohydrate intolerance (lactase, sucrose, sorbitol, fructose)
  Chronic gastrointestinal infection (amebiasis, giardiasis, *Clostridium difficile*)
  Chronic ischemic bowel
  Endocrine (diabetic neuropathy, hyperthyroidism, adrenal insufficiency)
  Fat intolerance
  Food additives (alcohol, caffeine)
  Inflammatory bowel disease
  Irritable bowel syndrome
  Laxative abuse
  Medications (antibiotics, magnesium antacids, antihypertensives, antiarrhythmics, antineoplastics)
  Paradoxical diarrhea (colon cancer)
  Previous surgery (pyloric bypass after truncal vagotomy, ileal resection, cholecystectomy)
  Radiation colitis
Less common causes
  Epidemic
  Fecal incontinence (not diarrhea by definition)
  Food allergy
  Hormone-producing tumors (gastrinoma, VIPoma, villous adenoma, carcinoid, medullary thyroid cancer)
  Infiltrative (scleroderma, amyloidosis, lymphoma)

Source: Adapted from Donowitz M, Kokke FT, Saidi R. Evaluation of patients with chronic diarrhea. *N Engl J Med* 1995;332:725–729, with permission.

EVALUATION

History

- *Organic disease* denotes actual pathology within the bowels; suggested by three or more of the following with 90% specificity (Donowitz et al., 1995):
  ⇒ Less than 3 months duration, nocturnal predominance, stool volume >400 g per day, abrupt onset, >10-pound weight loss, elevated erythrocyte sedimentation rate, anemia, low albumin level
- *Functional diarrhea* describes dietary, motility, and idiopathic causes.
  ⇒ Characterized by long duration of symptoms (>1 year), absence of weight loss or nocturnal diarrhea, and straining with defecation (Bytzer et al., 1990; Bertomeu et al., 1991)
- *Associated symptoms:* duration, frequency, high variability (IBS), nocturnal occurrence (absence favors IBS), abundant gas (IBS or malabsorption), cramping pain (absence favors secretory etiology), tenesmus (inflammation), incontinence (may be primary problem)
- *Relationship to food:* helps distinguish between osmotic and secretory diarrhea
  ⇒ Diarrhea that stops completely with fasting suggests unabsorbed carbohydrates, fatty acids, or bile acids, or surreptitious laxatives.
  ⇒ Secretory diarrhea does not or only partially terminates with fasting.
- *Characterization of stool; medications* (see Tables 40.3 and 40.4)

TABLE 40.3. CHARACTERIZATION OF STOOL

Large volumes (small intestine or proximal colon) vs. small volumes with urge to defecate (left colon or rectum)	Greasy, oily, rancid odor (steatorrhea)
	Nonbloody mucus (irritable bowel syndrome)
Rapid, watery consistency (secretory hormones)	Excessive flatus and "floating" stool
	Fecal soiling (incontinence consistent with anal sphincter disorder)

TABLE 40.4. MEDICATIONS

β-Blockers	5-Fluorouracil
Clindamycin	Clofibrate
Digoxin	Colchicine
Gemfibrozil	Diuretics
Penicillin derivatives	Lovastatin

- *Systemic symptoms:* fever, weight loss, rashes, and arthralgias
- *Travel history, sexual or physical abuse, and family history (inflammatory bowel disease [IBD]):* Anal sex predisposes to anal proctitis and human immunodeficiency virus (HIV).
- *Surgical history:* ileal resection, cholecystectomy, blind loops, fistulas, postgastrectomy dumping syndrome
- *Alcohol* can lead to pancreatic insufficiency after 10 to 20 years of use.
- *Other entities:* caffeine, heavy-metal toxins (lead, mercury, arsenic), endocrine disorders (diabetes mellitus, Addison's disease, hyperthyroidism)

Physical Examination

- *Nutritional depletion* leads to weight loss, cachexia, hypovolemia, cheilosis, glossitis, neuropathy, edema, and ecchymoses.
- *GI signs:* hepatomegaly, abdominal masses or tenderness, rectal examination for occult blood, fistula, or poor anal sphincter tone
- *Extraintestinal signs:* lymphadenopathy (Whipple's disease), arthritis (Whipple's disease, IBD)
- *Suggestive rashes:* erythema nodosum and pyoderma gangrenosum (IBD), flushing and telangiectasias (carcinoid), dermatitis herpetiformis (celiac disease), sclerodactyly (scleroderma)

Laboratory Data

- *May suggest etiology or chronicity of diarrhea, but rarely diagnostic* (see Tables 40.5 and 40.6)

TABLE 40.5. INITIAL LABORATORY WORKUP

Complete blood cell with differential (anemia, leukocytosis)	Electrolytes (metabolic imbalance, severe hypokalemia of villous adenoma)	Calcium (low in malabsorption)	Glucose (diabetes) Albumin Thyroid-stimulating hormone

TABLE 40.6. LABORATORY TESTS TO CONSIDER AFTER INITIAL EVALUATION

For osmotic malabsorption	For secretory diarrhea
Amylase	Calcitonin (thyroid medullary cancer,
Antiendomysial antibody or antigliadin (celiac	pancreatic adenoma)
disease)	Gastrin (Zollinger-Ellison syndrome).
Folic acid	Urine 5-hydroxyindole acetic acid for
Iron	carcinoid syndrome in patients with
Prothrombin time	flushing
Serum immunoelectrophoresis (α-1 antitrypsin	Vasoactive intestinal polypeptide
deficiency for protein-losing enteropathy)	(VIPoma)
Vitamin B$_{12}$ level	

- **Initial evaluation of stool** focuses on common causes of chronic diarrhea:
  - ⇒ *Stool leukocytes:* inflammatory process, such as invasive infection or colitis; rare white blood cells are normal finding.
  - ⇒ *Stool occult blood:* suggests inflammation; absence of concomitant leukocytes raises possibility of malignancy or acute ischemia.
  - ⇒ *Stool cultures:* low yield in chronic diarrhea of immunocompetent patients, more helpful in immunocompromised patients
  - ⇒ *Stool ova and parasites:* 60% to 85% sensitivity for *Giardia* and *Entamoeba* if three samples are collected (Donowitz et al., 1995). Enzyme-linked immunosorbent assay for *Giardia* antigen has specificity/sensitivity >90%.
  - ⇒ *Stool for Clostridium difficile toxin:* high sensitivity and specificity if three samples.
- **If above unrevealing, the following may be helpful in certain situations:**
  - ⇒ *Stool sudan stain:* qualitative detection of fat 90%
  - ⇒ *72-hour quantitative stool fat determination:* gold standard for fat malabsorption; diagnostic if stool fat content >6 g per day while on a 24-hour test diet of 100 g of fat
  - ⇒ *Stool or urine alkalinization:* (one drop of sodium hydroxide or potassium hydroxide "at the bedside") turns stool a pink color if it contains phenolphthalein, an ingredient in over-the-counter laxatives.
  - ⇒ *Stool volume:* <200 mL per day suggests fecal incontinence, rectal disease, or IBS. Stool volume >1 L per day indicates secretory diarrhea.
  - ⇒ *Stool osmolality and electrolytes:* Stool osmotic gap (measured stool osmolality − 2[sodium + potassium]) >125 mOsm/kg suggests osmotic diarrhea due to carbohydrates or magnesium-containing laxatives.
  - ⇒ *Stool pH:* pH <5.3 indicates carbohydrate (lactose or sorbitol) malabsorption; pH >5.6 makes carbohydrate malabsorption unlikely.

Endoscopy

- *Sigmoidoscopy with biopsy* indicated for blood or large numbers of stool leukocytes, or with severe systemic symptoms.
  - ⇒ Can help differentiate functional disorders (IBS; laxative use suggested by "melanosis coli" on histology) from organic disorders (IBD, pseudomembranous colitis).
- *Colonoscopy with biopsy* is alternative to sigmoidoscopy if there is concern for Crohn's disease, cancer, villous adenoma, or perhaps lymphocytic and collagenous colitis.

Radiology

- *Barium enema and upper GI series with small-bowel followthrough*
  - ⇒ Adjunct to endoscopy; better suited to detect anatomic abnormalities (fistulas and strictures)
  - ⇒ Thickened bowel indicates infiltrative diseases (cancer, lymphoma, Crohn's disease, Whipple's disease, and amyloidosis). Less invasive than colonoscopy, but less sensitive and does not allow for biopsy.

- *Computed tomography (CT):* Consider with malabsorptive diarrhea when concern for pancreatic cancer or chronic pancreatitis; can also identify other tumors, IBD.

TREATMENT

- Aim treatment at underlying process.
- *Diet:* Eliminate potential offenders, such as dairy products, sugar-free foods, or fat. Acute diarrhea is often followed by secondary lactose intolerance.
- *Antibiotics* can be used for suspicion of bacterial overgrowth; metronidazole for giardiasis, fluoroquinolone for bacterial diarrhea.
- *Cholestyramine* decreases diarrhea in patients with ileal resection <100 cm.
- *Antidepressants, fiber, and antispasmodics* treat IBS (see Chapter 41).
- *Clonidine,* an α_2-adrenergic agonist, is used for treatment of opiate withdrawal and diabetic diarrhea.
- *Octreotide:* long-acting synthetic somatostatin that can treat refractory secretory diarrhea (due to inhibition of hormone secretion) and HIV-related or chemotherapy-related chronic diarrhea
- *Pancreatic enzymes* are given in exocrine pancreas deficiency.
- Do not suppress symptoms if etiology is unknown, but in certain situations, it is reasonable to try **symptomatic therapy**; temporizing measure during evaluation.
  - ⇒ *Psyllium* increases bulk of stools.
  - ⇒ *Perianal hygiene:* Sitz baths (10 minutes two to three times per day), followed by gentle drying with absorbent cotton (instead of toilet paper); pads with witch hazel (Tucks); avoidance of soap (Desitin is an alternative); hydrocortisone creams (1%).
  - ⇒ *Opiate antimotility agents* (loperamide and diphenoxylate) decrease bowel motility but are contraindicated in IBD or infectious diarrhea, because of risk of toxic megacolon. May help in acute diarrhea and other colitis.

SELECTED REFERENCES

1. Avery ME, Snyder JD. Oral therapy for acute diarrhea—the underused simple solution. *N Engl J Med* 1990;323:891–894.
2. Bertomeu A, Ros E, Barragan V, et al. Chronic diarrhea with normal stool and colonic examinations: organic or functional? *J Clin Gastroenterol* 1991;13:531.
3. Binder HJ. The gastroenterologist's osmotic gap: fact or fiction? *Gastroenterology* 1992;103:702–704.
4. Bytzer P, Stokholm M, Andersen I, et al. Aetiology, medical history, and faecal weight in adult patients referred for diarrhea: a prospective study. *Scan J Gastroenterol* 1990;25:572.
5. Donowitz M, Kokke FT, Saidi R. Evaluation of patients with chronic diarrhea. *N Engl J Med* 1995;332:725–729.
6. Duncan A, Cameron A, Stewart MJ, et al. Diagnosis of the abuse of magnesium and stimulant laxatives. *Ann Clin Biochem* 1991;28:568–573.
7. Eherer AJ, Fordtran JS. Fecal osmotic gap and pH in experimental diarrhea of various causes. *Gastroenterology* 1992;103:545–551.
8. Everhart JE, ed. *Digestive disease in the United States: epidemiology and impact.* Bethesda, MD: National Institutes of Health; 1994. NIH publication 94-1447.
9. Fine KD, Fordtran JS. The effect of diarrhea on fecal fat excretion. *Gastroenterology* 1992;102:1936–1939.
10. Fine KD, Schiller LF. AGA guideline on the evaluation and management of chronic diarrhea. *Gastroenterology* 1999;116:1461.
11. Janda RC, Conklin JL, Mitros FA, et al. Multifocal colitis associated with an epidemic of chronic diarrhea. *Gastroenterology* 1991;100:458–464.
12. Levitt MD, Duane WC. Floating stools—flatus versus fat. *N Engl J Med* 1972;286:973–975.
13. Lynn RB, Friedman LS. Irritable bowel syndrome. *N Engl J Med* 1993;329:1940–1945.
14. Madoff RD, Williams JG, Caushaj PF. Fecal incontinence. *N Engl J Med* 1992;326:1002–1007.
15. Read NW, Krejs GJ, Read MG, et al. Chronic diarrhea of unknown origin. *Gastroenterology* 1980;78:264–271.
16. Ungar BL, Yolken RH, Nash TE, et al. ELISA-linked immunosorbent assay for the detection of *Giardia lamblia* in fecal specimens. *J Infect Dis* 1984;149:90–97.
17. Valdovinos MA, Camilleri M, Zimmerman BR. Chronic diarrhea in diabetes mellitus: mechanisms and an approach to diagnosis and treatment. *Mayo Clin Proc* 1993;68:691–702.

IRRITABLE BOWEL SYNDROME

INTRODUCTION

- Most common gastrointestinal (GI) condition encountered in general medical practice; 25% to 50% of outpatient referrals to gastroenterologists (Harvey et al., 1983; Talley et al., 1991)
- Seventh leading diagnosis made by all physicians
- Implicated as second most frequent cause of time lost from work, with economic impact in the United States estimated at $25 billion per year (Camilleri, 2001)

PATHOPHYSIOLOGY/CLINICAL PRESENTATION

- A biopsychosocial disorder arising from complex interaction of psychosocial factors, altered motility, and heightened sensory function of the intestine (Camilleri, 2001).
- Proposed mechanisms include abnormal colonic motility, heightened visceral sensation, psychological stress, and irritation of the small bowel or colon by substances such as lactose, bile acids, and food allergens (Camilleri, 2001).
- One single mechanism is unlikely to explain pathophysiology.
- More likely than controls to have childhood history of sexual or physical abuse. When compared with nonabused patients, patients with irritable bowel syndrome (IBS) have a lower pain threshold and greater frequency of psychiatric disorders (Lynn and Friedman, 1995).
- Symptoms: abdominal pain associated with altered bowel habits, specifically diarrhea, constipation, or alternating diarrhea and constipation; must be present for at least 3 months

DIFFERENTIAL DIAGNOSIS

- Colonic adenocarcinoma, villous adenoma, Crohn's disease, ulcerative colitis, ischemic colitis, chronic mesenteric vascular insufficiency, chronic idiopathic intestinal pseudoobstruction, fecal impaction, intermittent sigmoid volvulus, megacolon, giardiasis, lactase deficiency, endometriosis, depression, somatization, anxiety, panic disorder

EVALUATION

- Considered a **"diagnosis of exclusion"**
- No single biological marker can be used to make a definitive diagnosis; most symptoms have no specific physiologic explanation (Drossman, 1999).
- Manning et al. (1978) noted six symptoms more common in patients with IBS than in those with organic GI diseases (see Table 41.1).

TABLE 41.1. MANNING CRITERIA

1. Pain relief with bowel movement
2. More frequent stools with the onset of pain
3. Looser stools with the onset of pain
4. Passage of mucus
5. Sensation of incomplete evacuation
6. Abdominal distention, as evidenced by tight clothing or visible appearance

- Patients with IBS report higher frequencies of upper GI tract symptoms, including gastroesophageal reflux disease, noncardiac chest pain, globus sensation, heartburn, and dysphagia (Lynn and Friedman, 1993).
- In an effort to standardize the definition of IBS for research purposes, rigorous diagnostic criteria have been established (see Table 41.2). These criteria fail to include individuals with bowel dysfunction without pain as a primary feature.

TABLE 41.2. THE ROME II CRITERIA (DROSSMAN, 1999)

At least 12 wk or more, which need not be consecutive, in the previous 12 mo of abdominal pain or discomfort that has two of three features:
    Relief with defecation
    Onset associated with a change in the frequency of stool
    Onset associated with a change in form (appearance) of stool

- Goal of evaluating a patient with abdominal pain and altered bowel habits is to diagnose IBS while appropriately excluding other potential causes for symptoms (Lynn and Friedman, 1995). Table 41.3 outlines a simple approach toward the initial evaluation and management (Camilleri, 2001).

TABLE 41.3. A SIMPLIFIED APPROACH TOWARD THE INITIAL MANAGEMENT OF IRRITABLE BOWEL SYNDROME

1. Make the diagnosis
- Identify the Rome II/Manning criteria
- History and physical examination
- Complete review of medications
- Initial laboratories: complete blood cell count, SMA-7, erythrocyte sedimentation rate
- Initial stool studies: occult blood (everyone), ova and parasites (diarrhea predominant)
- Initial endoscopic procedures: flexible sigmoidoscopy (everyone), colonoscopy (age >40; positive family history of colon cancer or colon polyps)

2. Characterize the symptoms

Constipation	Diarrhea	Pain/gas/bloat

3. Review fiber intake and consider additional testing

No additional testing	H_2 breath test or lactose-free diet	KUB during pain

4. Therapeutic Trial

Increased dietary fiber	Antidiarrheal ±/− Antispasmodic	Antidepressant (low dose)

5. If symptoms persist, consider a gastroenterology referral for further evaluation

Note: KUB, Kidneys, ureters, bladder (plain frontal supine radiograph)

TREATMENT

- Cornerstone of treatment: A therapeutic physician–patient relationship is one that is nonjudgmental and reassuring, that establishes realistic expectations, and that involves the patient in treatment decisions.

- Adding fiber supplementation to the patient's diet and recommending avoidance of gas-forming foods (legumes) and foods or beverages sweetened with sorbitol or fructose will lead to symptomatic improvement in most patients. Two thirds will remain symptom free in 5 years (Lynn and Friedman, 1995).
- High placebo response rate (60%) for any drug used to treat IBS
- Additional specific drug therapy should be tailored to the predominant symptom (see Tables 41.3 and 41.4).
- Alosteron, a 5-HT$_3$ antagonist, was recently pulled from the market because of reported cases of ischemic colitis (Camilleri, 2001).
- A new agent about to receive Food and Drug Administration approval is Tegaserod, a partial 5-HT$_4$ agonist that increases orocecal transit in patients with constipation-predominant IBS (Prather et al., 2000). Most common side effects have been abdominal pain, diarrhea, nausea, flatulence, and headaches. Further clinical trials are currently underway.

TABLE 41.4. MEDICATIONS FOR IBS

Symptom Complex	Drug Type and Example (suggested starting dose)	Comment
Constipation-predominant IBS	Fiber supplements Wheat bran (1/2 cup to one bowl q.d., 10–30 g q.d.) Psyllium (1/2 to 1 tbsp q.d. to b.i.d.)	These interventions may be tried for any IBS symptom complex
Constipation-predominant IBS	Prokinetic agents Tegaserod (pending FDA approval) Domperidone (10–20 mg q.i.d. not available in United States	
Diarrhea-predominant IBS	Antidiarrheals Diphenoxylate (2.5–5 mg q.i.d.) Loperamide (2 mg b.i.d.) Cholestyramine (1/2 to one pck q.d.–b.i.d.)	
Pain-predominant IBS; chronic pain syndrome	Tricyclic antidepressants Amitriptyline (10–25 mg h.s.) Desipramine (50 mg h.s.)	Unlike the antidepressant effect, the anticholinergic and analgesic effects occur within 24–48 h
Pain-predominant IBS; prevention of post meal abdominal pain	Antispasmodics (anticholinergics) Tincture of belladonna (5–10 drops p.o. t.i.d.) Dicyclomine (10–20 mg t.i.d.-q.i.d.)	Side effects include decreased secretions, tachycardia, urinary retention, and pupillary dilation
Anxiety associated with IBS	Benzodiazepine-type anxiolytics	Use only for brief periods

Note: b.i.d., twice daily; FDA, Food and Drug Administration; h.s., at bedtime; IBS, irritable bowel syndrome; p.o., per os; q.d., every day; q.i.d., four times a day; t.i.d., three times a day.
Source: Adapted from Lynn RB, Friedman LS. Irritable bowel syndrome. *N Engl J Med* 1993;329: 1940, with permission.

RESOURCES

- International Foundation for Functional Gastrointestinal Disorders (publishes a quarterly newsletter with updates and fact sheets): PO Box 17864, Milwaukee, WI 53217; 888-964-2001
- National Digestive Disease Information Clearinghouse (distributes articles on IBS): 2 Information Way, Bethesda, MD 20892-570; 301-654-3810
- Internet sites:

    Irritable Bowel Self-Help Group: http://www.ibsgroup.org
    Center for Digestive Health and Nutrition: http://www.gihealth.com/Articles/Articles.html
    International Foundation for Functional Gastrointestinal Disorders: http:/execpc.com/iffgd.

SELECTED REFERENCES

1. Accarino A, Azpiroz F, Malagelada. Selective dysfunction of mechanosensitive intestinal afferents in irritable bowel syndrome. *Gastroenterology* 1995;108:636.
2. Camilleri M. Gastrointestinal disorders and the Rome II process. *Gut* 1999;45[Suppl II]:II1–II5.
3. Camilleri M. Management of the irritable bowel syndrome. *Gastroenterology* 2001;120:652–668.
4. Drossman DA. The functional in the irritable bowel syndrome: a 5-year prospective study. *Lancet* 1987;1:963.
5. Drossman DA. The Rome criteria process: diagnosis and legitimization of irritable bowel syndrome. *Am J Gastroenterology* 1999;94(10):2803.
6. Harvey RF, Salih SY, Read AE. Organic and functional disorders in 2000 gastroenterology outpatients. *Lancet* 1983;1:632.
7. Lefkowitz M. The 5-HT$_4$ receptor partial agonist Tegaserod improves abdominal discomfort/pain and normalizes altered bowel function in irritable bowel syndrome (IBS). Poster presentation at the annual meeting of the American College of Gastroenterology; 1999; Phoenix, Arizona.
8. Lynn RB, Friedman LS. Irritable bowel syndrome. *N Engl J Med* 1993;329:1940.
9. Lynn RB, Friedman LS. Irritable bowel syndrome: managing the patient with abdominal pain and altered bowel habits. *Med Clin North Am* 1995;79:373.
10. Manning AP, Thompson WG, Heaton KW, et al. Towards positive diagnosis of the irritable bowel syndrome. *Br Med J* 1978;2:653.
11. Prather C, Camilleri M, Zinsmeister AR, et al. Tegaserod accelerates orocecal transit in patients with constipation-predominant irritable bowel syndrome. *Gastroenterology* 2000;188:463.
12. Talley NJ, Zinsmerister AR, Van Dyke C, et al. Epidemiology of colonic symptoms and irritable bowel syndrome. *Gastroenterology* 1991;101:927.
13. Whitehead WE, Palsson OS. Is rectal pain sensitivity a biological marker for irritable bowel syndrome; psychological influences on pain perception. *Gastroenterology* 1998;115:1263.
14. Whitehead WE. Psychosocial aspects of function gastrointestinal disorders. *Gastroenterol Clin North Am* 1996;25:21.

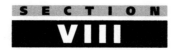

SECTION VIII

HEMATOLOGY

42

ANEMIA

INTRODUCTION

- Defined as reduction in volume of red blood cells (RBCs) per 100 mL of blood (hematocrit <42% in men, <37% in women); hemoglobin level (<13 g/dL in men, <12 g/dL in women); or RBC count (<4.70 × 1,012/L in men, <4.15 × 1,012/L in women).
- Affects 3.4 million Americans (2.1 younger than age 45 years); women are more frequently affected than men.

PATHOPHYSIOLOGY/CLINICAL PRESENTATION

- Normal RBC lifespan is about 120 days; three primary mechanisms for anemia:
  ⇒ *Decreased production:* Bone marrow unable to replace those cells normally lost
  ⇒ *Increased destruction:* RBC lifetime shortened beyond the bone marrow's ability to compensate
  ⇒ *Acute or chronic blood loss:* Bone marrow unable to compensate rapidly; iron deficiency often develops when chronic.
- Symptoms depend on chronicity: acute anemia symptomatic at higher hematocrit level than slowly developing anemia (to which the body has physiologically adapted)

DIFFERENTIAL DIAGNOSIS

- Generally classified by morphology (see Table 42.1)
- Two or more processes may coexist (e.g., iron deficiency and vitamin B_{12} deficiency), complicating interpretation of the mean corpuscular volume; some etiologies may not clearly fall within one category (e.g., anemia of chronic disease; myelodysplastic syndrome).

TABLE 42.1. DIFFERENTIAL OF ANEMIA BY MORPHOLOGY

Microcytic (MCV <80)	Normocytic (MCV 80-100)	Macrocytic (MCV >100)
Iron deficiency	Any early anemia	Megaloblastic: vitamin B_{12} or folate deficiency
Thalassemia	Acute blood loss	Liver disease
Anemia of chronic disease	Anemia of chronic disease	Drugs (AZT, hydoxyurea, chemotherapy, etc.)
Sideroblastic anemia	Chronic renal insufficiency	Alcohol
	Hemolysis	Myelodysplastic syndrome
	Bone marrow suppression/invasion	
	Myelodysplastic syndrome	
	Hypothyroidism/hypopituitarism	

Note: MCV, mean corpuscular volume; AZT, azidothymidine.
Source: Adapted from Schrier SL. Approach to the patient with anemia. Up to date, 2001, with permission.

EVALUATION

History

- Symptoms of anemia:
  - ⇒ Initially occur with physiologic stress: palpitations, shortness of breath, muscle cramps, decreased exercise tolerance
  - ⇒ Progress to at-rest symptoms: weakness, fatigue, dyspnea, dizziness; patients with coronary disease may develop angina or congestive heart failure
  - ⇒ Acute blood loss causes symptoms of hypovolemia in addition to anemia; less well tolerated
- Personal or family history of anemia and blood transfusions; ethnic background (sickle cell, glucose-6-phosphate dehydrogenase [G6PD] deficiency in African Americans, thalassemias in Mediterranean, Asian, pernicious anemia in Northern Europeans)
- Dietary habits: vegetarian, "tea and toast," alcohol intake
- Menstrual history, including pregnancies (lose 300 to 700 mg of iron per pregnancy)
- History of bleeding/blood loss, including both overt and occult gastrointestinal (GI) loss (stool color, bowel habits)
- Associated disorders: neurologic, glossitis with vitamin B_{12} deficiency; easy bruising, fevers, bone pain with multiple myeloma or lymphoproliferative disorders
- Medical history: renal failure, chronic infections, connective tissue disorders, coagulopathy, small-bowel or gastric surgery/malabsorption; medication use including aspirin, nonsteroidal antiinflammatory drugs, potentially myelosuppressive drugs

Physical Examination

- Vital signs: tachycardia, tachypnea, orthostatic hypotension
- Hematologic: pallor, bruising, petechiae, lymphadenopathy, hepatosplenomegaly, bony pain
- GI: rectal examination, guaiac status, jaundice (not sensitive or specific)

Laboratory (Tables 42.3 through 42.6 for Specific Anemias)

- Complete blood cell count to evaluate white blood cells and platelets; red blood cell (RBC) indices to classify anemia as microcytic, macrocytic, or normocytic
- Reticulocyte count (%): measure of immature RBCs, assesses appropriateness of bone marrow response.
  - ⇒ Reticulocyte production index (RPI) = absolute reticulocyte ÷ maturation time
  - ⇒ Correct for patient's level of anemia (absolute reticulocyte = % reticulocyte × [patient hematocrit ÷ 45]), earlier release of reticulocytes into periphery with more severe anemia (reticulocyte maturation time: 1 for hematocrit 40% to 45%, 1.5 for 35% to 40%, 2 for 25% to 34%, 2.5 for 15% to 24%).
  - ⇒ RPI >2.0% indicates appropriate bone marrow response to anemia; implicates RBC loss or destruction as primary etiology.
- Iron studies, ferritin if microcytic/normocytic or multifactorial (see Table 42.2); vitamin B_{12}/folate levels if macrocytic/normocytic

TABLE 42.2. INTERPRETATION OF IRON STORES

	Serum Ferritin	Serum Iron	Total Iron-Binding Capacity	% Transferrin Saturation	RDW
Iron-deficiency anemia	Low	Low	High	Low (often <9%)	High
Thalassemia minor	Normal/high	Normal/high	Normal	Normal	Normal/high
Anemia of chronic disease	Normal/high	Low	Low	10–20%	Normal
Sideroblastic anemia	Normal/high	High	Normal	High	Normal
Lead poisoning	Normal	Variable	Normal	High	Normal
Normal values	Men: 30–300 ng/mL Women: 15–200 ng/mL	30–160 μg/dL	228–428 μg/dL	20–40%	11–14%

- Further testing in selected circumstances: SPEP (serum protein electrophoresis) (multiple myeloma); erythropoietin level; erythrocyte sedimentation rate; hemoglobin electrophoresis (hemoglobinopathy); Coombs test (autoimmune hemolysis); lactate dehydrogenase, bilirubin, haptoglobin (hemolysis)
- Peripheral smear: red cell size; spherocytes (immune-mediated hemolysis); schistocytes (microangiopathic hemolytic anemia); teardrop cells (myelophthisis); bite cells (G6PD deficiency); Howell-Jolly bodies (asplenia); hypersegmented neutrophils (vitamin B_{12}, folate deficiency)
- Bone marrow biopsy: not generally helpful for diagnosis; indications include pancytopenia, immature cells (blasts) or suggestion of myelodysplasia on peripheral smear, monoclonal gammopathy, unexplained anemia despite careful workup

TREATMENT

- Specific therapy varies depending on underlying etiology; anemia is a sign of an underlying process which must be identified and treated (see Tables 42.3 through 42.6).

TABLE 42.3 MICROCYTIC ANEMIAS (MCV <80, RPI <2.0%, INDICATING INADEQUATE RBC PRODUCTION)

	Etiologies	Diagnosis	Treatment
IDA	—Blood loss (menstruation, bleeding, parasites) —Poor absorption	—Peripheral smear: microcytic, hypochromic RBCs —Red cell distribution width increased —Increased platelets —Ferritin low: diagnostic if <12 μg/L; may be elevated due to inflammation (check ESR) —Transferrin saturation <9% diagnostic —TIBC high in IDA, low in ACD —Mentzer index (MCV/RBC no.) >13; (<13 suggests thalassemia) —Bone marrow biopsy (gold standard for iron stores, rarely necessary)	—Most idiopathic IDA due to gastrointestinal bleeding: colon cancer in men or postmenopausal women until proven otherwise; mandates colonoscopy/esophagogastroduodenoscopy —Consider oral contraceptives to minimize blood loss in menstruating women —FeSO₄ 325 mg p.o t.i.d. between meals —Reticulocyte count rises within 1 wk —Hematocrit rises within 1 mo —Treat for 6 mo to replete iron stores
ACD	—Low erythropoietin; impaired iron utilization —Inflammation: rheumatoid arthritis, inflammatory bowel disease, chronic infection, malignancy	—Microcytic or normocytic RBCs —Ferritin elevated, iron and TIBC decreased —Transferrin saturation 10–20% —Erythropoietin level low —Bone marrow biopsy for iron stores if unable to differentiate from IDA	—Treat underlying etiology —Recombinant erythropoietin injections, transfuse p.r.n. if symptomatic —Iron may be detrimental given already increased iron stores
Sideroblastic anemia	—Rare disorders of ineffective erythropoiesis with elevated iron stores —Hereditary form presents in childhood —Acquired may be primary (myelodysplatic syndrome) or secondary (lead, drugs, porphyria, cancer, rheumatoid arthritis, pyridoxine deficiency)	—Normocytic, normochromic and microcytic, hypochromic RBCs —Elevated transferrin saturation, ferritin; normal TIBC —Consider checking lead level —Bone marrow biopsy: Perinuclear iron deposits in erythroid precursors (ringed sideroblasts)	—Hereditary form may respond to pyridoxine (50–200 mg/d) —Transfusions p.r.n. —Desferrioxamine to chelate excess iron
Thalassemia	—Hereditary, due to defective synthesis of α- or β-globin; severity depends on number of genes affected —α-Thalassemia common in Asia, Africa, β-thalassemia seen in Mediterranean populations	—Microcytic hypochromic; teardrop forms, target cells, basophilic stippling in severe forms —Mentzer index (MCV/RBC cell no.) <13 —Ferritin/transferrin saturation normal to elevated —Hemoglobin electrophoresis normal in alpha trait (molecular diagnosis required); increased Hb A₂ (4–8%) and Hb F (1–5%) in beta trait	—Genetic counseling critical for those with α- or β -thalassemia trait contemplating pregnancy; if both partners carry trait, may result in more serious disease, including hydrops fetalis

Note: ACD, anemia of chronic disease; ESR, erythrocyte sedimentation rate; Hb, hemoglobin; IDA, iron deficiency anemia; MCV, mean corpuscular volume; p.o., per os; p.r.n., when necessary; RBC, red blood cell; RPI, reticulocyte production index; TIBC, total iron-binding capacity; t.i.d., three times a day.

● Normocytic anemias: Early stages of *any* anemia can be normocytic.
● Critical to identify hemolytic anemias and acute bone marrow processes rapidly: Check smear and reticulocyte count early.

TABLE 42.4.   NORMOCYTIC ANEMIAS WITH ELEVATED RETICULOCYTOSIS (RPI > 2%): HEMOLYTIC ANEMIAS

	Etiology	Diagnosis	Treatment
Microangiopathic hemolytic anemia	TTP/HUS, DIC, artificial valve, pre-eclampsia, antiphospholipid antibody syndrome, malignant hypertension, vasculitis, malaria, *Babesia*	Schistocytes on smear, with hemoglobinuria/hemosiderinuria	Treat underlying etiology when possible
Coombs test–positive hemolytic anemia	Autoimmune, IgG mediated; SLE, lymphoma, drugs (penicillins, sulfas, NSAIDs, quinine)	Spherocytes on smear, + direct Coombs test	Discontinue offending drugs; immunosuppression/splenectomy often needed
Coombs test–negative hemolytic anemia	IgM mediated: mycoplasma, EBV, lymphoma or autoimmune disease Donath-Landsteiner antibody: paroxysmal cold hemoglobinuria, syphilis	Spherocytes; cold agglutinins	Usually mild; keep patient warm; rarely, immunosuppressives Treat underlying lymphoproliferative disease
Sickle cell disease	Due to Hb S, which polymerizes in hypoxic conditions	—Normocytic, normochromic RBCs; sickle and target cells, nucleated RBCs, basophilic stippling, Howell-Jolly bodies —Hb electrophoresis shows Hb S	—Supportive care for crises —Exchange transfusions for acute chest syndrome, central nervous system symptoms —Vaccinations for functional asplenia
Glucose-6-phosphate dehydrogenase deficiency	—Wide variety of X-linked mutations distributed worldwide —Hemolytic crises triggered by drugs (sulfas, vitamin K analogues, nitrofurantoin), infections, fava beans	—Heinz bodies, bite cells, and spherocytes on smear —Laboratory evidence of hemolysis	—Supportive; transfusions p.r.n.; hemodialysis may be required for renal failure —Avoid oxidative drugs, which trigger hemolysis

Note: DIC, disseminated intravascular coagulation; EBV, Epstein-Barr virus; Hb, hemoglobin; HUS, hemolytic—uremic syndrome; IgG, immunoglobulin G; IgM, immunoglobulin M; NSAID, nonsteroidal antiinflammatory drug; p.r.n., when necessary; RBC, red blood cell; RPI, reticulocyte production index; SLE, systemic lupus erythematosus; TTP, thrombotic thrombocytopenic purpura.

TABLE 42.5.   NORMOCYTIC ANEMIA WITH INAPPROPRIATELY LOW RETICULOCYTOSIS (RPI <2%): SUPPRESSED BONE MARROW

	Etiology	Diagnosis	Treatment
Myelophthisic anemias	—Replacement or infiltration of bone marrow —Leukemia, multiple myeloma, lymphoma, metastatic carcinoma, disseminated tuberculosis, histoplasmosis	—Teardrop cells and leuko-erythroblastosis (nucleated RBCs, left-shifted myeloid elements) —Bone marrow biopsy	—Treat underlying disease, if possible —Hematology involvement
Myelodysplastic syndromes	—Clonal disorders of hematopoietic stem cell leading to ineffective erythropoiesis	—Smear: normocytic or macrocytic RBCs, bilobed neutrophils, hypogranular platelets, micromegakaryocytes, left-shifted, hypogranular myeloid elements —Bone marrow biopsy: dysplasia of one or more lineages, ineffective erythropoiesis, increased blasts	—Stage dependent: supportive care, differentiation or chemotherapy, bone marrow transplant; hematology involved —Often progresses to AML (>30% blasts)

(continued)

TABLE 42.5. *(continued)*

	Etiology	Diagnosis	Treatment
Aplastic anemia	—Bone marrow failure —Radiation, chemotherapy, benzene, arsenic, EtOH, viral infections, drugs (carbamazepine, cephalosporins, nonsteroidal anti-inflammatory drugs, sulfas) —Pure red cell aplasia (drugs, parvovirus infection)	—Pancytopenia —Bone marrow biopsy	—Discontinue potential drug causes —Treatment per hematology, including limited transfusions, growth factors, immunosuppression, bone marrow transplant
Anemia of chronic renal insufficiency	—Low erythropoietin levels	—Normocytic normochromic RBCs, burr cells —Erythropoietin level	—Erythropoietin 4,000 units s.c. 3x/wk, transfusions p.r.n. —Iron repletion —Monitor serum ferritin level (goal 50–100 μg/L)
Human immunodeficiency virus–associated anemia	Low erythropoietin level, bone marrow suppression by human immunodeficiency virus, opportunistic pathogens, Azidothymidine (macrocytic anemia)	Normocytic normochromic RBCs	—Erythropoietin —Transfusions p.r.n.

Note: p.r.n., when necessary; RBC, red blood cell; s.c., subcutaneously.

TABLE 42.6. MACROCYTIC ANEMIAS[a]

	Etiology	Diagnosis	Treatment
Vitamin B_{12} deficiency (often MCV > 115)	—Pernicious anemia, gastrectomy atrophic gastritis, pancreatic insufficiency, blind loop syndrome with bacterial overgrowth, dysfunction of terminal ileum, *Diphyllobothrium latum* infection, genetic deficiencies (intrinsic factor, transcobalamin II), inadequate intake (vegans; B_{12} stores adequate for 3 yr)	—Smear: macroovalocytes, hypersegmented PMN —Neurologic symptoms (loss of memory, subacute combined degeneration); anorexia; nausea —Serum B_{12} level < 100 pg/mL, elevated serum methylmalonic acid, homocysteine levels —Shilling test: defines gastric vs. ileal etiologies of B_{12} malabsorption	—Replete with B_{12} 100—1,000 μg/d for 3–7d. —Weekly and then monthly subcutaneous injections of 100 μ (for life)
Drugs	—EtOH, AZT, methotrexate, trimethoprim-sulfa, hydroxyurea, pentamidine, pyrimethamine	Medical history, macrocytic smear	Discontinue medication
Folate deficiency (often MCV > 115)	—Decreased intake —Increased utilization (pregnancy, hemolytic anemia, exfoliative skin disease) —Celiac sprue (malabsorption) —Drugs (accelerated metabolism) —Alcohol (impaired metabolism of folate)	—Symptoms: anorexia, nausea, diarrhea, depression, neurologic abnormalities like B_{12} deficiency —Neural tube defects —Decreased serum and erythrocyte folate —Homocysteinemia without high methylmalonic acid	—Folate supplementation before pregnancy —Folate 1 mg p.o. q.d for 6 wk —may unmask B_{12} deficiency (check level after 2 wk)

[a] *Other etiologies include* hypothyroidism, liver disease, myelodysplastic syndromes, and reticulocytosis.
Note: AZT, azidothymidine; MCV, mean corpuscular volume; PMN, polymorphonuclear; p.o., per os; q.d., every day.

SELECTED REFERENCES

1. Beutler E. The common anemias. *JAMA* 1988;259:2433.
2. Camitta BM, Storb R, Thomas ED. Aplastic anemia: pathogenesis, diagnosis, treatment and prognosis. *N Engl J Med* 1982;306:645.
3. Carmel R. Prevalence of undiagnosed pernicious anemia in the elderly. *Arch Intern Med* 1996;156:1097–1100.
4. Crosby W. Who needs iron? *N Engl J Med* 1977;297:543.
5. Erslev AJ. Erythropoietin. *N Engl J Med* 1991;324:1339.
6. Fry J. Clinical patterns and course of anemias in general practice. *Br Med J* 1961;2:1732.

7. Hershko C, Vitells A, Braverman DZ. Causes of iron deficiency anemia in an adult inpatient population: effect of diagnostic workup on etiologic distribution. *Blut* 1984;49:347–352.

8. Hillman R. Red blood cell disorders. In: Hillman R, ed. *Hematology in clinical practice: a guide to diagnosis and management.* New York: McGraw-Hill, 1995:1–230.

9. Rodak B. Hematopathology: erythrocyte disorders. In: Rodak B, ed. *Diagnostic hematology.* Philadelphia: WB Saunders, 1995:171–287.

10. Sadeghi S, Skelton T. Systematic approach to evaluation of anemia in the adult population. *Turnaround Times* 1996;5(4):1–12.

11. Scadden DT, Zon LI, Groopman JE, et al. Pathophysiology and management of HIV-associated hematologic disorders. *Blood* 1989;74:1455.

12. Wood M, Elwood P. Symptoms of iron deficiency anemia: a community survey. *Br J Prev Soc Med* 1966;20:117.

ANTICOAGULATION IN PRIMARY CARE

ANTICOAGULATION FOR ATRIAL FIBRILLATION

Introduction

- Atrial fibrillation (AF) causes 75,000 strokes per year (14% of all strokes); increases stroke rate by five times; most common cause of systemic embolism (Wolf et al., 1978; Flegel et al., 1987).
- Incidence doubles with each decade of life; overall prevalence 0.95%; affects 4% of people older than 60 years and 9% older than 80 years (Go et al., 2001; Narayan et al., 1997).

Pathophysiology

- AF-associated thromboemboli likely multifactorial, including hemodynamic stasis of atria (particularly left atrial appendage) and possible AF-associated hypercoagulable state (Narayan et al., 1997).

Evaluation

Risk Factors for Embolism (Albers et al., 2001)

- American College of Chest Physicians guideline for stroke risk with concomitant AF (Albers et al., 2001):
  - ⇒ **High-risk factors:** prior stroke, prior transient ischemic attack (TIA)/systemic embolus, history of hypertension, poor left ventricular function, age older than 75 years, rheumatic mitral valve disease, prosthetic valve
  - ⇒ **Moderate-risk factors:** age 65 to 75 years, diabetes mellitus, coronary artery disease with preserved left ventricular function
- Paroxysmal atrial fibrillation (PAF) carries same stroke risk as persistent AF and should be treated similarly, as should atrial flutter due to coexisting PAF (AF Investigators, 1994; Hart et al., 2000).
- Risk of stroke in nonvalvular AF has been stratified by age and concomitant risk factors (see Table 43.1).

TABLE 43.1. ANNUAL STROKE RATE IN PATIENTS WITH ATRIAL FIBRILLATION

Age (yr)	Placebo		Warfarin	
	No Risk Factors	One or More Risk Factors[a]	No Risk Factors[a]	One or More Risk Factors[a]
<65	1.0%	4.9%	1.0%	1.7%
65–75	4.3%	5.7%	1.1%	1.7%
>75	3.5%	8.1%	1.7%	1.2%

[a] Risk factors include hypertenstion, diabetes, prior stroke/transient ischemic attack.
Source: From Atrial Fibrillation Investigators. Risk factors for stoke and efficacy of antithrombotic therapy in atrial fibrillation. Analysis of pooled data from five randomized controlled trials. *Arch Intern Med* 1994;154: 1449–1457, with permission

- AF in setting of rheumatic heart disease increases stroke risk 17 times and should be considered a separate epidemiologic entity (Narayan et al., 1997).

Treatment

Anticoagulation

- **Warfarin** (see Table 43.2): Trials have shown 2.7% absolute risk reduction of stroke risk with warfarin, 68% relative risk reduction (Hart et al., 1999).
- Recommended for individuals with any major risk factor or more than one moderate-risk factor. Consensus international normalized ratio (INR) target is 2.0 to 3.0 (Hylek et al., 1996; Albers et al., 2001).

TABLE 43.2. WARFARIN ANTICOAGULATION

Initiation of therapy	Initiate with 5 mg/d over 1–4 d (5 mg vs. 10 mg starting dose may provide better/safer antithrombotic effect with reduced risk of bleeding complications) (Harrison et al., 1997). Early increase in prothrombin time reflects reduction of factor VII levels (shortest half-life), although true antithrombosis is not achieved until factor II synthesis is inhibited (occurs around day 5) (Zivelin et al., 1993). Standard practice is to overlap warfarin with heparin for minimum 4–5 d when rapid anticoagulation is necessary (Hyers et al., 2001). International normalized ratio (INR) is usually checked daily until therapeutic ≥2 consecutive days, followed by monitoring two to three times/wk for 1–2 wk, then less often (depending on stability of results). If INR is stable, monitoring can be reduced to every 4 wk (Ansell et al., 2001).
Management of elevated INR	INR may fluctuate due to dietary changes in vitamin K intake, changes in warfarin absorption, changes in warfarin metabolism from drug interactions, patient compliance. Guidelines for managing elevated INR are based on consensus (no reliable randomized trials to compare strategies) (Ansell et al., 2001). INR 2.0–3.0 takes ~4–5 d to normalize (White et al., 1995); in patients without significant bleeding with INR 5.0–9.0, skip next one to two doses and consider 1–2.5 mg oral vitamin K (Crowther et al., 2001); for INR> 9.0, hold warfarin and give 3–5 mg oral vitamin K with resumption of warfarin once INR is therapeutic. For serious bleeding give fresh frozen plasma and 10 Mg intravenous vitamin K by slow infusion. Note: Response to vitamin K is unpredictable and may lead to warfarin resistance.
Interactions	Multiple medication interactions have been documented with warfarin (Hirsh et al., 2001). Drugs shown to potentiate warfarin include amiodarone, cotrimoxazole, erythromycin, fluorquinolones, and omeprazole, among others. Drugs that inhibit warfarin metabolism include barbiturates, carbamazepine, and β-lactam antibotics such as dicloxacillin and nafcillin.
Complications of therapy	**Bleeding:** In Intitial trials, use of warfarin was complicated by high rate of intracranial hemorrhage, but many cases occurred with target INR > 3.0. Subsequent studies with target INR 2.0–3.0 found lower bleeding rates (Levine et al., 2001). Intracranial hemorrhage occurs from 0.1–0.5% per year with 46% mortality rate (Levine et al., 2001); subdural hemorrhage may also occur and carries 20% mortality (Hylek and Singer, 1994). Risk of hemorrhage greatly increases with INR > 4.0. With INR > 6.0, 8.8% of patients have been found to seek medical attention for abnormal bleeding over a 2 wk follow-up period (Hylek et al., 2000). **Skin necrosis:** Rarely, warfarin-induced necrosis can occur in fatty areas such as breasts, pannus, buttocks, typically between days 3–10 of therapy; more common in women and patients with protein C deficiency (Bauer, 1993).

- **Aspirin monotherapy:** 325 mg daily is often recommended for patients with nonvalvular AF younger than 65 years without risk factors, or for patients with contraindications to anticoagulant therapy. In lone AF (no evidence of clinical heart disease), risks of anticoagulation with warfarin are felt greater than potential benefits. However, early anecdotal evidence suggests that all patients without contraindications to anticoagulation may benefit from warfarin.
- Patients with only one moderate-risk factor may receive either warfarin or aspirin (clinical judgment).

Anticoagulation Before and After Cardioversion

- See Chapter 7.

ANTICOAGULATION FOR VALVULAR HEART DISEASE

Introduction

- Due to risk of stroke, anticoagulation recommendations exist for mechanical/bioprosthetic heart valves and for rheumatic mitral regurgitation (see Table 43.3).
- Signs of thromboembolism include TIA, visceral infarcts, compromised peripheral perfusion.

TABLE 43.3. ANTICOAGULATION FOR VALVULAR HEART DISEASE

Valve Abnormality	Risk or Thromboembolism	Recommended Anticoagulation
Mechanical heart valve(s)	0.1–5.7% per patient-year. Clinical predictors of embolic events include multiple prosthetic valves, mitral valve location, caged-ball—type valve, atrial fibrillation, age >70, depressed left ventricular systolic function.	Lifelong anticoagulation with international normalized ratio (INR) 2.5–3.5 (Cannegieten et al., 1994, 1995; Stein et al., 2001).
Bioprosthetic heart valve(s)	0.2–2.6% per year. Risk highest during first 3 mo after valve insertion.	Anticoagulation with INR 2.0–3.0 during first 3 mo (highest risk); patients with history of thromboembolism should be treated for minimum 3–12 mo; patients with atrial fibrillation should be treated indefinitely (Ionescu, 1982; Stein et al., 2001).
Rheumatic mitral disease	~20% incidence of clinically detectable embolism during course of disease (higher than other common nonprosthetic valvular abnormalities). Risk greatly increased by coexisting atrial fibrillation or if mitral stenosis is present; risk increased by older age, lower cardiac index, left atrial diameter >55 mm.	Warfarin anticoagulation with INR target 2.0–3.0 for patients with coexisting history of embolism or paroxysmal/chronic atrial fibrillation (Salem et al., 2001); warfarin should be strongly considered for patients in normal sinus rhythm with atrial diameter >55 mm.

ANTICOAGULATION FOR VENOUS THROMBOEMBOLISM

Introduction

- About 250,000 patients hospitalized with deep venous thrombosis (DVT) or pulmonary embolism (PE) in the United States each year (Goldhaber, 1998; Weinmann and Salzman, 1994).
- Mortality high for PE, even with treatment (15% at 3 months) (Goldhaber et al., 1999).

Evaluation

Risk Factors

- Venous stasis (secondary to bed rest, immobility, congestive heart failure, obesity, venous obstruction), older age, trauma, orthopedic surgery (particularly involving lower extremities), pregnancy, hypercoagulable states, malignancy
- **Oral contraceptives (OCs):** Patients taking lower dose estrogen OCs containing 30 to 40 μg of ethynylestradiol still have risk of venous thrombosis three to six times greater that of than nonusers (Vandenbroucke et al., 2001). However, absolute risk is low (3 to 4 per 10,000 per-

son-years). For women with factor V Leiden mutation who use OCs, the Heart and Estrogen/Progestin Replacement Study showed a relative risk of 2.7 for women taking postmenopausal estrogen (Grady et al., 2000).

- **Activated protein C resistance/factor V Leiden:** Most common genetic predisposition with prevalence of 3% to 7% among white subjects. Found in 20% to 30% of patients with venous thrombosis. For homozygous individuals, risk is increased 80-fold (Rosendaal, 1999).
- **Prothrombin G20210A mutation:** threefold increased risk of venous thromboembolism; prevalence of 2% to 5% among white subjects (Poort et al., 1996).
- **Other mutations:** antithrombin III deficiency, protein C/protein S deficiencies, antiphospholipid antibody syndrome, hyperhomocystinemia, dysfibrinogenemia, plasminogen deficiency, elevated factor VIII levels (Rosendaal, 1999; Kyrle et al., 2000)

Treatment

Goals

- Minimize clot propagation, embolization, and recurrence.
- **Proximal DVT:** Should be treated aggressively because of propensity to embolize to lung. Initial treatment is with heparin (unfractionated or low molecular weight) with conversion to warfarin for longer term therapy (see Table 43.2) (Hyers et al., 2001). Heparin and warfarin should be overlapped for minimum 4 to 5 days, and heparin continued until the INR exceeds 2.0 on two consecutive measurements.
- **Localized calf DVT:** Lower risk of proximal extension and should be followed with serial lower extremity Doppler studies over 7 to 14 days, to assess for development of proximal extension.

Pharmacotherapy

- Low-molecular-weight heparin (LMWH): Used more commonly than unfractionated heparin for DVT (Hirsch et al., 2001b; Hyers et al., 2001).
  ⇒ Advantages over unfractionated heparin: predictable dose response (obviates need for laboratory monitoring); longer half-life (allowing for periodic injections and outpatient use); slightly lower risk of heparin-induced thrombocytopenia. Advantages are largely attributable to decreased binding of LMWH to circulating/cellular proteins.
  ⇒ Dosing: LMWH is dosed by weight. Patients who are obese or pregnant or who have renal failure should have anti-Xa levels monitored. For twice-daily dosing, anti-Xa should be measured 4 hours after subcutaneous injection; target therapeutic range is 0.6 to 1.0 IU/mL. In daily dosing, target range is 1.0 to 2.0 IU/mL.
  ⇒ Contraindications: Patients with possible need for urgent surgery may not be appropriate candidates, because there is no adequate means of reversing LMWH anticoagulant effect. Randomized trials of LMWH have excluded patients with renal failure, so use in this setting has not been fully studied.

Duration of Treatment

- Risk of recurrence after 6 months of treatment for idiopathic DVT is about 9% per year (Schulman et al., 1995). Risk of recurrence after second episode is 21% in patients treated for 6 months and 3% in patients treated indefinitely (Schulman et al., 1997).
- Optimal duration of anticoagulant therapy in different clinical settings is under investigation. Current recommendations include 3 months of anticoagulation for patients with reversible or time-limited risk factors; 6 months of anticoagulation for first episode of idiopathic venous thrombosis (Hyers et al., 2001).
- For recurrent idiopathic venous thrombosis or patients with continuing risk factors (cancer, certain inherited hypercoagulable states such as anticardiolipin antibody syndrome), treatment for ≥12 months is recommended. Duration of therapy continues to be individualized for patients with factor V Leiden mutation, hyperhomocystinemia, and other hypercoagulable states (Hyers et al., 2001).

ANTICOAGULATION FOR HEART FAILURE

Introduction

- Patients with a low ejection fraction (EF) may be predisposed to formation of thrombi.
- Retrospective analyses have correlated increasing stroke rates with decreasing EFs in patients with an EF <35% to 40%.

Treatment

- Recommendations for anticoagulation are not well formulated due to conflicting data between trials.
- In a retrospective study of patients with symptomatic/asymptomatic left ventricular dysfunction, use of warfarin was correlated with reductions in heart failure mortality, all-cause mortality, and hospitalization (Al-Khadra et al., 1998).

SELECTED REFERENCES

1. Albers GW, Dalen JE, Laupacis A, et al. Antithrombotic therapy in atrial fibrillation. *Chest* 2001;119: 194S–206S.
2. Al-Khadra AS, Salem DN, Rand WM, et al. Warfarin anticoagulation and survival: a cohort analysis from the Studies of Left Ventricular Dysfunction. *J Am Coll Cardiol* 1998;31:749–753.
3. Ansell J, Hirsh J, Dalen J, et al. Managing oral anticoagulant therapy. *Chest* 2001;119:22S–38S.
4. Atrial Fibrillation Investigators. Risk factors for stroke and efficacy of antithrombotic therapy in atrial fibrillation. Analysis of pooled data from five randomized controlled trials. *Arch Intern Med* 1994;154:1449–1457.
5. Bauer KA. Coumarin-induced skin necrosis. *Arch Dermatol* 1993;129:766.
6. Cannegieter SC, Rosendaal FR, Briet E. Thromboembolic and bleeding complications in patients with mechanical trial heart valve prostheses. *Circulation* 1994;89:635–641.
7. Crowther MA, Julian J, McCarty D, et al. Treatment of warfarin-associated coagulopathy with oral vitamin K: a randomised controlled trial. *Lancet* 2000;356:1551–1553.
8. Flegel KM, Shipley MJ, Rose G. Risk of stroke in non-rheumatic atrial fibrillation. *Lancet* 1987;1:526–529.
9. Ginsberg JS. Management of venous thromboembolism. *N Engl J Med* 1996;335:1816–1829.
10. Go AS, Hylek EM, Philips KA, et al. Prevalence of diagnosed atrial fibrillation in adults. National implications for rhythm management and stroke prevention: the Anticoagulation and Risk Factors in Atrial Fibrillation (ATRIA) Study. *JAMA* 2001;285:2370–2375.
11. Goldhaber SZ. Pulmonary embolism. N Engl J Med 1998; 339:93–104.
12. Goldhaber SZ, Visani L, De Rosa M. Acute pulmonary embolism: clinical outcomes in the International Cooperative Pulmonary Embolism Registry. *Lancet* 1999;353:1386–1389.
13. Grady D, Wenger NK, Herrington D, et al. Postmenopausal hormone therapy increases risk for venous thrombembolic disease. The Heart and Estrogen/progestin Replacement Study. *Ann Intern Med* 2000;132: 689–696.
14. Harrison L, Johnston M, Massicotte MP, et al. Comparison of 5-mg and 10-mg loading doses in initiation of warfarin therapy. *Ann Intern Med* 1997;126:133–136.
15. Hart RG, Benavente O, McBride R, et al. Antithrombotic therapy to prevent stroke in patients with atrial fibrillation: a meta-analysis. *Ann Intern Med* 1999;131:492–501.
16. Hart RG, Pearce LA, Rothbart RM, et al. Stroke with intermittent atrial fibrillation: incidence and predictors during aspirin therapy. *J Am Coll Cardiol* 2000;35:183–187.
17. Hirsh J, Dalen JE, Anderson DR, et al. Oral anticoagulants: mechanism of action, clinical effectiveness, and optimal therapeutic range. *Chest* 2001a;119:8S–21S.
18. Hirsh J, Warkentin TE, Shaughnessy SG, et al. Heparin and low-molecular-weight heparin: mechanism of action, pharmacokinetics, dosing, monitoring, efficacy and safety. *Chest* 2001b;119:64S–94S.
19. Hyers TM, Agnelli G, Hull RD, et al. Antithrombotic therapy for venous thromboembolic disease. *Chest* 2001;119:176S–193S.
20. Hylek EM, Chang YC, Skates SJ, et al. Prospective study of the outcomes of ambulatory patients with excessive warfarin anticoagulation. *Arch Intern Med* 2000;160:1612–1617.
21. Hylek EM, Singer DE. Risk factors for intracranial hemorrhage in outpatients taking warfarin. *Ann Intern Med* 1994;120:897–902.
22. Hylek EM, Skates SJ, Sheehan MA, et al. An analysis of the lowest effective intensity of prophylactic anticoagulation for patients with nonrheumatic atrial fibrillation. *New Eng J Med* 1996;V335:540–546.
23. Kyrle PA, Minar E, Hirschl M, et al. High plasma levels of factor VIII and the risk of recurrent venous thromboembolism. *N Engl J Med* 2000;343;457–462.
24. Levine MN, Raskob G, Landefeld S, et al. Hemorrhagic complications of anticoagulant treatment. *Chest* 2001;119:108S–121S.
25. Narayan, et al. Atrial fibrillation. *Lancet* 1997;350:943–950.
26. Poort SR, Rosendaal FR, Reitsma PH, et al. A common genetic variation in the 3′-untranslated region of the

prothrombin gene is associated with elevated plasma prothrombin levels and an increase in venous thrombosis. *Blood* 1996;88:3698–3703.

27. Rosendaal FR. Venous thrombosis: a multicausal disease. *Lancet* 1999;353:1167–1173.

28. Salem DN, Daudelin DH, Levine HJ, et al. Antithrombotic therapy in valvular heart disease. *Chest* 2001;119:207S–219S.

29. Schulman S, Granqvist S, Holmstrom M, et al. The duration of oral anticoagulant therapy after a second episode of venous thromboembolism. The Duration of Anticoagulation Trial Study Group. *N Engl J Med* 1997;336:393–398.

30. Schulman S, Rhedin AS, Lindmarker P, et al. A comparison of six weeks with six months of oral anticoagulant therapy after a first episode of venous thromboembolism. Duration of Anticoagulation Trial Study Group. *N Engl J Med* 1995;332:1661–1665.

31. Stein PD, Alpert JS, Bussey HI, et al. Antithrombotic therapy in patients with mechanical and biologic prosthetic heart valves. *Chest* 2001;119:220S–227S.

32. Vandenbroucke JP, Rosing J, Bloemenkamp KW, et al. Medical progress: oral contraceptives and the risk of venous thrombosis. *N Engl J Med* 2001;344:1527–1535.

33. Weinmann EE, Salzman EW. Deep-vein thrombosis. *N Engl J Med* 1994;331:1630–1641.

34. White RH, McKittrick T, Hutchinson R, et al. Temporary discontinuation of warfarin therapy: changes in the international normalized ratio. *Ann Intern Med* 1995;122:40–42.

35. Wolf PA, Dawber TR, Thomas H, et al. Epidemiologic assessment of chronic atrial fibrillation and risk of stroke: the Framingham study. *Neurology* 1978;28:973–977.

36. Zivelin A, Rao LV, Rapaport SI. Mechanism of the anticoagulant effect of warfarin as evaluated in rabbits by selective depression of individual procoagulant vitamin-K dependent clotting factors. *J Clin Invest* 1993; 92:2131–2140.

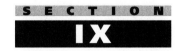

MUSCULOSKELETAL

MUSCULOSKELETAL EXAMINATION

HISTORY AND REVIEW OF SYSTEMS

- Acute versus chronic symptoms
- History of significant trauma
- Character of the pain: nocturnal, with activity or at rest, radiation, aggravating and alleviating factors
- Distribution and location of the joint complaints:
  ⇒ Monoarticular/oligoarticular/polyarticular
  ⇒ Symmetric versus asymmetric
  ⇒ Large versus small joints
  ⇒ Myalgia versus arthralgia versus arthritis
- Signs of infection/inflammation: erythema, warmth, fever, swelling
- Neurologic symptoms: burning/shooting pain, paresthesias, dermatomal versus peripheral distribution, sensory loss or changes, weakness (focal or diffuse)
- Constitutional symptoms: fatigue, fever, malaise, anorexia, weight loss
- Morning stiffness: if present, how long until "you're as loose as you'll get?"
- Raynaud's phenomenon
- Skin rashes, psoriatic lesions, subcutaneous nodules on extensor surfaces, oral or nasal lesions, hair loss
- Collect past medical, surgical and psychiatric histories.
- Review medications and allergies.

PHYSICAL EXAMINATION (SEE LATER SECTIONS FOR INDIVIDUAL JOINTS)

- Observe gait and posture.
- Examine above and below the joint of concern.
- Palpate each joint: Assess for effusions, active and passive range of motion, internal/external rotation, flexion/extension, abduction/adduction. Palpate bursae and other periarticular structures.
- Tenderness helps localize, not quantify, pain.
- If constitutional symptoms present, assess skin, head and neck for oral and nasal ulcers; lymphadenopathy; chest for crackles; cardiovascular for rubs, murmurs and pulses; abdomen for hepatosplenomegaly.

HANDS AND WRISTS

- *Deformities in rheumatoid arthritis (RA):* ulnar deviation, swan neck deformity (metacarpophalangeal [MCP] flexion, proximal interphalangeal [PIP] hyperextension, distal interphalangeal [DIP] flexion), boutonniere deformity (PIP flexion, DIP hyperextension).
- *Deformities in osteoarthritis (OA):* Heberden nodes (enlargement of the DIP joints), Bouchard nodes (enlargement of PIP joints)

- *De Quervain's tenosynovitis:* tenosynovitis of radial aspect of the wrist; pain over radial styloid aggravated by making a fist
  ⇒ *Finkelstein's test:* Ulnar deviation of the wrist with hand held as fist with thumb inside causes pain over inflamed tendons and synovium.
- *Carpal tunnel syndrome:* paresthesias, numbness, and pain in distribution of the median nerve in hand caused by median nerve entrapment at the wrist
  ⇒ *Phalen's test:* Placing wrists in position of maximal flexion for 45 seconds causes numbness and pain.
  ⇒ *Tinel's sign:* Percussion of the median nerve at the wrist causes tingling in digits.
- *Dupuytren's contracture:* thickening and contracture of the palmar fascia with flexion deformity, most commonly of the ring finger; etiology unknown (genetic component; also associated with epilepsy, diabetes, alcoholism, and pulmonary disease)

ELBOWS

- *Olecranon bursitis:* chronic/sterile or acute/infected; can be aspirated and sent for culture
- *Medial epicondylitis (golfer's elbow):* pain with resisted adduction forearm and palpation over medial epicondyle
- *Lateral epicondylitis (tennis elbow):* pain with hand grip on resisted rotation of forearm, palpation of extensor carpi radialis over lateral epicondyle

SHOULDERS

- *Rotator cuff tear:* rotator cuff comprised of the four "SITS" muscles (supraspinatus, infraspinatus, teres minor, subscapularis); supraspinatus tendon most frequently torn. Symptoms: pain with lifting arm over head, weakness, muscle atrophy. Magnetic resonance imaging (MRI) rules out large, full-thickness tear requiring surgical repair.
- *Subacromial bursitis/bicipital tendonitis/rotator cuff tendonitis:* Impingement of acromion, the coracoacromial ligament, acromioclavicular (AC) joint, rotator cuff muscles, or biceps tendon. Gradual-onset pain in lateral or anterior shoulder, worse with activity, occasional crepitus, or feeling of "catch." Treat with nonsteroidal antiinflammatory drugs (NSAIDs), rest, stretching exercises, corticosteroid injections (subacromial bursa, bicipital tendon sheath).
- *Glenohumeral instability (shoulder dislocation):* Generalized laxity or recurrent trauma. Head of humerus dislocates anteriorly or posteriorly from glenoid fossa. Pain with abduction and external rotation (throwing position). Visible on anteroposterior (AP) lateral and axillary lateral or a transscapular "Y"-view radiograph.
- *Polymyalgia rheumatica:* Prominent shoulder and hip myalgias and tenderness, usually painful, but full range of motion. Elevated erythrocyte sedimentation rate (ESR). Very responsive to low-dose prednisone.
- *AC joint separation:* Usually the result of a fall onto the acromion with arm tucked in to side. Tenderness over palpated AC joint with an obvious deformity in high-grade injury. AP shoulder film to confirm widening of the AC joint. Treat with sling, orthopedic referral if high-grade injury.
- *Adhesive capsulitis (frozen shoulder):* Insidious-onset pain and decreased range of motion, usually in the nondominant shoulder. May occur after an injury or inflammation. Associated with diabetes mellitus and hypothyroidism; most common in women ages 40 to 65 years. Treated with NSAIDs and physical therapy.

HEAD AND NECK

- *Temporomandibular joint (TMJ) syndrome:* Arthralgias and myofascial joint pain associated with bruxism (grinding of teeth at night). Treat with NSAIDs, dental referral for nighttime biteplate.
- *Temporal arteritis:* Tender, thickened temporal arteries, with headache, visual loss, and/or claudication of jaw. Associated with elevated ESR; seen in patients older than 60 years. Diagnosed

with temporal artery biopsy; responds to high-dose steroids. May develop in patients with PMR (polymyalgia). May require urgent treatment (see Chapter 49).

- *Costochondritis:* Pain and tenderness, without swelling, of costochondral junctions. Tietze syndrome: more rare, associated with swelling over costochondral junction. Treat with NSAIDs, rest.
- *Cervical arthritis (cervical spondylosis):* Seen in OA and RA; caused by bony spurs, disc herniation, buckling or protrusion of the interlaminar ligaments. Pain with motion, stiffness, and paraspinal muscle spasm frequent; may cause headaches and radiation of pain to arms. Treat with NSAIDs, neck collar, physical therapy, check C-spine x-ray for stability.

HIPS

- *OA:* loss of cartilage in hip joint associated with obesity, prior infection, trauma, age. Gradual onset of pain radiating to groin; initially only with activity. Loss of internal rotation first, progresses to limitations with flexion and extension and antalgic gait.
  - ⇒ *Trendelenburg test:* swaying of the trunk to the side of weak hip abductor muscles; patient viewed from the back, asked to flex knee in standing position
  - ⇒ Treatment: NSAIDs, weight loss if needed, orthopedics for hip replacement if persistent symptoms
- *Trochanteric bursitis:* tenderness over the lateral hip, increased discomfort at night and after periods of inactivity. Treat with NSAIDs, steroid injections, and rest.
- *Avascular necrosis of the hip:* necrosis of trabecular bone in femoral head. Risk factors: corticosteroids, alcohol, RA, lupus, previous trauma, myeloproliferative diseases, sickle cell disease. Presents with dull ache in the groin or buttock; discomfort with rotation and abduction, antalgic gait. MRI needed to detect osteonecrosis without collapse. Refer to orthopedics for surgical intervention.
- *Hip fracture (femoral neck or intertrochanteric):* Presents with inability to walk/pain after a fall; leg held in externally rotated, abducted, and shortened position. Risk factors: age, female sex, osteoporosis, dizziness, medication changes, peripheral neuropathy. Surgical correction is usually necessary.

KNEES

- *Popliteal cyst (Baker's cyst):* Patient complains of ache and fullness in popliteal area. Patients with RA are prone to cyst rupture with fluid dissection distally into calf muscles. Treat with NSAIDs, orthopedics referral if persistent.
- *Prepatellar bursitis (housemaid's knee):* chronic and sterile, secondary to repeated trauma such as working on knees, or acute and septic, particularly with penetrating injury. Differentiate prepatellar bursitis (dome-shaped swelling over patella but no intraarticular effusion, preserved range of motion) from intraarticular knee infection. Once infection is ruled out, treat with NSAIDs, rest, and steroid injection.
- *Anterior cruciate ligament (ACL) tear:* secondary to acute twisting injury to the knee; significant effusion, pain and difficulty walking
  - ⇒ *Anterior drawer test:* With patient lying supine and knee at 90-degree flexion, sit on the patient's foot, grasp the proximal tibia, and pull anteriorly with both hands; instability of tibia beneath femur if no sharp endpoint.
  - ⇒ Usually requires arthroscopic surgical repair.
- *Meniscal tear:* Traumatic or degenerative tear of medial or lateral meniscus; may occur alone or in association with cruciate ligament injuries, usually with a twisting injury. Acute event followed by insidious onset swelling and stiffness with sensation of "popping" or "clicking" with use.
- *Osgood-Schlatter disease (patellar tendonitis):* Anterior knee pain, with one primary tender spot. Overuse syndrome exacerbated by climbing stairs, squatting, jumping. Treat with NSAIDs and rest.
- *Chondromalacia patella:* anterior knee pain worse after prolonged sitting or climbing stairs. Pain, crepitus, and sticking sensation caused by damage to articular surface of the patella. Af-

fects women more than men, associated with weight gain. Treat with knee brace, NSAIDs, and rest. If symptoms persist, refer to orthopedics.

FEET AND ANKLES

- *Achilles tendonitis:* inflammation of tendon can be insertional (at bone–tendon interface of calcaneus) or noninsertional (4 to 5 cm proximal to the insertion). Insidious pain in the Achilles area, worse with exercise, tender to palpation. The Achilles tendon occasionally ruptures with acute stress; requires orthopedic repair. Otherwise, treat with NSAIDs and rest.
- *Plantar fasciitis:* plantar heel pain at site of plantar fascia insertion into medial calcaneal tuberosity. Bilateral plantar fasciitis associated with seronegative spondyloarthropathies. Treatment: heel cups, comfortable shoes, NSAIDs, refrain from exercise. Refer to podiatry or orthopedics if symptoms persist.
- *Charcot joint (diabetic foot):* Sensory polyneuropathy causes damage and destruction of joint with multiple nonhealing fractures, skin breakdown, infection, and irreversible deformity. Best treatment is prevention with careful foot care in diabetic patients.
- *Tarsal and metatarsal deformities:* common in RA, OA, women more than men due to tight-fitting shoe wear. *Hallux valgus* (lateral deviation of the great toe at the metatarsophalangeal [MTP] joint causing a painful prominence on the medial aspect of the first MTP joint); *mallet toe* (flexion of the DIP); *hammer toe* (extension of the MTP and flexion of the PIP); *claw toe* (extension at the MTP, flexion at the PIP and DIP). Refer to orthopedics or podiatry.
- *Ankle sprain:* most commonly acute inversion injury with damage to lateral collateral ligaments of ankle, pain, swelling, ecchymosis, and loss of function. Recovers with rest, ice, compression, elevation ("RICE"), and NSAIDs.

BACK

- *Degenerative spondylolisthesis:* Slippage of a vertebral body (often L4-5 or L5-S1) onto the one below it, causing disc narrowing and degeneration; low back pain exacerbated by bending, twisting, and lifting. Rule out neurologic defect on examination, diagnosis confirmed by LS spine films. May cause chronic, disabling pain. Treat with NSAIDs, physical therapy.
- *Spinal stenosis (neurogenic claudication):* Narrowing of spinal canal causes buttock, posterior thigh and calf pain worst after standing or walking, relieved by sitting or stooping (flexing spine). Decreased knee and ankle reflexes on examination, preserved arterial pulses. Usually due to age-related degenerative spondylolisthesis and enlargement of the facet joints, which causes nerve entrapment, visible on MRI. Treat with NSAIDs; refer to pain service or surgery for uncontrolled symptoms.
- *Lumbar radiculopathy (sciatica):* Irritation of (most commonly) L5 or S1 nerve roots by herniated nucleosis pulposus. Pain is dermatomal, worse with flexion and use, radiates from buttocks to posterior or posterolateral leg, ankle or foot. Straight-leg raise reproduces symptoms in 80% to 90%. Peak incidence in patients in their 40s. NSAIDs, rest, physical therapy; imaging only if symptoms do not improve with conservative therapy.
- *Sacroiliitis:* Onset usually before age 30 years; presents with recurrent bouts of low back pain and stiffness, worse after rest; eventual ossification, bridging syndesmophytes, and complete fusion of the vertebral column (bamboo spine) if untreated. Associated with human leukocyte antigen B27; seen with ankylosing spondylitis, Reiter's syndrome, reactive arthritis, psoriatic arthritis, and inflammatory bowel disease (IBD)–associated arthritis. Sacroiliac joint x-rays may reveal erosions or reactive sclerosis. Treat with NSAIDs; physical therapy is key.
- *Osseous back pain:* Presents as constant pain unrelated to position, with point tenderness over involved vertebrae; due to metastatic tumor, bacterial or tuberculous osteomyelitis or compression fracture. Neurologic deficits may represent cord compression or cauda equina syndrome. Plain films may reveal destruction, fracture, or mass; obtain in any patient with red flag symptoms (see Chapter 46).

ARTHROCENTESIS

- *Diagnostic:* undiagnosed acute monoarthritis; febrile patient with arthritis; rule out septic arthritis and examine for crystals to make diagnosis of crystal-induced arthropathy (gout, pseudogout).
- *Therapeutic:* For joint fluid evacuation, injection of corticosteroids or anesthetics.
- Contraindications to steroid injection: possible joint infection; septic patient; marked osteoporosis or joint instability; blood-clotting disorder.
- Fluid analysis: *noninflammatory fluid*
  ⇒ Pale, yellow, clear, viscous, nonclotting
  ⇒ White blood cell count (WBC) <2,000/mm^3, polymorphonuclear leukocyte (PMN) count <65%
  ⇒ Gram stain and cultures negative
  ⇒ OA, trauma, chronic gout or pseudogout, systemic lupus erythematosus (SLE), scleroderma
- Fluid analysis: *inflammatory fluid*
  ⇒ Greenish, gray, cloudy, decreased viscosity, clots on standing
  ⇒ WBC >2,000/mm^3, PMNs >65% (acute gout can have up to 100,000 WBCs/mm^3, but if WBC >100,000/mm^3 most likely bacterial infection)
  ⇒ Gram stain and cultures positive in septic arthritis
  ⇒ RA, psoriatic arthritis, ankylosing spondylitis, acute gout or pseudogout, Reiter syndrome, IBD-associated arthritis, bacterial infection, viral infection, fungal infection, mycobacterial infection, SLE, polymyositis, scleroderma

SELECTED REFERENCES

1. American College of Rheumatology Ad Hoc Committee on Clinical Guidelines. Guidelines for the initial evaluation of the adult patient with acute musculoskeletal symptoms. *Arthritis Rheum* 1996;39:1–8.
2. Baker DG, Schumacher HR. Acute monoarthritis. *N Engl J Med* 1993;329:1013–1020.
3. Boden SD, David DO, Dina T, et al. Abnormal magnetic resonance scans of the lumbar spine in asymptomatic subjects: a prospective investigation. *J Bone Joint Surg* 1990;72A:403.
4. Daltroy LH, Iversen MD, Larson MG, et al. A controlled trial of an educational program to prevent low back injuries. *N Engl J Med* 1997;337:332.
5. Hoppenfeld S. *Physical examination of the spine and extremities.* New York: Appleton-Croft, 1976.
6. Katz J, Katz N. Lumbar spine disease. In: *Treatment of rheumatic disease.* WB Saunders, 1994.
7. Klippel JH, Dieppe P. *Practical rheumatology.* London: Times Mirror, 1995.
8. Kolba KS. The approach to the acute joint and synovial fluid examination. *Prim Care* 1984;11:211–218.
9. Pinals RS. Polyarthritis and fever. *N Engl J Med* 1994;330:769–774.
10. Snider RK. *Essentials of musculoskeletal care.* American Academy of Orthopedic Surgeons, 1997.

ARTHRITIS: OSTEOARTHRITIS, RHEUMATOID ARTHRITIS, GOUT

OSTEOARTHRITIS

Introduction

- Present in 10% to 20% of people older than 65 years; responsible for >30% of all office visits to primary care doctors

Pathophysiology/Clinical Presentation

- Defined by cartilage degeneration and bone hypertrophy at articular margins.
- Risk factors: age, female gender, race, genetic factors, joint trauma, repetitive stress, obesity, prior inflammatory joint disease

Evaluation

History

- Insidious onset of articular stiffness, gelling after inactivity, morning stiffness, decreased range of motion and function; commonly affects hips, knees, spine (lumbar and cervical), hands (distal interphalangeal [DIP] joints, carpometacarpal joints)

Physical Examination

- Crepitus and tender spots around joint margins, bony enlargement, not warm or swollen (inflammation is not an important part of pathogenesis)
  ⇒ Hip: antalgic gait, loss of internal rotation, loss of flexion/extension
  ⇒ Cervical spondyloses: Bony spurs, buckling of interlaminar ligaments causes pain with motion, paraspinal muscle spasm, headaches, and radiation of pain to arms.
  ⇒ Spinal stenosis: Enlargement of facet joints of lumbosacral spine entraps nerve roots and leads to buttock/posterior thigh and calf pain.

Laboratory Data

- Synovial fluid analysis only needed when diagnosis is unclear.
- *X-rays:* Narrowing of joint space, subchondral sclerosis and cyst formation, marginal osteophytes. No correlation between severity of radiographic findings and clinical symptoms.

Treatment

Nonpharmacologic

- Strength training: quadriceps strengthening in patients with knee osteoarthritis (OA)
- Physical therapy: training on safe exercise methods and ways to compensate for arthritis

- Patient education: self-management programs (e.g., Arthritis Foundation Self-Management Program)
- Weight loss: clear correlation between obesity and knee arthritis. Even moderate weight loss anecdotally improves arthritis symptoms.
- Canes: Often underutilized in knee/hip disease; should be held in the opposite hand.
- Medial taping of the patella: Symptom relief in knee OA
- Cervical collar/traction: Soft cervical collar worn 24 hours a day has benefit in C-spine OA but takes several weeks for symptom improvement. Cervical traction can also be helpful.
- Diathermy: ultrasound to bring heat into the joint before exertion; no benefit over exercise alone in trials

Pharmacologic

- Acetaminophen: first-line agent; effective for mild to moderate disease at doses up to 1,000 mg four times a day (q.i.d.)
- Nonsteroidal antiinflammatory drugs (NSAIDs): better in more severe disease (Dieppe, 1993)
  ⇒ COX-2–specific agents: equal though not superior efficacy; lesser risk of gastrointestinal (GI) bleeding; significantly increased cost. In patients with risk factors for GI bleeding (age older than 65 year, oral glucocorticoid use, history of ulcer disease, anticoagulants, high-dose NSAIDs, concurrent use of aspirin) then either a COX-2 agent or an NSAID with a gastroprotective agent (H_2-blocker or proton pump inhibitor) is appropriate.
- Tramadol: synthetic opioid analogue that does not appear to induce addiction (unscheduled). Fifty mg q.i.d. for patients who failed NSAIDs or have a contraindication (American College of Rheumatology, 2000).
- Glucosamine: 1,500 mg every day (q.d.) as effective or slightly better than NSAIDs in multiple randomized controlled trials; preliminary evidence that it slows disease progression
- Chondroitin sulfate: 1,200 mg q.d. may have synergistic effect with glucosamine; trials are underway.
- Topical methyl salicylate creams: poor evidence; benefit may be from systemic absorption.
- Capsaicin: Extract of chili peppers with topical analgesic properties has modest benefit.
- Intraarticular glucocorticoids: No good trials, but widely used and anecdotally effective, particularly in knees when the joints are painful and swollen.
- Hyaluronic acid injections: New option for knee OA unresponsive to conservative therapy; >50% efficacy, but good data not available. Mechanism unknown (effect longer than life of injected medication). Expensive.

Surgery

- Arthroscopic: optimal use controversial; no well-controlled trials evaluating arthroscopy (joint lavage and debridement appear equal in efficacy). Many patients report significant relief, although placebo effect is possible.
- Joint replacement: indicated for radiologic evidence of disease with moderate to severe, persistent pain inadequately controlled with nonsurgical options.

RHEUMATOID ARTHRITIS

Introduction

- Prevalence 1% in adult populations worldwide; increases with age (>10% of patients older than 65 years).
- More than twice as common in women

Pathophysiology/Clinical Presentation

- Frequently debilitating, destructive polyarthritis involving a chronic, symmetric, sterile, erosive synovitis of peripheral joints, commonly including proximal interphalangeal (PIP) joints, MCP joints, wrists, knees, ankles, metatarsophalangeal (MTP) joints, and the cervical spine.

- Underlying etiology unknown, although genetic factors contribute: incidence is higher in patients with a positive family history and/or class II major histocompatibility complex DR1 and DR4.

Evaluation

History/Physical Examination (Table 45.1)

- Systemic symptoms: Fatigue may dominate early clinical presentation; fever, weight loss in severe cases.
- Joint immobilization, muscle spasm/shortening, bone/cartilage destruction, joint deformities: ulnar deviation; swan neck deformity (MCP flexion, PIP hyperextension, DIP flexion); boutonniere deformity (PIP flexion, DIP hyperextension); cock-up deformities; subluxations of the MTP heads in the feet
- Rheumatoid nodules (20% to 30% of patients): subcutaneously along tendon sheaths, in bursae, and areas subjected to mechanical pressure; also found in lung, pleura, pericardium, sclera.
- Pulmonary findings: interstitial lung disease (fibrosis of bases more than apices); pleural effusions (characteristically low glucose)
- Cardiac findings: pericarditis, pericardial effusion, aortitis
- Ophthalmologic findings: keratoconjunctivitis, sicca syndrome, episcleritis, scleritis
- Vascular findings: Raynaud's phenomenon, small nailfold infarcts, palpable purpura, leukocytoclastic vasculitis

Laboratory/Radiology

- High erythrocyte sedimentation rate (ESR) and C-reactive peptide, increased globulin, decreased complement levels during periods of active disease. Anemia of chronic disease common. Positive rheumatoid factor (levels correlate only loosely with disease activity).
- Plain films: erosions, deformities, and periarticular decalcification of bone

TABLE 45.1. 1987 REVISED AMERICAN COLLEGE OF RHEUMATOLOGY DIAGNOSTIC CRITERIA[a]

Morning stiffness of at least 1 hr
Arthritis in more than three joints simultaneously (soft tissue swelling or joint effusions)
Hand joint arthritis
Simultaneous symmetric joint involvement
Rheumatoid nodules: subcutaneous nodules over extensor surfaces/bony prominences
+ Rheumatoid factor
Radiographic changes consistent with rheumatoid arthritis

[a] One to four symptoms must be present for at least 6 wk; a physician must observe two to five of the above signs. Need four of seven criteria; sensitivity 91–94%, specificity 89%.

Treatment

- *Patient education:* rest, exercise, management of symptoms, disease course
- *Physical therapy:* Maintain range of motion, muscle strength; teach joint protection.
- *NSAIDs:* first-line treatment of rheumatoid arthritis
- *Low-dose glucocorticoids:* rapid symptom relief; may retard progression of bony erosions.
- *Slow-acting/disease-modifying antirheumatic drugs (DMARDs)* decrease the destructive capacity of the disease.
  ⇒ Methotrexate, gold, D-penicillamine, antimalarials (retinal toxicity), sulfasalazine
  ⇒ 1 to 6 months for full efficacy; may use two agents if monotherapy fails.
- *Intraarticular glucocorticoids:* transitional relief (supplements other therapies)
- *Immunosuppressive therapies:* for patients who fail DMARDs (azathioprine, cyclophosphamide)

- *Anti-tumor necrosis factor*-α (TNF-α) drugs (Weinblatt et al., 1999; Lipsky, 2000; Bathon, 2000):
  ⇒ Promising new agents slow disease progression at a rate equal to or better than methotrexate, minimal side effects, although some reports of reactivation tuberculosis. Average cost $10,000 to $12,000 a year.
  ⇒ Etanercept: TNF-α type II receptor immunoglobulin G1 fusion protein; twice-weekly subcutaneous injections.
  ⇒ Infliximab: chimeric monoclonal antibody against TNF-α; every 1 to 2 months intravenously.
  ⇒ Exact indications, dosing regimen, and use in combination with methotrexate still unclear. Currently used in DMARDs-refractory patients.

GOUT

Introduction

- Ten times more common in men than women; peak incidence in the fifth decade. Prevalence in the United States is 8.4 per 1,000 individuals (Lawrence et al., 1998); most common cause of inflammatory arthritis in men older than 30 years.

Pathophysiology/Clinical Presentation

- Metabolic disease caused by abnormal deposition of urate (monosodium urate monohydrate).
- Gouty arthritis characterized by severe attacks of acute or recurrent articular and periarticular arthritis and by microtophi. Hyperuricemia in itself does not necessitate treatment.
- Risk factors: obesity, hypertriglyceridemia, diabetes mellitus, food or alcohol excess, surgery, infection, diuretics, dehydration

Evaluation

- *Acute gouty arthritis:* Painful, monoarticular arthritis of feet, ankles, or knees. Podagra is involvement of the great toe MTP joint. Severe inflammatory response (pain, warmth, erythema) within hours; patients may have fever, elevated white blood cell count and ESR.
- *Intercritical gout:* asymptomatic intervals between attacks; physical examination unremarkable unless tophi are present, but urate crystals can be aspirated from previously affected joints in 70% of these patients.
- *Tophi:* Nodular deposits of urate crystals that lead to a foreign body reaction; typically appear after 10 years of gouty arthritis; may be found in Heberden nodes, bursae, Achilles tendons, pinna of the ear.
- *Chronic gouty arthritis:* May cause gross deformities, functional loss, and disability.
- *Urate nephrolithiasis:* Occurs in about 20% of patients with gout; more likely to occur in patients with increased urate excretion, low urine pH, or family or personal history of urate calculi.

Diagnosis

- Joint aspiration:
  ⇒ More than 85% sensitive in acute attack, less so in intercritical periods; distinguishes gout from other crystal-induced arthritides (calcium pyrophosphate dihydrate, calcium hydroxyapatite, calcium oxalate).
  ⇒ Polarized microscopy shows bright yellow, needle-shaped, negatively birefringent (parallel to the axis marked on polarizer) monosodium urate crystals, either intracellular or extracellular.
  ⇒ Cloudy fluid, with 20,000 to 100,000 leukocytes/mm^3, mostly neutrophils.
  ⇒ **Cultures are critical**; infection may coexist with an acute attack, or a septic joint may masquerade as gout.
- Tophi aspiration: Urate crystals within tophi are diagnostic.

- Historical/clinical diagnosis (less specific):
  ⇒ Classic history of monoarticular arthritis with asymptomatic intercritical periods
  ⇒ Hyperuricemia
  ⇒ Resolution of symptoms with colchicine therapy

Laboratory/Radiographs

- Serum urate levels useful long term, not helpful in acute attack. 24-hour urine for uric acid guides prophylactic therapy.
- Affected joints demonstrate soft tissue swelling, "punched-out" erosions with sclerotic margins, calcifications.

Treatment

- *Asymptomatic hyperuricemia:* no treatment (except for patients undergoing chemotherapy who are at risk for acute nephropathy)
- *Acute gouty arthritis:*
  ⇒ Colchicine: when the diagnosis is in question (specific response aids diagnosis) or in patients who cannot take NSAIDs. Dose is 0.6 mg orally every hour until improvement, side effects (GI), or ten doses. Some rheumatologists now recommend 0.6 mg p.o. b.i.d. rather than loading dose.
  ⇒ NSAIDs: first line with established diagnosis. Use highest approved dose of either indomethacin (traditional NSAID used for gout) or other NSAIDs until there is resolution.
  ⇒ Intraarticular glucocorticoids: if the above are contraindicated (renal disease), or in monoarticular disease
  ⇒ Oral steroids: if the above are ineffective or contraindicated
- *Intercritical/chronic gout:*
  ⇒ Lifestyle changes: Decrease alcohol; avoid dehydration (including diuretic induced) and foods high in purine (meats, beans, peas, spinach, beer).
  ⇒ Probenecid/sulfinpyrazone: For underexcretors (24-hour urine uric acid <800 mg per day). Avoid in those with renal insufficiency or a history of any kind of nephrolithiasis.
  ⇒ Allopurinol: Blocks conversion of purines to urate; used for overproducers or patients with tophaceous gout.
  ⇒ Lifelong treatment with antigout prophylaxis is not indicated in patients with infrequent episodes.
  ⇒ An acute decrease in uric acid levels may precipitate a gouty attack, so treatment medications should be given as prophylactic medications are started.
  ⇒ Titrate the medications to a goal uric acid level of 5.0 to 6.0; combination therapy is sometimes required. Watch for multiple-drug interactions.

SELECTED REFERENCES

1. American College of Rheumatology. Guidelines for monitoring drug therapy in rheumatoid arthritis. *Arthritis Rheum* 1996;39: 723–731.
2. American College of Rheumatology. Guidelines for the management of rheumatoid arthritis. *Arthritis Rheum* 1996;39:713–722.
3. American College of Rheumatology. Recommendations for the medical management of osteoarthritis of the hip and knee. *Arthritis Rheum* September 2000;43(9).
4. Bathon MB. A comparison of etanercept and methotrexate in patients with early rheumatoid arthritis. *N Engl J Med* 2000;343:1586–1593.
5. Bradley JD. Comparison of an anti-inflammatory dose of Ibuprofen, an analgesic dose of ibuprofen and acetaminophen in the treatment of patients with osteoarthritis of the knee. *N Engl J Med* 1991;325:87–91.
6. Dieppe P, Basler HD, Chard J, et al. Knee replacement surgery for osteoarthritis: effectiveness, practice variations, indications, and possible determinants of utilization. *Rheumatology* 1999;38(1):73–83.
7. Dieppe P. A two-year placebo-controlled trial of non-steroidal anti-inflammatory agents in osteoarthritis of the knee. *Br J Rheum* 1993;35:595–600.
8. Emmerson BT. The management of gout. *N Engl J Med* 1996;334:445–451.
9. Katz J, Katz N. Lumbar spine disease in treatment of rheumatic disease. WB Saunders, 1994.
10. LaPrade RF, Swiontkowski MF. New horizons in the treatment of osteoarthritis of the knee. *JAMA* 1999; 281(10):876–878.

11. Lawrence RC, Helmick CG, Arnett FC, et al. Estimates of the prevalence of arthritis and selected musculoskeletal disorders in the United States. *Arthritis Rheum* 1998;41:778.

12. Lipsky PE. Infliximab and methotrexate in the treatment of rheumatoid arthritis. *N Engl J Med* 2000; 343: 1594–1602.

13. Matteson EL. Current treatment strategies for rheumatoid arthritis. *Mayo Clin Proc* 2000;75:69–74.

14. Pittman JR, Bross MH. Diagnosis and management of gout. *Am Fam Phys* 1999;59(7):1799–1806.

15. Schumacher HR. Crystal-induced arthritis: an overview. *Am J Med* 1996;100(2A):2A, 46S–52S.

16. Terkeltaub R. Gout: epidemiology, pathology and pathogenesis. In: Schumacher HR, ed. *Primer on the rheumatic diseases,* 10th ed. Atlanta, GA: Arthritis Foundation, 1993:209–213.

17. Weinblatt ME, Kremer JM, Bankhurst AD, et al. A trial of etanercept, a recombinant tumor necrosis factor receptor: Fc fusion protein, in patients with rheumatoid arthritis receiving methotrexate. *N Engl J Med* 1999;340(4):253–259.

46

ACUTE LOW BACK PAIN

INTRODUCTION

- Spinal and paraspinal symptoms in the lumbosacral region; may be acute (duration <2 to 4 weeks), subacute (<12 weeks), or chronic (>12 weeks).
- 60% to 90% of individuals have an episode of low back pain (LBP) during their life. Equal incidence in men and women, with onset usually between ages 30 and 50 years.
- The annual societal cost of back pain in the United States is between $20 and $50 billion; common cause of disability and lost work in patients younger than 45 years; most common reason for visits to orthopedists and neurosurgeons; second most common reason for problem visits to generalists.

PATHOPHYSIOLOGY

- Etiology unknown in up to 85% of cases, attributed to musculoligamentous injuries. Good prognosis (75% to 90% of patients report spontaneous improvement within 1 month), although recurrence is common.
- Occasionally, LBP represents a serious underlying problem that must be identified.
- Risk factors: physically demanding occupations, cigarette smoking, obesity, psychosocial issues
- Findings associated with poor outcomes: history of chronic pain, depression, substance abuse, litigation or disability compensation, job-related or home stress

DIFFERENTIAL DIAGNOSIS (TABLE 46.1)

TABLE 46.1. DIFFERENTIAL DIAGNOSIS OF LOW BACK PAIN (LBP)

Musculoligamentous injuries >70% cases of LBP	Partial tears, overuse and inflammation of muscle fibers/distal ligaments cause local tenderness, usually without injury to nerve roots. Includes degenerative processes of discs, usually age related.
Disc herniation ~4% cases LBP	Compression and irritation of lower lumbar and upper sacral nerve roots are most commonly due to a posterior-lateral disc herniation.
Spinal stenosis ~3% cases of LBP	Narrowing of the central canal or lateral recesses of the canal, typically an age-related degenerative process.
Cauda equina syndrome 0.04% cases of LBP	Compression of the nerve roots of the cauda equina due to a space-occupying lesion (central disc herniation, tumor, abscess).
Vertebral compression fracture 4% cases of LBP	Pathologic, spontaneous fractures in patients with severe osteoporosis, long-term steroid use or lytic bone metastases; only occur with trauma in normal bone.
Anatomic anomalies (scoliosis, spondylolisthesis) 3%	Forward subluxation of one vertebral body over another, usually L4-5, L5-S1.

(continued)

TABLE 46.1. *(continued)*

Neoplasm 0.7% cases of LBP	Multiple myeloma the most common primary; metastases more common overall (lung, breast, prostate, gastrointestinal or genitourinary; renal cell and thyroid cause lytic lesions).
Infection 0.01% cases of LBP	Vertebral osteomyelitis, epidural abscess, septic discitis, shingles, paraspinal abscess.
Inflammatory arthritis 0.3% cases of LBP	Ankylosing spondylitis, inflammatory bowel disease, psoriatic arthritis, Reiter's syndrome.
Visceral conditions (referred or direct pain) 2% cases of LBP	*Pelvic disease:* endometriosis, prostatitis, pelvic inflammatory disease, mittelschmerz, ectopic pregnancy *Renal disease:* nephrolithiasis, pyelonephritis *Vascular disease:* aortic aneurysm *Gastrointestinal disease:* inflammatory bowel disease, diverticulitis, retrocecal appendicitis, peptic ulcer disease, cholecystitis, pancreatitis

EVALUATION

Identify Red Flags to Evaluate for Serious Systemic/Visceral Diseases

- *Cancer:* personal/family history of cancer, unexplained weight loss, failure of conservative therapy. Pain is insidious in onset, nonpositional, and frequently worse at night. Intraspinal tumors present like disc herniation but at a higher vertebral level with progression despite conservative treatment.
- *Spinal infections:* recent or ongoing urinary or skin infections, indwelling catheter, or injection drug use. Fever not common, but concerning when present (specific). Pain tends to be dull and continuous.
- *Compression fractures:* significant trauma, age older than 50 years, corticosteroid use, osteoporosis. Acutely painful with local radiation across back.
- *Ankylosing spondylitis:* morning stiffness, improvement with exercise, onset at age younger than 40 years, slow onset, pain for at least 3 months
- *Vascular or visceral etiologies:* Pain not related to activity, worse when lying down or not positional, night pain, presence of atherosclerotic risk factors, gastrointestinal or genitourinary symptoms

Identify Neurologic Compromise

- *Sciatica:* sharp, burning pains radiating down lateral or posterior aspect of one or both legs to below the knee (usually foot or ankle); may include dermatomal sensory loss/paresthesias and localized motor weakness. Indicative of nerve root irritation (98% involve L5 or S1 roots); history of sciatica is 95% sensitive for disc herniation
- *Cauda equina syndrome:* a medical emergency involving spinal cord compression, with progression of symptoms from pain to motor/sensory dysfunction to loss of bowel/bladder control, ending in paralysis
  ⇒ Symptoms: leg or foot weakness/numbness, saddle anesthesia, difficulty with or decreased urination (urinary retention 90% sensitive, 95% specific), bowel problems
- *Spinal stenosis:* leg pain with standing, walking ("neurogenic claudication"), or any activity in which the back is extended; relieved by positions in which the back is flexed, such as sitting

Physical Examination

- Inspect for symmetry, posture, and flexibility, along with hyperkyphosis, hyperlordosis, and scoliosis.
  ⇒ Spasm, abnormal posture, flattening of lordosis, and splinting (asymmetry) often indicate muscular etiology, although lower disc herniation may also cause paraspinal muscle spasm.
  ⇒ Severe guarding of lumbar motion may indicate infection, fracture, or tumor.
  ⇒ Flexion (bending forward) limited by paraspinal muscle spasm and spondylosis; extension (leaning backward) limited by nerve root compression or spinal stenosis.

- Palpation: Assess pain severity, spinal versus paraspinal location, lumbosacral junction for step-off indicative of spondylolisthesis. Hypersensitivity to light touch indicates psychologic overlay.
- Tests for sciatica:
  ⇒ Straight-leg raise (SLR): Hip flexion with the knee extended while seated or supine; sensitive but not specific for nerve root irritation. A positive response is pain below the knee, elicited between 15° and 45°, increased with ankle dorsiflexion. Contralateral pain with SLR more specific but less sensitive.
  ⇒ Postures: Sitting stretches sciatic nerve (L5, S1—passes posterior to hip) but not the femoral nerve (L2, L3, L4—passes anterior to hip).
- Neurologic evaluation: elicit signs of disc herniation (see Table 46.2)

TABLE 46.2. NERVE ROOT INNERVATION

Root	Motor	Sensory	Reflex
L-2	Iliopsoas	Anterior thigh, groin	None
L-3	Quadriceps	Inner thigh/anterior knee	Patellar
L-4	Quadriceps	Inner leg/ankle	Patellar
L-5	Ankle dorsiflexion	Dorsum of foot	None
S-1	Ankle plantarflexion	Lateral plantar foot	Achilles

  ⇒ Cauda equina syndrome: diminished anal sphincter tone, saddle anesthesia, unilateral/bilateral sciatica. Babinski sign may be positive in cord compression.
- Waddell's signs suggest psychological overtones (predict chronic course of pain)
  ⇒ Tenderness unrelated to anatomic structures, superficial (light touch), or widespread
  ⇒ Inconsistent performance of seated versus supine SLR test
  ⇒ Pain on simulated axial loading (top of head) or spine rotation
  ⇒ Neurologic deficits without physiologic or anatomic explanation
  ⇒ General overreaction during examination

Laboratory/Radiologic Studies

- Radiologic abnormalities do not correlate well with symptoms; common in asymptomatic patients (about 30% of patients younger than 30 years, nearly all patients older than 60 have disc degeneration). Imaging occasionally indicated:
  ⇒ *Plain films of the lumbar spine (anteroposterior [AP] and lateral):* risk factors for vertebral fracture (trauma, chronic steroid use, osteoporosis), no improvement with 1 month of conservative therapy
  ⇒ *Computed tomography:* Evaluate bony abnormalities and lumbar disk herniation (after a month of persistent symptoms).
  ⇒ *Magnetic resonance imaging (MRI):* Evaluate for spinal stenosis, cord compression, osteomyelitis, epidural abscess.
  ⇒ *Bone scan:* Screen for osteomyelitis, although MRI is equally effective.
- Laboratory evaluation: Screen for tumors/infection (complete blood cell count, erythrocyte sedimentation rate, urinalysis) if history and physical examination warrant.

TREATMENT

- The following treatment strategy is recommended for patients in whom the cause of acute LBP is either nonspecific or likely disc disease, and in whom serious systemic disease has been excluded.
- *Patient education* regarding natural history and prognosis: Symptoms are usually self-limited and further testing is rarely indicated, although patients with sciatica may have a longer recovery time. Printed patient information is helpful.

- *"Usual activity:"* equal or improved outcomes with usual activity as tolerated, rather than bed rest or back-mobilizing exercises. Limiting prolonged sitting, avoiding twisting or unassisted lifting, and early low-stress aerobic activity, particularly walking, may hasten recovery.
- *Medications:* NSAIDs or acetaminophen (on a regular schedule) are usually sufficient pain relief; co-morbid conditions and side effects may limit their use. No definitive studies have supported the use of muscle relaxants: Use should be limited to a few days. Narcotics should be avoided.
- *Physical therapy:* May hasten recovery for patients whose symptoms do not improve with 2 weeks of conservative treatment, but no change in outcomes at 3 months. Physical therapy and chiropractic manipulation appear to offer only marginal benefit, if any, over patient education and are not cost-effective.
- Therapies of unclear or unproven benefit are available for patients with acute and chronic symptoms:
  ⇒ Acupuncture: for acute symptoms; equivocal data
  ⇒ Massage: for acute symptoms; very safe
  ⇒ Steroid injections: Used for chronic symptoms, although there is little supporting evidence.
  ⇒ Transcutaneous electrical nerve stimulation and biofeedback may be helpful on a case-by-case basis for chronic symptoms; few randomized data.
- Referral for surgical evaluation (neurosurgery or orthopedics):
  ⇒ Cauda equina syndrome: immediate referral/imaging
  ⇒ Sciatica: Consider nerve root decompression if severe and disabling sciatica persists for over 4 to 6 weeks.
  ⇒ Spinal stenosis: Consider surgery after 3 months if there is associated disability or pain.
- Referral to neurology:
  ⇒ Patients with moderate or severe leg pain, with equivocal or absent nerve root findings, and who have failed conservative treatment.

SELECTED REFERENCES

1. Atlas SJ, Deyo RA. Evaluating and managing acute low back pain in the primary care setting. *J Gen Intern Med* 2001;16:120–131.
2. Bigos S. *Clinical practice guideline number 14: acute low back problems in adults: assessment and treatment.* Rockville, MD: US Dept of Health and Human Services, Agency for Health Care Policy and Research; December 1994. AHCPR publication 95-0642.
3. Cherkin DC, Deyo RA, Battie M, et al. A comparison of physical therapy, chiropractic manipulation, and provision of an educational booklet for the treatment of patients with low back pain. *N Engl J Med* 1998; 339:1021–1029.
4. Deyo RA, Weinstein JN. Low back pain. *N Engl J Med* 2001;344:363–370.
5. Malmivaara A, Hakkinen U, Aro T, et al. The treatment of acute low back pain—bed rest, exercises, or ordinary activity? *N Engl J Med* 1995;332(6):351–355.
6. Powell MC, Wilson M, Szypryt P, et al. Prevalence of lumbar disc degeneration observed by magnetic resonance in symptomless women. *Lancet* 1986;2:1366–1367.
7. Skargren EI, Oberg BE, Carlsson PG, et al. Cost and effectiveness analysis of chiropractic and physiotherapy treatment for low back and neck pain. *Spine* 1997;22:2167–2177.
8. Vroomen P, deKrom MC, Wilmink JT, et al. Lack of effectiveness of bed rest for sciatica. *N Engl J Med* 1999;340:418–423.

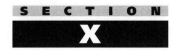

DERMATOLOGY

BENIGN SKIN CONDITIONS: PSORIASIS, ACNE VULGARIS, ROSACEA, WARTS, ECZEMA, TINEA, URTICARIA

PSORIASIS

Introduction

- Seen in 2% of people with European ancestry (Stern, 1997); positive family history in 30% of cases.
- Presentation ranges from asymptomatic localized plaques to uncomfortable generalized lesions; onset typically in patients in their 20s.

Pathophysiology/Clinical Presentation

- Shortened keratinocyte cell cycle: epidermal transit time reduced from 30 to 45 days to 3 days, preventing normal cell maturation and keratinization
- Psoriatic lesions: erythematous, sharply demarcated plaques, covered by silvery scales; commonly found on elbows, knees, lower back, buttocks, scalp, genitalia, and intertriginous areas; nail pitting or yellow-brown subungual discoloration seen in 50% of patients
- Flares: May be precipitated by stress, medications (β-blockers, lithium, nonsteroidal antiinflammatory drugs, interferon-α (IFN-α), and progesterone), streptococcal infections, human immunodeficiency virus (HIV), ethanol, or sunburn.

Treatment

- *General recommendations*
  ⇒ Avoid hot showers; moisturize skin with petroleum jelly after bathing.
  ⇒ Control itching with antihistamines as needed.
  ⇒ Scalp: antidandruff or tar-based shampoo, followed by steroid preparation, (e.g. fluocinolone acetonide or betamethasone valerate). Some patients may prefer one vehicle (mousse, lotion, solution) over another.
  ⇒ Careful sun exposure may be helpful.
- *Mild psoriasis:* (<10% body surface area [BSA]):
  ⇒ Topical vitamin D twice daily (calcipotriene ointment 0.005%) or topical steroids (hydrocortisone 1% on face and groin; fluocinolone acetonide 0.025% or fluocinonide 0.05% elsewhere)
  ⇒ New vitamin D analogue maxacalcitol may be superior to calcipotriene (Lebwohl, 2000).
- *Moderate psoriasis* (10% to 50% body surface area [BSA]): Dermatology-guided ultraviolet light therapy (ultraviolet B [UVB] or oral administration of psoralen and subsequent exposure to long-wavelength ultraviolet A [PUVA]).
- *Severe psoriasis* (>50% BSA): UVB and PUVA combined with oral agents (etretinate, methotrexate, hydroxyurea) to restore keratinocyte differentiation. Methotrexate for psoriatic arthritis.

- *Combination therapy:* more effective than any agent or modality alone (e.g., calcipotriene with halobetasol, calcipotriene with psoralen and PUVA, tazarotene gel with UVB or topical steroids, retinoids and UVB or PUVA) (Lebwohl, 2000).
- *Novel therapies:* Oral cyclosporine microemulsion and injectable inhibitors of T-cell activation show promise in trials.

ACNE VULGARIS

Introduction

- Common disorder with highest incidence in teenage years, decreasing in adulthood.

Pathophysiology/Clinical Presentation

- Retained stratum corneum of the pilosebaceous follicle ruptures due to pressure of increased sebum/keratin production and proliferation of *Propionibacterium acnes* (Usatine and Quan, 2000).
- Noninflammatory lesions: closed comedones are white 1- to 2-mm micropapules (whiteheads). Follicles that open onto the skin become open comedones (blackheads).
- Inflammatory lesions: erythematous papules, pustules, cysts, or abscesses caused by comedo wall leak or rupture
- Face, neck, chest, upper back, and upper arms most commonly affected; exacerbated by trauma (harsh scrubs or tight clothing), stress, oil-based makeup, genetics, androgens, and some medications (steroids, lithium, isoniazid) (Usatine and Quan, 2000).

Treatment

- *General:* Avoid oil-based products (glycerine soaps instead). Apply medication broadly, beyond just affected areas. Patients must be aware that weeks or months of therapy may be needed for results.
- *Comedonal (obstructive, noninflammatory):*
  ⇒ Topical tretinoin (Retin-A) 0.025% cream (dry skin) or 0.01% gel (oily skin) qhs increase slowly. Adapalene 0.01% gel (oily skin) or cream (dry skin) is less irritating than tretinoin, which may cause dryness/redness.
  ⇒ Other agents better tolerated than tretinoin but less effective, such as salicylic acid (Brown and Shalita, 1998), benzoyl peroxide, azelaic acid (Azelex), and alphahydroxy acids (Usatine and Quan, 2000).
- *Mild papulopustular:* Benzoyl peroxide (2.5% to 10%) or topical antibiotics (erythromycin or clindamycin as pads, gels, solutions, or lotions), alone or in combination, daily or twice daily. Tretinoin, adapalene (Differin), azelaic acid, and oral antibiotics are also effective (Usatine, 2000).
- *Moderate papulopustular:*
  ⇒ Benzoyl peroxide and topical antibiotics remain first line.
  ⇒ Comedones: tretinoin, adapalene, or azelaic acid useful. Systemic antibiotics (tetracycline, doxycycline, or minocycline) are also helpful for inflammatory component.
  ⇒ Ortho-TriCyclen improves acne (Usatine and Quan, 2000), possibly a class effect of oral contraceptives.
- Severe (nodulocystic) acne: isotretinoin 1 mg/kg per day for 4–5 months. Given teratogenicity, women must give consent, undergo pregnancy tests, and use two forms of birth control.

ROSACEA

Introduction

- Episodic reddening of the face and neck skin with concurrent, centrofacial acneform eruption with papules and pustules, but no comedones.
- Commonly presents between the ages of 40 to 50; more prevalent in women but less severe.

Pathophysiology/Clinical Presentation

- Not well understood: Hypotheses include a relationship to the *Demodex* mite or *Helicobacter pylori* infection.
- Presents as recurrent erythema in the middle third of the face. Symptoms occur after stimuli (spicy food, alcohol, sun exposure) but may progress to persistent redness, acneiform lesions without comedones, or rhinophyma (hypertrophied, bulbous nose).

Treatment

- Avoid hot food and drinks, alcohol, sunlight, and extreme temperatures.
- Metronidazole gel 0.75% (MetroGel) or cream 0.1% (Noritate) twice daily for 9 weeks improves papules and reduces relapse; topical erythromycin and clindamycin or oral tetracycline are also effective.
- Surgical treatment of rhinophyma is highly successful (Thiboutot, 2000).

WARTS

Introduction

- Intraepithelial tumors of the skin caused by infection of basal keratinocytes by human papillomavirus (HPV) (Fazel et al., 1999); prevalence highest among children (20% of school-age children).
- Multiple subtypes of warts: *verruca vulgaris* (70% of cutaneous warts), *verruca plantaris* (plantar warts), *verruca plana* (flat warts seen on face, neck, arms), *condylomata acuminata* (sexually transmitted, associated with HPV-6 or HPV-11 in 90% of cases), and *flat condyloma* (vaginal cervix, associated with HPV-16, -18, -31, -33, and -35, frequently premalignant) (Fazel et al., 1999)

Pathophysiology/Clinical Presentation

- HPV penetrates the epithelium and proliferates in keratinocyte nuclei. Although viral DNA remains in the basal keratinocytes, copies are carried in cells that migrate toward the stratum spinosum (Fazel et al., 1999).
- Each wart has a typical appearance depending on body site; incubation is 2 to 3 months, and more than 60% of cases will resolve spontaneously within 2 years.

Treatment

- **Cryotherapy** (application of liquid nitrogen) is the mainstay treatment of all warts. Other therapies for specific types of warts:
  ⇒ *Verruca vulgaris:* Salicylic acid/lactic acid (Duofilm or occlusal HP) cures 60% to 80% of warts if applied at night for 12 weeks after soaking and filing the warts.
  ⇒ *Verruca plana:* cryosurgery, electrodesiccation, topical tretinoin, laser removal, topical 5-fluorouracil (5-FU) (Fazel et al., 1999)
  ⇒ *Verruca plantaris:* salicylic acid, electrodesiccation, or cryosurgery (Fazel et al., 1999)
  ⇒ *Condylomata acuminata:* monthly topical application of 25% podophyllum (Podofilox); 3 consecutive days Podofilox 0.5% applied topically with 4 days off, repeated over a 4-week cycle; imiquimod gel (Aldara) three times a week for 1 month; cryotherapy; 5-FU cream; laser surgery; electrodesiccation; curettage; surgical excision; interferons (Fazel et al., 1999). Patients must be counseled to use condoms.

ECZEMA

Introduction

- A chronic, pruritic inflammation of the epidermis and dermis, with onset in childhood (90% by age 6) and symptoms improving with age; adult onset should raise concern for systemic immunocompromise (Leung, 2000).

Pathophysiology/Clinical Presentation

- Proposed mechanisms: altered vascular response to stimuli such as heat, cold, foods, and histamines; cytokine mediation; epidermal inflammation; genetics (Leung, 2000). Immunoglobulin E (IgE)–mediated hypersensitivity reaction may be involved, but not definitively established.
- Lesions are ill defined, erythematous patches, with scales and erosions that lichenify with scratching; *Staphylococcus aureus* superinfection is common.
- In infants, lesions may be oozing papules or vesicles seen on chest, face, scalp, and extensor surfaces; lesions in older patients are more typically found on flexor surfaces.

Treatment

- Avoid stress and temperature extremes, including hot showers; hydrate skin with bland emollients.
- Topical steroids: fluocinolone acetonide 0.025% or fluocinonide 0.05% on trunk/extremities, hydrocortisone 1% on face/groin for 2-week blocks (minimizes atrophy) (Leung, 2000).
- Tacrolimus (Protopic) ointment 0.1% twice daily, a nonsteroidal topical immunomodulator: effective without causing atrophy (Fleischer, 1999).
- Systemic antihistamines for severe pruritus; antipruritic lotions or baths (Aveeno, Sarna)
- Novel therapies for refractory cases: recombinant IFN-γ, phosphodiesterase inhibitors, cyclosporine, intravenous immunoglobulin, and leukotriene antagonists all under investigation.

TINEA

Introduction

- Superficial fungal infection of the skin precipitated by moisture, warmth, poor hygiene (shared bathrooms), certain medications, or immune dysfunction (HIV, renal failure, diabetes).

Pathophysiology/Clinical Presentation

- Lesions are caused by the infection of dead keratinocytes by dermatophytes such as *Trichophyton rubrum*, *Trichophyton mentagrophytes*, and *Microsporum canis*.
- Annular scaling plaques on a raised, centrifugally expanding border with central clearing (ring lesions) characteristic everywhere except scalp and nails.
- Confirm clinical diagnosis by direct microscopy with potassium hydroxide preparation (visible hyphae).
- Tinea infections generally named by body location: tinea pedis (feet), tinea manuum (hands), tinea cruris (groin), tinea corporis (body), tinea capitis (scalp), tinea barbae (beard), tinea faciei (face), onychomycosis (nails), and tinea versicolor (pityriasis versicolor: pink or tan macules on the upper trunk, caused by *Malassezia furfur* infection of stratum corneum [Rupke, 2000]). Tinea incognito is the atypical appearance of incompletely treated tinea (Rupke, 2000).

Treatment

- Topical antifungals: for mild to moderate skin cases with no hair or nail involvement
  ⇒ Clotrimazole (Lotrimin), miconazole (Micatin), ketoconazole (Nizoral), and econazole (Spectazole) are equally effective azoles, which inhibit fungal cell membrane synthesis. Newer azoles have not proven superior (Rupke, 2000).
  ⇒ Tinea pedis responds to clotrimazole 1% cream applied twice daily for 4 weeks. Tinea corporis responds to miconazole or clotrimazole applied twice daily for 2 to 3 weeks (Rupke, 2000).
- Selenium sulfate 2.5% (Selsun) or zinc pyrithione (Head and Shoulders) shampoo: 10 to 14 daily applications, left on for 10 minutes and then rinsed off, effective for mild cases
- Systemic therapy: extensive lesions, failure of topical treatment, hair/nail infections
  ⇒ Skin: ketoconazole (200 mg daily) or itraconazole (100 mg daily for 7 to 14 days)
  ⇒ Nails: Lamisil (250 mg daily) or Sporanox (100 mg daily for 3 to 6 months); recurrence common

URTICARIA

Introduction

- Roughly 20% of the general population will experience an urticarial reaction (hives) at some point.
- Acute urticaria of <30 days' duration is characterized by large, transient wheals; chronic urticaria, more common in women, is often idiopathic.
- Both acute and chronic urticaria can be associated with angioedema, a swelling of the dermis and subcutaneous tissues, often in the head and neck threatening the airway (Fitzpatrick et al., 1997).

Pathophysiology/Clinical Presentation

- Multiple mechanisms: IgE-mediated; complement; autoimmune disease; histaminergic release by physical stimuli (cold, pressure, sun exposure), food, or exercise (Fitzpatrick et al., 1997)
- Chronic urticaria: Rule out systemic diseases such as lupus, vasculitis, and lymphoma. Patients with symptoms >6 weeks need a chest x-ray, complete blood cell count, erythrocyte sedimentation rate, urinalysis, and liver and renal function tests (Fitzpatrick et al., 1997).
- Hives: transient, pruritic, edematous papules, and plaques that change over hours

Treatment

- Avoid triggers: foods (shellfish, nuts, strawberries are frequent culprits), physical stimuli
- Pruritus: topical menthol 1% aqueous cream or oral H_1-blockers (Allegra, Zyrtec, or hydroxyzine)
- Doxepin: antidepressant with H_1 activity, effective for chronic symptoms with co-morbid depression.
- Refractory cases: H_2-blocker for 4 to 6 weeks may help prevent recurrence.
- Severe, chronic cases: systemic corticosteroids (prednisone 40 to 60 mg daily with a rapid taper). There may also be a role for systemic immunoglobulin (O'Donnell, 1998).

SELECTED REFERENCES

1. Brown SK, Shalita A. Acne vulgaris. *Lancet* 1998;351:1871–1876.
2. Dahl MV, Katz HI, Krueger GG, et al. Topical metronidazole maintains remissions of rosacea. *Arch Dermatol* 1998;134:679–683.
3. Fazel N, Wilczynski S, Lowe L, et al. Clinical, histopathological, and molecular aspects of cutaneous human papillomavirus infections. *Dermatol Clin* 1999;17:3.
4. Fitzpatrick TB, Johnson RA, Wolff K, et al. *Color atlas and synopsis of clinical dermatology.* New York: McGraw-Hill, 1997.
5. Fleischer AB. Atopic dermatitis: role of tacrolimus ointment as a topical noncorticosteroidal therapy. *J Allergy Immunol* 1999;104:3.
6. Lebwohl M. Advances in psoriasis therapy. *Dermatol Clin* 2000;18:1.
7. Leung DYM. Atopic dermatitis: new insights and opportunities for therapeutic intervention. *J Allergy Clin Immunol* 2000;105:5.
8. O'Donnell BF. Intravenous immunoglobulin in autoimmune chronic urticaria. *Br J Dermatol* January 1998; 138(1):101–106.
9. Rupke SJ. Fungal skin disorders. *Primary Care Clin Office Pract* 2000;27:2.
10. Stern RS. Psoriasis. *Lancet* 1997;350:349–353.
11. Thiboutot DM. Acne and rosacea: new and emerging therapies. *Dermatol Clin* 2000;18:1.
12. Usatine RP, Quan MA. Pearls in the management of acne: an advanced approach. *Primary Care Clin Office Pract* 2000;27:2.

48

SKIN CANCERS

INTRODUCTION

- 47,700 new melanomas and >1 million nonmelanoma skin cancers (NMSCs) are diagnosed each year (Greenlee et al., 2000; Miller and Weinstock, 1994).
- Current lifetime risk of developing a melanoma in the United States is 1 in 75 (Greenlee et al., 2000).

PATHOPHYSIOLOGY (TABLE 48.1)

- Risk factors for skin cancer:
  ⇒ Idiosyncratic: fair skin, changing pigmented lesion, multiple typical nevi, atypical nevi, freckling, personal/family history of melanoma
  ⇒ Environmental: excessive sunlight exposure in childhood, arsenic ingestion, immunosuppression, therapeutic use of long wavelength ultraviolet (UV) radiation (e.g., PUVA [oral administration of *p*soralen and subsequent exposure to long-wavelength *UV l*ight] used to treat psoriasis)
- Risk factors for squamous cell carcinoma (SCC) and basal cell carcinoma (BCC) versus melanoma (Elwood et al., 1985):
  ⇒ NMSCs: continuous sun exposure (total dose); for example, farmers and fishermen
  ⇒ Melanoma: intermittent intense exposure (severe sunburns); for example, "weekend sun worshipers"
- Primary prevention: Majority of lifetime UV exposure is before adulthood (Marks, 1988).
  ⇒ Routine use of a sunscreen with a sun protection factor of 15 (SPF-15) to high-exposure sites decreased incidence of SCC in Australia (Green et al., 1999), and use of an SPF-30 sunscreen decreased nevi formation in children (Gallagher et al., 2000).
  ⇒ Counsel patients to *minimize sun exposure* between 10 a.m. and 4 p.m.; use adequate amounts of *sunscreen with at least an SPF of 15*; use hats, sunglasses, and protective clothing.

TABLE 48.1. DIFFERENTIAL DIAGNOSIS OF SKIN CANCER

	Appearance	Treatment	Comments
Seborrheic keratoses	Multiple, elevated, round papules, horn, cysts, irregular surface, "stuck on" appearance	Surgery or cryotherapy, if desired for cosmetic reasons	Seen on face, trunk, and arms; common and benign
Actinic (solar) keratoses	Well defined, light brown, erythematous flat lesions, irregular surface with adherent, keratotic consistency	Cryotherapy (98.8% cure rate), superficial curettage, electrodesiccation, CO_2 laser, topical fluorouracil	Premalignant lesion. 0.01% progress to squamous cell carcinoma (SCC) if untreated; seen on sun-exposed areas; biopsy large lesions to rule out SCC

(continued)

TABLE 48.1. *(continued)*

	Appearance	Treatment	Comments
Bowen's disease	Resembles localized patch of psoriasis or dermatitis		SCC in situ
Keratoacanthoma	Solitary lesion with central keratin plug	Conservative management, surgical excision, curettage, electrodesiccation, or fluorouracil injection	Sun-damaged skin during the sixth and seventh decades of life; 6–12 mo follow up and full skin examination indicated

EVALUATION

Nonmelanoma Skin Cancers

Basal Cell Carcinoma

- Most common skin cancer: lifetime risk 28% to 33%; 75% of NMSC (Miller and Weinstock, 1994)
- **Risk factors:** cumulative sun exposure, red/blonde hair, blue/green eyes, fair skin, freckling, actinic keratoses, outdoor occupation, older age, low socioeconomic status, immunosuppression, hereditary skin cancer syndromes
- **Clinical features:** translucent/pearly papules with raised areas covered by thin epidermis and telangiectasias; as lesions enlarge, central ulceration with formation of peripheral, rolled border may occur. Typically indolent and slow growing; 80% occur on head and neck. Suspicious lesions need biopsy.
- **Types:** nodular, pigmented, ulcerative, superficial (seen on trunk), sclerosing

Squamous Cell Carcinoma

- 20% of NMSC, with rising incidence. Average presentation at age 60 years; men more than women. May arise de novo or from actinic keratoses (up to 60%) (Marks et al., 1988).
- **Risk factors:** cumulative sun exposure, prior trauma or burn, frostbite, ionizing radiation, PUVA therapy, chemical carcinogens, human papillomavirus (HPV) types 16, 18, and 31, immunosuppression, chronic inflammation, fair skin, hereditary skin cancer syndromes, arsenic exposure
- **Clinical features:** asymptomatic hyperkeratotic papule, nodule, or plaque. Common in sun-exposed areas: head or neck (50% to 60%), hands, forearms, upper trunk, lower leg, mucous membranes. Suspicious lesions need biopsy.

Malignant Melanoma

- Seventh most common cancer in the U.S.; rising incidence (Rigel, 1996). Median age at diagnosis 53 (Koh, 1991); highest risk in Caucasians.
- **Risk factors:** family history (especially first degree relative), congenital or dysplastic nevi, fair skin, blond or red hair, blue eyes, antecedent blistering sunburn, immunosuppression, xeroderma pigmentosum.
- **Clinical features:** arise in pigmented cells of skin, mucous membranes, and eye. ABCDE's of melanoma recognition 95% sensitive; 5% of melanomas nonpigmented (Healsmith et al., 1994) (see Table 48.2)
  ⇒ Presenting symptoms may include pruritus, tenderness, bleeding, or ulceration of an existing lesion.
  ⇒ *Hutchinson's sign:* periungual pigmentation associated with a subungual streak, highly suspicious for melanoma. Nail-plate destruction is also suggestive.

TABLE 48.2. THE *ABCDEs* OF MELANOMA RECOGNITION

Asymmetry	Irregular lesions more concerning than symmetric round to oval lesions
Border irregularity	Notched or irregular borders
Color variation	Irregular pigmentation (different colors within the same lesion)
Diameter	Nevi larger than 6 mm need evaluation
Enlargement	Enlargement over time worrisome

- Subtypes
  - ⇒ *Superficial spreading melanoma:* 70% of cases; occurs during sixth and seventh decades at sites of intermittent sun exposure (legs and backs of women, backs of men). Enlarging, small, pigmented lesion is completely curable in radial growth phase (in situ lesion), but vertical growth phase (may see nodule within plaque) has dermal invasion.
  - ⇒ *Nodular melanoma:* 15% of cases; encompasses amelanotic melanomas. Occurs at sites of intermittent intense sun exposure. Darkly pigmented dome-shaped nodules that may ulcerate and bleed. Amelanotic variants lack pigment and appear as flesh-colored, pink, or erythematous nodules with surrounding halo. Poor prognosis.
  - ⇒ *Lentigo maligna melanoma:* 5% of cases; common in elderly patients. Arise on severely sun-damaged skin as in situ irregular macules with varying hues of dark brown, black, and blue. Prolonged horizontal growth phase: appearance of elevated nodule suggests onset of vertical growth and worse prognosis.
  - ⇒ *Acral lentiginous melanoma:* 10% of cases; predominant subtype among blacks, Asians, and Hispanics. Hyperpigmented blue/black macules with irregular borders arising on palms, soles, and nail beds.
- **Diagnosis:** Excision biopsy must be performed for diagnostic and prognostic purposes.
- **Staging:** based on depth of lesion and extent of metastasis (TNM staging):
  - ⇒ Breslow's classification: tumor thickness to deepest penetration (<0.85 mm, 0.85 to 1.7 mm, 1.7 to 3.6 mm, >3.6 mm); correlates with prognosis.
  - ⇒ Clark's level of invasion: I (confined to epidermis, melanoma in situ); II (penetrates into papillary dermis); III (fills papillary dermis); IV (invades reticular dermis); V (subcutaneous tissue or deeper)
- **Physical examination:** total body skin examination; lymph node palpation
- **Laboratory/radiologic studies:** complete blood cell count, liver function tests, and chest x-ray. Suspected metastatic disease warrants computed tomographic scan of chest/abdomen/pelvis, bone scan, and brain magnetic resonance imaging (lung, liver, brain most common metastatic sites).

TREATMENT

Basal Cell Carcinoma

- **Resection options:** primary resection; curettage and electrodesiccation; Mohs surgery (microscopically controlled excision with immediate pathologic inspection to ensure clear margins); radiotherapy; cryotherapy; laser excision; 5-fluorouracil (5-FU) chemotherapy implants (experimental)
- **Prognosis:** cure rates 90% to 99%; 5% to 10% local recurrence rate, lowest with Mohs excision (1% to 6%). Recurrence risk increases with tumor size, location (highest at eyes, nose, and ears), histologic invasion, resection margin <5 mm.
  - ⇒ Significant chance of local recurrence or second primary NMSC, increased risk for melanoma; frequent skin examinations are warranted.
  - ⇒ Metastatic disease is very rare (<1%).

Squamous Cell Carcinoma

- **Resection options:** surgical excision; Mohs surgery; radiotherapy (primarily in older patients or in an effort to preserve function; combined with surgery for high-risk lesions); diathermy; cryosurgery (for in-situ lesions only).
- Chemotherapy: Reserved for metastatic disease.
- **Prognosis:** >90% surgical cure, varies depending on site.
  - ⇒ Increased risk recurrent NMSCs, as with BCC
  - ⇒ Metastatic disease in 3% of cases, with a 5-year survival rate between 14% and 39%

Malignant Melanoma

- **Excision** with adequate margins (0.5 cm for in situ; 1 to 3 cm for invasive lesions)
  - ⇒ *Elective lymph node dissection:* controversial; indicated if lymph node metastases clinically apparent. No survival advantage in patients with melanomas <1 mm or >4 mm thick (Day and Lew, 1985).
  - ⇒ *Sentinel node biopsy:* Recommended for patients with intermediate and thick melanomas (>1 mm). Identifies for biopsy the first lymph node in the primary drainage basin via pigment or radiolabeling, with node dissection only if the sentinel node is positive. False-negative rate <1% (Morton et al., 1992).
- **Adjuvant therapy**
  - ⇒ Stage II or III: IFN-α associated with a 9-month prolongation in disease-free survival and a 1-year prolongation in overall survival (Kirkwood et al., 1996)
  - ⇒ Stage IV: Combination chemotherapy/radiation yields partial response rates of 15% to 35% (Legha et al., 1996).
  - ⇒ Promising recent results for melanoma vaccines in advanced disease
- *Prognosis:* dependent on stage at diagnosis (see Table 48.3)

TABLE 48.3. PROGNOSIS OF MELANOMA ACCORDING TO INVASION DEPTH AND STAGING (JOHNSON ET AL., 1995)

Primary Lesion Thickness	5-yr Survival
<0.85 mm	98%
+ regression	90–95%
0.85–1.69 mm	80–90%
(+) Nodes	70–75%
1.70–33.65 mm	70–75%
(+) nodes	45–50%
>3.65 mm	25–35%
(+) nodes	0–20%

- *Follow-up:* Educate about "ABCDE's" (see Table 48.2); frequent self-examinations
  - ⇒ For in situ lesions: biannual office visits for 1 year, then annually
  - ⇒ For all other lesions: office visits every 3 months for 2 years, every 6 months for 3 years, and then annually. Recurrence after 10 years is not uncommon. Some experts recommend yearly chest x-rays; other studies only as indicated by symptoms or signs.

SELECTED REFERENCES

1. Day CL, Lew RA. Malignant melanoma prognostic factors 7: elective lymph node dissection. *J Dermatol Surg Oncol* 1985;11:233.
2. Elwood JM, Gallagher RP, Hill GB, et al. Cutaneous melanoma in relation to intermittent and constant sun exposure—the Western Canada Melanoma Study. *Int J Cancer* 1985;35:427.
3. Fleming ID, Cooper JS, Henson DE, et al., eds. *AJCC (American Joint Committee on Cancer) cancer staging manual,* 5th ed. Philadelphia: Lippincott–Raven Publishers, 1997.
4. Gallagher RP, Rivers JK, Lee TK, et al. Broad-spectrum sunscreen use and the development of new nevi in white children. *JAMA* 2000;283:2955.

5. Green A, Williams G, Neale R, et al. Daily sunscreen application and betacarotene supplementation in prevention of basal-cell and squamous-cell carcinomas of the skin: a randomised controlled trial. *Lancet* 1999;354:723.

6. Greenlee RT, Murray T, Bolden S, et al. Cancer statistics, 2000. *CA Cancer J Clin* 2000;50:7.

7. Healsmith MF, Bourke JF, Osborne JE, et al. An evaluation of the seven-point checklist for the early diagnosis of cutaneous malignant melanoma. *Br J Dermatol* 1994;130:48.

8. Johnson TM, Smith JW, Nelson BR, et al. Current therapy for cutaneous melanoma. *J Am Acad Dermatol* 1995;32:689.

9. Kirkwood JM, Strawderman MH, Ernstoff MS, et al. Interferon alfa-2b adjuvant therapy of high-risk resected cutaneous melanoma: The Eastern Cooperative Oncology Group trial EST 1684. *J Clin Oncol* 1996;14:7.

10. Koh HK. Cutaneous melanoma. *N Engl J Med* 1991;325:171.

11. Legha SS, Ring S, Bedikian A, et al. Treatment of metastatic melanoma with combined chemotherapy containing cisplatin, vinblastine and dacarbazine and biotherapy using interleukin-2 and interferon-alpha. *Ann Oncol* 1996;7:827.

12. Marks R. Role of childhood in the development of skin cancer. *Aust Paediatr J* 1988;24:337.

13. Marks R, Rennie G, Selwood TS. Malignant transformation of solar keratoses to squamous cell carcinoma. *Lancet* 1988;1:795.

14. Miller DL, Weinstock MA. Nonmelanoma skin cancer in the United States: incidence. *J Am Acad Dermatol* 1994;30:774.

15. Morton DL, Wen DR, Wong JH, et al. Technical details of intraoperative lymphatic mapping for early stage melanoma. *Arch Surg* 1992;127:392.

16. Rhodes AR, Weinstock MA, Fitzpatrick TB, et al. Risk factors for cutaneous melanoma. *JAMA* 1987;258:3146.

17. Rigel DS, Friedman RJ, Kopf AW. The incidence of malignant melanoma in the United States: issues as we approach the 21st century. *J Am Acad Dermatol* 1996;34:839.

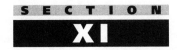

SECTION
XI

NEUROLOGY/OPTHAMOLOGY

49

HEADACHE

INTRODUCTION

- Affects nearly 75% of all Americans annually, although only about 5% seek medical help.
- Two thirds of patients list headache as a major symptom in visits to physicians' offices or emergency rooms.

PATHOPHYSIOLOGY/CLINICAL PRESENTATION (TABLE 49.1)

- Sensation of headache comes from meninges, skin, periosteum, subcutaneous tissue, muscles, intracranial blood vessels, nasal and sinus mucosa, delicate structures in eyes and ears, cranial nerves (II, III, V, IX, X), and nerve roots C1–3. All other elements of the brain lack pain receptors.
- Headache is commonly caused by mechanical traction on the above structures.
- Headaches are subdivided into primary (no identifiable cause) and secondary (identifiable underlying process).

DIFFERENTIAL DIAGNOSIS (TABLE 49.1)

TABLE 49.1. DIFFERENTIAL DIAGNOSIS OF HEADACHE IN THE AMBULATORY SETTING

Diagnosis	Onset and Time Course	Character and Location	Physical Findings	Laboratory Data	Mainstay Rx
Migraine	Rapid course, sometimes preceded by aura, lasts a few hours (sometimes 1–2 d)	Severe, throbbing, incapacitating, holo- or hemicranial, similar to previous episodes	Visual symptoms, photophobia, nausea and vomiting, phonophobia. More common in women	Noncontributory	Over-the-counter analgesics, Reglan, triptan, or ergotamine preparations (see Tables 49.3 and 49.4)
Tension	Gradual onset, can last days	Steady ache often in occipital/neck area, also frontal/ bitemporal, bilateral, similar to previous events	Tenderness to firm palpation of affected area, may notice tense musculature; anxiety, depression	Noncontributory	NSAIDs/COX-2 inhibitors, acetaminophen, tricyclic antidepressments
Cluster	Rapid onset, at the same time every day, lasting hours, in clusters lasting weeks to months	Unilateral severe, throbbing orbital pain, similar to previous episodes	Ptosis, miosis, lacrimation, unilateral eye injection, rhinorrhea, (Horner's without anhidrosis); 4:1 male:female ratio	Noncontributory	Ergotamine preparations triptans, 100% O_2, lidocaine methysergide, verapamil
SAH	Sudden, explosive, "thunderclap" May have had preceding "sentinel headaches"	Severe diffuse headache becoming more occipital, "worst headache of my life"	Nausea, vomiting, LOC at pain onset, meningismus (stiffness on flexion), subhyaloid hemorrhages, Δ MS	CT:(+) in ~90% LP:RBCs or xanthochromia	Neurosurgery referral; Control blood pressure; prevent vasospasm

(continued)

TABLE 49.1. *(continued)*

Diagnosis	Onset and Time Course	Character and Location	Physical Findings	Laboratory Data	Mainstay Rx
Carotid-vert dissection	Sudden onset, pulsatile	Unilateral, anterior (or post) neck and face pain radiating to ipsilateral ear	Oculoparesis, Horner's, focal deficits, pulsatile tinnitus, visual symptoms	MRI/MRA (or CT angiogram)	Anticoagulation; consider surgery
Sinus thrombosis	Gradual, progressive, unrelieved by conventional therapy	May begin unilaterally → sagittally; more common in postpartum period	Possible cranial nerve findings; no venous pulsations on fundus examination	MRV or CT (I⊕) LP: ↑ OP, RBCs	Anticoagulation; hypercoagulability workup
Mass lesion: tumor, AVM, abscess, SDH	Gradual, progressive over days or weeks, worse upon awakening	Dull constant headache, diffuse or localized, may wax and wane, new type of headache	Focal neuro signs, papilledema; signs of trauma (subdural hematoma) or endocarditis (abscess)	CT scan (⊕) MRI	Resection, evacuation or radiation depending on etiology
Meningitis	In general, rapid onset in bacterial or viral, gradual in mycobacterial or fungal, evolving over 24 h	Severe diffuse headache with occipital predominance, different from previous headaches	Fever, confusion, lethargy, meningismus, positive Kernig, positive Brudzinski's, photophobia	LP mandatory; ↑ WBCs	Treat infection Empiric: vanco + ceftriaxone in adults, community acquired
Systemic infection	Acute or gradual onset parallels underlying illness	Diffuse, generally mild, similar to previous febrile episodes	Fever, neck tenderness on flexion/lateral motion, but no rigidity	May have ↑serum WBC but LP is (–)	Treat underlying infection
HTN	Hypertensive crises, eclampsia, adrenal tumors, drug induced	Dull, pounding, similar to previous episodes of poor BP control	↑ BP, retinal hemorrhages and exudates, papilledema	Noncontributory	Treat the high blood pressure
Temporal arteritis	Gradual onset, progressive, mostly in patients >55	Dull ache over temporal artery area, unilateral, new type of headache	Tender to palpation of superficial temporal artery area, sudden blindness	↑ESR; temporal artery Bx a must	Initiate empiric high-dose steroid Rx as soon as possible
Pseudotumor cerebri	Gradual onset, progressive	Severe, diffuse headache; Most patients are obese and female	Papilledema; may have cranial nerve VI palsies; otherwise, a normal examination	NI CT and MRI LP:↑ OP, nl CSF	Serial LPs; prednisone, acetazolamide, furosemide
Acute glaucoma	Rapid or gradual, can wax and wane or be fulminant	Severe, boring ache centered in the eye, h/o narrow angle glaucoma	Globe injected and firm, pupil fixed and dilated	Tonometry	Ophthalmology referral
Acute sinusitis	Gradual onset, progressive	Dull ache, throbbing, behind eye or teeth over involved sinus	Concurrent URI or allergy, purulent nasal discharge, sinus tenderness	CT sinuses	Appropriate antibiotics; decongestants
Trigeminal neuralgia	Sudden onset, each attack lasts seconds to minutes	Searing, lancinating pains in distribution of trigeminal nerve	Small trigger zones on lips, gums or below nose; 2:1 female:male ratio	Noncontributory	Tegretol or Neurontin; consider surgical referral
TMJ pain	Gradual onset, progressive	Severe TMJ ache, pain on chewing	Tenderness in TMJ area	Noncontributory	Oral surgery referral
Dentalgia	Sudden/gradual onset, progressive	Severe dull ache around affected tooth	Tender to tooth palpation, gingivitis	Panorex	Dental referral
Cervical vertebral pathology	Gradual onset, progressive	Sharp radiating pains, occipitocervical, may be similar to previous episodes	Neck tender to palpation and all movement; neck and torso move together; radicular pain; signs of radiculopathy in UE, myelopathy in LE	X-ray of C-spine MRI for radiculopathy or myelopathy	PT, cervical collars, NSAIDs/COX-2 inhibitors; neurosurgical referral if disc herniation or cord compression

Note: AVM, arteriovenous malformation; BP, blood pressure; Bx, biopsy, COX-2, cyclooxygenase 2; CSF, cerebrospinal fluid; CT, computed tomography; DHE, dihydroergotamine; Dx, diagnosis; ESR, erythrocyte sedimentation rate; HTN, hypertension; LE, lower extremities; LP, lumbar puncture; MRI, magnetic resonance imaging; MRA, magnetic resonance angiography; MRV, magnetic resonance venography; MS, mental status; NSAID, nonsteroidal antiinflammatory drug; PT, physical therapy; RBC, red blood cell; Rx, therapy; TMJ, temporomandibular joint; UE, upper extremities; URI, upper respiratory infection; WBC, white blood cell.

EVALUATION (TABLE 49.1)

History

- Look for *red flags*, which suggest serious intracranial pathology; benign headaches are by far the most common (see Table 49.2).
- *Intensity or quality:* Seldom are objective enough to suggest a diagnosis. Exceptions: "The worst headache of my life" suggests subarachnoid hemorrhage; throbbing with an arterial pulse suggests a vascular etiology.
- *Onset, duration, and previous headache history*
- Identify *triggering factors:* foods (red wine, ripened cheeses, cured meats, monosodium glutamate, caffeine, alcohol); medications (nitrates, antihypertensives, nonsteroidal antiinflammatory drugs [NSAIDs], H$_2$-blockers, trimethoprim-sulfamethoxazole [Bactrim]); cough; menses; exercise; sexual intercourse; withdrawal from caffeine or analgesics
- Concomitant *medical conditions/symptoms:* fever, hypertension, sleep apnea, nasal discharge, history of malignancy, history of endocarditis
- *Family history* of headaches
- *Focal neurologic deficits:* concerning, although migraines frequently have neurologic prodrome

TABLE 49.2. "RED FLAGS" (RAMIREZ-LASSEPAS ET AL., 1997)

Onset after age 55
Onset of new or different headache
Worst headache ever experienced
Subacute headache with a progressive course
Occipitonuchal location
Associated neurologic deficits

Physical Examination

- Vital signs
- *Head and face:* Identify trauma, sinus tenderness, "trigger points" in trigeminal neuralgia, clicking/tenderness at the temporomandibular joint [TMJ], temporal artery tenderness.
- *Fundoscopic examination:* Confirm papilledema in syndromes of increased intracranial pressure.
- *Ears, nose, mouth, and throat:* Rule out inflammation of mucosal surfaces.
- *Neck:* Assess rigidity, Kernig's and Brudzinski's signs, range of motion, palpation of spinous processes and paraspinal musculature, and auscultation over the carotids.
- *Complete neurologic examination:* mental status, cranial nerves, visual fields, strength in the major muscle groups, sensory function, deep tendon reflexes, coordination, gait/balance. Abnormal findings on neurologic examination are associated with intracranial pathology.

Diagnostic Testing

- History of similar headaches, normal vital signs, intact mental status, supple neck, absence of neurologic deficits: Initiate empiric therapy without further testing.
- *Laboratory studies:* Guided by initial evaluation, including complete blood cell count if suspected infection, erythrocyte sedimentation rate if considering temporal arteritis, toxicology screen for impaired mental status.
- *Neuroimaging* (computed tomography [CT] and/or magnetic resonance imaging [MRI]): any suspicion for intracranial pathology (subarachnoid hemorrhage, mass lesions, sinusitis, carcinomatous meningitis, Chiari malformation). MRI can better visualize infratentorial and spinal lesions; magnetic resonance angiography can preclude angiography in diagnosis of aneurysms and arterial dissection.
- Special diagnostic procedures: *lumbar puncture* for suspected meningitis or suspected subarachnoid hemorrhage with normal CT scan (also helpful in diagnosing carcinomatous meningitis and pseudotumor cerebri); *temporal artery biopsy* for possible temporal arteritis
- Referral to specialists for specific conditions indicated in Table 49.1

TREATMENT (TABLE 49.1)

- Varies depending on the headache; treatment and prophylaxis of migraine are detailed in Tables 49.3 and 49.4.
- Chronic use of ergotamine preparations, NSAIDs, acetaminophen, and opioid analgesics can lead to rebound headaches.

TABLE 49.3 SOME DRUGS FOR TREATMENT OF MIGRAINE

Drug[a]

Excedrin (acetaminophen [250 mg], ASA [250 mg], caffeine [65 mg])
Midrin (acetaminophen [325 mg], isometheptene [65 mg], dichloralphenazone [100 mg])
Fiorinal (ASA [325 mg], caffeine [40 mg], butalbital [50 mg])
Fioricet (acetaminophen [325 mg], caffeine [40 mg], butalbital [50 mg])
DHE 45 (dihydroergotamine)
Cafergot (ergotamine [1 mg], caffeine [100 mg])
Imitrex (sumatriptan)
Zomig (zolmitriptan)
Amerge (naratriptan)
Maxalt (rizatriptan) (patients on propranolol should halve dose)
Axert (almotriptan)

[a] Only one well-known brand name is provided for each category.
Source: Modified from *Drugs of choice from The Medical Letter*, 1997: 98–99, and *The Medical Letter*, 1998: 97, with permission.

TABLE 49.4. SOME DRUGS FOR PREVENTION OF MIGRAINE

Propranolol (*Inderal*) (can use long-acting form for daily dosing)
Timolol (*Blocadren*)
Metoprolol (*Lopressor*)
Atenolol
Amitriptyline (*Elavil*)
Nortriptyline (*Pamelor*)
Verapamil (*Calan*) (can use sustained-release form for daily dosing)
Valproate

RESOURCES

- American Council for Headache Education: 19 Mantua Road, Mount Royal, NJ 08096-3172; phone, 856-423-0258; fax, 856-423-0082; e-mail, achehg@talley.com; www.achenet.org
- National Headache Foundation: 428 W. St. James Place, 2nd floor, Chicago, IL 60614-2750; phone, 888-NHF-5552, 312-388-6399; fax, 773-525-7357; www.headaches.org

SELECTED REFERENCES

1. Baumel B. Migraine: a pharmacologic review with newer options and delivery modalities. *Neurology* 1994;44[Suppl 3]:S13–S17.
2. Cady RK, Wendt JK, Kirchner JR, et al. Treatment of acute migraine with subcutaneous sumatriptan. *JAMA* 1991;265:2831–2835.
3. Couch JR. Headache to worry about. *Med Clin North Am* 1993;77:141–167.
4. Dalessio DJ. Diagnosing the severe headache. *Neurology* 1994;44[Suppl 3]:S6–S12.
5. Evans RW. Diagnostic testing for the evaluation of headaches. *Neurol Clin* 1996;14:1–26.
6. Frishberg BM. The utility of neuroimaging in the evaluation of headache in patients with normal neurologic examinations. *Neurology* 1994;44:1191–1197.

7. International Headache Society. Classification and diagnostic criteria for headache disorders, cranial neuralgias and facial pain. *Cephalalgia* 1998;8[Suppl 7]:1–96.
8. Kloster R, Nestvold K, Vilming ST. A double-blind study of ibuprofen versus placebo in the treatment of acute migraine attacks. *Cephalalgia* 1992;12:169–171.
9. Ramirez-Lassepas M, Espinosa CE, Cicero JJ, et al., Predictors of intracranial pathologic findings in patients who seek emergency care because of headache. *Arch Neurol* 1997;54:1506–1509.
10. Skyhoj-Olsen T, Friberg L, Lassen NA. Ischemia may be the primary cause of the neurologic deficits in classic migraine. *Arch Neurol* 1987;44:156–161.
11. Welch KMA. Drug therapy of migraine. *N Engl J Med* 1993;329:1476–1483.
12. Welch KMA, Darnley D, Simkins RT. The role of estrogen in migraine: a review and hypothesis. *Cephalalgia* 1984;4:227–236.

DEMENTIA

INTRODUCTION

- Affects 15% to 20% of people older than 65 years; prevalence increases to 45% in people older than 80 years. Annual U.S. expenditure of $123 billion to treat patients with dementia.
- Estimated life expectancy from symptom onset is 5 to 9 years; median survival only 3.3 years in one recent study (Wolfson et al., 2001).
- Alzheimer's disease (AD) most common; affects 4 million Americans, accounts for 70% of dementia.

DIFFERENTIAL DIAGNOSIS/CLINICAL PRESENTATION

- Some decline in cognitive function, known as age-associated memory impairment, may be seen in normal aging; it does not interfere with work or social abilities.
- *Diagnostic and Statistical Manual of Mental Disorders,* fourth edition (*DSM-IV*), criteria for dementia: demonstration of a decline in memory; impairment of at least one other domain of cognitive function:
  ⇒ Aphasia, or difficulty with any aspect of language
  ⇒ Apraxia, or impaired ability to perform motor tasks despite intact motor function
  ⇒ Agnosia, or impaired object recognition despite intact sensory function
  ⇒ Executive dysfunction, or difficulty in planning, organizing, sequencing, or abstracting
- *Delirium* differs from dementia: Onset is acute or subacute (hours to days); course often fluctuates; level of consciousness and particularly attention is impaired.
- When possible, establishing a precise etiology/diagnosis allows more focused treatment and accurate estimation of prognosis (see Tables 50.1 and 50.2).

TABLE 50.1. ETIOLOGIES OF DEMENTIA

Vascular	Multiinfarct dementia, diffuse white matter disease
Infectious	Human immunodeficiency virus, neurosyphilis, progressive multifocal leukoencephalopathy, Creutzfeldt-Jakob disease, tuberculosis, sarcoidosis, Whipple's disease
Neoplastic	Primary or metastatic cancer, paraneoplastic syndrome
Degenerative	Alzheimer's disease, Pick's disease, Lewy body dementia, Parkinson's disease, progressive supranuclear palsy, amyotrophic lateral sclerosis, cortical-basal degeneration, multiple sclerosis
Inflammatory	Vasculitis
Endocrine	Hypothyroidism, adrenal insufficiency, Cushing's syndrome, hypo/hyperparathyroidism, renal or liver failure
Metabolic	Thiamine deficiency (Wernicke's encephalopathy), B_{12} deficiency, inherited enzyme defects
Toxins	Alcoholic amnestic syndrome, alcoholic dementia, drugs/medication effects, heavy metals, dialysis dementia (aluminum)
Trauma	Dementia pugilistica, chronic subdural hemorrhages, postanoxic injury
Other	Normal pressure hydrocephalus (posthemorrhagic, posttraumatic, postmeningitic)

TABLE 50.2. SELECTED DEMENTIAS

Alzheimer's disease (AD)	—Primary risk factors: age, family history. Up to 50% of individuals with first-degree relative with AD affected by age 90. ApoE ε4 associated with increased risk for common late-onset AD. —Definitive diagnosis based on autopsy data, but "probable" AD based on evaluation of dementia (motor impairment, diminished ADLs, family history, cerebral atrophy on CT).
Vascular dementia	—10–20% cases of dementia. —May result from single infarct, multiple infarcts, or white matter ischemia. Any stroke yields a ninefold increased risk for dementia. —Characterized by stepwise progression of cognitive deficits, +/- sensory or motor deficits.
Dementia with Lewy bodies	—Dementia plus one of the following: detailed visual hallucinations, signs of parkinsonism, altered attention/alertness. —Lewy bodies found in 15–25% of patients who have undergone autopsy.
Frontotemporal dementia (Pick's disease)	—Slowly progressive dementia, difficult to distinguish from AD. —Early behavioral disturbances (disinhibition, irritability) and language impairment.
Normal pressure hydrocephalus	—"Magnetic gait" (patient's feet appear glued to the floor); urinary incontinence, and dementia (in that order); impaired concentration and mild memory deficits. —Diagnosis rests on improvement following serial lumbar punctures (30 ml each).

Note: ADL, activities of daily living; CT, computed tomography

EVALUATION

History

- Input from family members and/or caregivers is essential; patient may be unaware or ashamed of cognitive deficits and/or behavioral changes.
- *Dementia-related symptoms:* onset (insidious vs. acute); progression of mental impairments (steady vs. episodic), duration (1 to 2 years before evaluation suggests AD; <6 months suggests other etiology); pattern of cognitive deficits; patient's functional status (ability to perform activities of daily living [ADL]).
- *Other historical features:* personal/family history of stroke or cancer; medications (anticholinergic, antihypertensive, psychotropic, analgesic, sedative-hypnotic); trauma/falls; incontinence; weight loss; fevers; depression; alcohol use; hypoxic events.

Physical Examination

- Vital signs, carotids, thyroid, cardiac, lymph nodes
- Neurologic examination:
  ⇒ Evidence of previous strokes (hemiparesis, hemisensory loss, visual field cuts)
  ⇒ Loss of vibratory or joint position sense
  ⇒ Extrapyramidal motor symptoms: rigidity, slowness
  ⇒ Tremor, asterixis, gait abnormalities
  ⇒ Primitive reflexes, including palmar grasp, palmomental reflex, snout reflex, and glabellar tap
  ⇒ Mini-Mental State Examination (MMSE): Document findings, not just MMSE score (see Table 50.3)
  ⇒ Supplemental mental status examination (see Table 50.4).

TABLE 50.3. MINI-MENTAL STATUS EXAMINATION

Task	Instructions	Scoring	Total possible
Date orientation	"Tell me the date."	One point each for year, season, date, day of week, month	5
Place orientation	"Where are you?"	One point each for state, county, town, building, floor/room	5

(continued)

TABLE 50.3. *(continued)*

Task	Instructions	Scoring	Total possible
Register three objects	Name three objects, ask patient to repeat them.	One point for each correctly repeated	3
Attention and calculation	Ask the patient to count backwards from 100 by 7. Stop after 5 answers. (Or ask patient to spell "world" backwards)	One point for each correct answer or letter	5
Recall three objects	Ask the patient to recall the registered objects.	One point for each correct object	3
Naming	Point to watch, ask "what is this?" Repeat with a pencil.	One point for each correct answer	2
Repeating a phrase	Ask patient to say, "No ifs, ands, or buts."	One point if succesful on first try	1
Verbal commands	Give the patient a piece of paper, and say "Take this paper in your right hand, fold it in half, and put it on the floor."	One point for each correct action (out of three total)	3
Written commands	Show the patient a piece of paper with the words "close your eyes."	One point if the patient's eyes close	1
Writing	Ask the patient to write a sentence.	One point if the sentence has subject, verb, and makes sense	1
Construction	Ask the patient to copy a pair of intersecting pentagons.	One point if the figure has ten corners, two intersecting lines	1
		Total number of points	30

Source: From Folstein MF, Folstein SE, McHugh PR, "Mini-Mental State"; a practical method of grading the cognitive state of patients for the clinician. *J Psychiatr Res* 1975; 12: 189–A8, with permission.

TABLE 50.4. SUPPLEMENTAL MENTAL STATUS TESTING FOR PATIENTS WITH DEMENTIA

Domain	Test
Memory	Recall name and address: "Jane Smith, 18 Sullivan Street, San Francisco." Recall three unusual words: "red ball, mailman, fear." Six-word list learning with selective reminding, prompting on recall
Language	Naming parts: "Shirt: collar, sleeve, cuff; watch: band, face, crystal." Complex commands (try to include commands that cross the midline): "With your right thumb, touch your left ear after you point to the ceiling." Word list: "In 1 minute, name all the vegetables you can think of."
Praxis	"Show me how you would peel a banana."
Visuospatial	"Draw a clock face with numbers, and mark the hands to say 8:10."
Judgment/reasoning	"How is a peach like a grape?" "How is a house different from an apartment?"
Attention/concentration	"Repeat the months of the year in reverse order, starting with December."

Source: From Geldmacher DS, Whitehouse PJ. Evaluation of dementia. *N Engl J Med* 1996; 335: 330–336, with permission.

Laboratory Studies

- Electrolytes, glucose, blood urea nitrogen, creatinine, liver function tests, complete blood count, thyroid function, vitamin B_{12}, rapid plasma reagin
- Brain imaging (without contrast) optional, particularly if evaluation suggests AD; can be useful to rule out subdural hematoma, hydrocephalus, stroke, or tumor
- Additional investigations: if the initial workup is uninformative, a particular diagnosis is suspected, or the presentation is atypical for AD. Particularly important in young patients with rapid progression of dementia (see Table 50.5)

TABLE 50.5. ADJUNCTIVE TESTS IN DEMENTIA WORKUP

Test	Indication	Value
Neuropsychological testing	Patient's deficits are mild or difficult to characterize	Sensitivity of the Mini-Mental State Examination for dementia is poor, particularly in highly educated or intelligent patients (compensate for deficits).
Lumbar puncture	Known or suspected cancer, immunosuppression, suspected CNS infection or vasculitis, hydrocephalus by CT, age <55, rapid or atypical course	Helps rule out infection, cancer, NPH, etc.
MRI with gadolinium	Any focal or atypical findings on neurologic examination	More sensitive for tumor, stroke.
EEG	Suspected toxic-metabolic encephalopathy, partial complex seizures, Creutzfeldt-Jacob disease	Look for diffuse slowing (encephalopathy) vs. focal seizure activity.
HIV testing	Risk factors or opportunistic infections	Up to 20% of patients with HIV may develop dementia.
Heavy metal screening, and ceruloplasmin	Possible history of exposure or reasons to suspect Wilson's disease	

Note: CNS, central nervous system; CT, computed tomography; EEG, electroencephalogram; HIV, human immunodeficiency virus; MRI, magnetic resonance imaging.

TREATMENT

- *Educate and support patient and family:* Diagnosis often devastating; refer early to community agencies such as Alzheimer's Association. Intensive family education and counseling can delay patient placement into a nursing home by up to 1 year (Mittelman et al., 1996).
- *Ensure patient safety:* Discuss relinquishing driver's license, lock use, and Alzheimer's Association "safe return" program to prevent wandering.
- *Address legal issues:* Family member should assist with finances (co-signing bills); patient should be advised to complete legal documents (wills, estate planning, healthcare proxy, code status, and other end-of-life papers) in a timely fashion.
- *Discuss options for short-term and long-term care:* Early options include adult day care, respite care, home health aides, outreach services, homemakers (mostly not Medicare services); nearly three fourths of patients will eventually require care at a long-term facility.
- *Address behavioral problems:* wandering, screaming, incontinence, aggression, psychosis; pharmacologic therapy should be initiated when appropriate (for depression, anxiety, psychosis).
- Remember to care for the caregiver.

Medications for Alzheimer Disease

- Donepezil (Aricept): acetylcholinesterase inhibitor; 4.1% improvement in cognitive assessment scores in one study (Rogers et al., 1998)
  - ⇒ Restores level of function to that which was present 6 to 12 months earlier; does not stop deterioration.
  - ⇒ Start with 5 mg orally everyday (q.d.) at bedtime; may increase to 10 mg after 1 month. Many experts recommend a 6-month trial with precognitive and postcognitive measures.
  - ⇒ Adverse reactions in up to 14% (increased cholinergic tone): nausea, diarrhea, vomiting, insomnia; contraindicated in sick sinus syndrome. No significant effect on metabolism/binding of other drugs.
- Vitamin E: One trial showed that 2,000 IU q.d. resulted in increased time to primary endpoint (death/institutionalization/loss of ADL/severe dementia) but no improvement in measures of cognition (Sano et al., 1997). Higher MMSE score in placebo group flawed this study; difference only noted after an adjustment was made.
- Ginkgo extract: *Gingko biloba* stabilized cognitive/social function in those with AD or multi-infarct dementia at 1-year follow-up (Le Bars et al., 1997).
- Statins: Potentially biased case–control study showed a 0.29 relative risk of first-time dementia diagnosis for those prescribed statins (Jick et al., 2000). A large, double-blind, randomized, controlled trial of statin effect on cognitive decline is due in 2002.

- Other possible therapies: nonsteroidal antiinflammatory drugs (used for 2 years or longer), estrogen both associated with a decreased risk of development of AD (relative risk, 0.4). Randomized trials of propentofylline and idebenone have shown small improvements on Alzheimer cognitive assessment scales.

RESOURCES

- Alzheimer's Association: 800-272-3900
- American Geriatrics Society: 212-308-1414
- Alzheimer's Disease Education and Referral Center: 800-438-4380; http://www.alzheimers.org/ir.html

SELECTED REFERENCES

1. Amar K, Wilcock G. Vascular dementia. *BMJ* 1996;312:227–231.
2. Berg L, McKeel DW, Miller JP, et al. Clinicopathologic studies in cognitively healthy aging and Alzheimer's disease: relation of histologic markers to dementia severity, age, sex, and apolipoprotein E genotype. *Arch Neurol* 1998;55:326–335.
3. Corey-Bloom J, Thal LJ, Galasko D, et al. Diagnosis and evaluation of dementia. *Neurology* 1995;45:211–218.
4. Erkinjuntti T, Ostbye T, Steenhuis R, et al. The effect of different diagnostic criteria on the prevalence of dementia. *N Engl J Med* 1997;337:1667–1674.
5. Folstein MF, Folstein SE, McHugh PR. Mini-Mental State: a practical method of grading the cognitive state of patients for the clinician. *J Psychiatr Res* 1975;12:189–198.
6. Geldmacher DS, Whitehouse PJ. Evaluation of dementia. *N Engl J Med* 1996;335:330–336.
7. Jick H, Zornberg GL, Jick SS, et al. Statins and the risk of dementia. *Lancet* 2000;356:1627–1631.
8. Kaye JA. Diagnostic challenges in dementia. *Neurology* 1998;51:S45–S52.
9. Le Bars PL, Katz MM, Berman N, et al. A placebo-controlled, double-blind, randomized trial of an extract of *Ginkgo biloba* for dementia. North American EGb Study Group. *JAMA* 1997;278:1327–1332.
10. Mayeux R, Sano M. Treatment of Alzheimer's disease. *N Engl J Med* 1999;341:1670–1679.
11. Mittelman MS, Ferris SH, Shulman E, et al. A family intervention to delay nursing home placement of patients with Alzheimer disease. A randomized controlled trial. *JAMA* 1996;276:1725–1731.
12. Price RW. Neurological complications of HIV infection. *Lancet* 1996;348:445–452.
13. Rogers SL, Farlow MR, Doody RS, et al. A 24-week, double-blind, placebo-controlled trial of donepezil in patients with Alzheimer's disease. *Neurology* 1998;50:136–145.
14. Sano M, Ernesto C, Thomas RG, et al. A controlled trial of selegiline, alpha-tocopherol, or both as treatment for Alzheimer's disease. The Alzheimer's Disease Cooperative Study. *N Engl J Med* 1997;336:1216–1222.
15. Small GW, Rabins PV, Barry PP, et al. Diagnosis and treatment of Alzheimer disease and related disorders. Consensus statement of the American Association for Geriatric Psychiatry, the Alzheimer's Association, and the American Geriatrics Society. *JAMA* 1997;278:1363–1371.
16. Stern Y, Tang MX, Albert MS, et al. Predicting time to nursing home care and death in individuals with Alzheimer disease. *JAMA* 1997;277:806–812.
17. Stewart WF, Kawas C, Corrada M, et al. Risk of Alzheimer's disease and duration of NSAID use [see Comments]. *Neurology* 1997;48:626–632.
18. Tang MX, Jacobs D, Stern Y, et al. Effect of oestrogen during menopause on risk and age at onset of Alzheimer's disease. *Lancet* 1996;348:429–432.
19. Wolfson C, Wolfson DB, Asgharian M, et al. A reevaluation of the duration of survival after the onset of dementia. *N Engl J Med* 2001;344:1111–1116.

51

DIZZINESS

INTRODUCTION

- Accounts for 8 million annual U.S. patient visits (Sloane, 1989)
- Wide variety of disparate etiologies, no definitive laboratory or imaging tests

DIFFERENTIAL DIAGNOSIS (TABLE 51.1)

TABLE 51.1. DIFFERENTIAL DIAGNOSIS

	Vertigo	Presyncope	Disequilibrium	Lightheadedness
Description	Illusion of motion	Impending LOC	Unsteadiness	Anxiety
Complaint	"My head is spinning."	"I might pass out."	"My balance is off."	"I'm just dizzy."
	"The room is whirling."	"I'm going to faint."	"I'm going to fall."	"I'm giddy."
Etiology	Peripheral	Cardiac	Motion sickness	Hyperventilation
	Benign positional vertigo	Vasovagal	Multiple sensory deficits	Panic attack
	Ménière's syndrome	Carotid sinus hypersensitivity	(e.g., diabetes mellitus)	Major phobias
	Vestibular neuronitis	Arrhythmias	Cerebellar dysfunction	Anxiety
	Acute labyrinthitis	Obstructive hypertrophic	Extrapyramidal disorders	Somatization
	Posttraumatic	cardiomyopathy	Seizure disorder	Chronic
	Hypothyroidism		Drug intoxications	vestibulopathy
				Hyperthyroidism
	Central	Systemic	Posterior fossa tumors	
	Acoustic neuroma	Hypovolemia	Chronic vestibulopathy	
	Posterior fossa tumors	Drug induced		
	Cerebellar dysfunction	Anemia		
	Brainstem ischemia	Thyroid dysfunction		
	Multiple sclerosis	Hypoglycemia		
	Basilar migraine			

LOC, loss of consciousness.

EVALUATION

Goals

- Classify the patient's symptomatology as belonging to one of four major etiologic groups (Table 51.1).
- Distinguish benign from ominous causes of dizziness.

History

- Helps establish the diagnosis in about 75% of patients:
    ⇒ Explain symptoms without the word dizzy.
    ⇒ Elicit history of *"illusion of motion,"* either patient or surroundings (spinning, whirling, similar to getting off a merry-go-round).
    ⇒ Distinguish between the sensation of fainting (impending loss of consciousness) and *falling* (imbalance, unsteadiness).

⇒ Hearing loss, tinnitus, ear fullness
⇒ Circumstances causing dizzy spells (head turning, standing, straining/Valsalva maneuver)
⇒ Duration/pattern of episodes
⇒ Associated symptoms (diplopia, perioral numbness, hearing symptoms, palpitations)
⇒ Co-morbid conditions (heart disease, arrhythmias, diabetes, anemia, thyroid disease, multiple sclerosis, migraine headaches, Parkinson's disease, trauma, stress, psychiatric disorders)
⇒ List of medications and other drugs (see below)
● Distinguish central versus peripheral causes (see Tables 51.2 and 51.3):
⇒ Nausea/vomiting: peripheral vertigo
⇒ Gait imbalance: central vertigo
⇒ Auditory symptoms: lesion of the labyrinth or the eighth nerve
⇒ Ipsilateral facial numbness/weakness or limb ataxia: lesion of the cerebellopontine angle
⇒ Other neurologic deficits: brainstem or cerebellar lesions

TABLE 51.2. VERTIGO OF PERIPHERAL ORIGIN (INVOLVING THE VESTIBULAR SYSTEM)

Benign positional vertigo	Experienced upon head motion or change of position while lying or standing. Lasts few seconds; accompanied by nausea and vomiting (without hearing loss or tinnitus).
	Diagnosis by Dix-Hallpike maneuver (latent onset of rotatory nystagmus with vertical component beating toward forehead, of short duration and fatigable).
	Caused by dislodging and coalescing of otoconia from utricle or saccule, which then lie in a semicircular canal (usually posterior) and cause sensation of motion.
Ménière's Syndrome (endolymphatic hydrops	Four typical symptoms: dizziness with sensation of motion, sensorineural hearing loss, tinnitus, and ear fullness. Attacks are often violent, can last up to several hours.
	Diagnosis made clinically; chronic remissions and relapses. Magnetic resonance imaging to rule out acoustic neuroma.
	Caused by distention of endolymphatic system from insufficient resorption or overproduction; contributes to endolymphatic hydrops from rupture of membranes and mixing of endolymph and perilymph.
Ototoxic drugs	Include the aminoglycosides, nonsteroidal antiinflammatory drugs, cinchona alkaloids (quinine, quinidine), loop diuretics, alcohol, and cisplatinum.
	Act *peripherally* in causing unsteadiness of gait and oscillopsia, although seldom cause true vertigo.
Vestibular neuronitis/acute labyrinthitis	An upper respiratory tract infection or influenza-like syndrome may precede vestibular neuronitis. Symptoms usually come on suddenly and resolve gradually. While Ménière Syndrome is recurrent, vestibular neuronitis is not.
Posttraumatic	Symptomatic medications can be helpful; surgery is sometimes indicated. Spontaneous resolution common.

TABLE 51.3. VERTIGO OF CENTRAL ORIGIN (WITHIN THE NEURAXIS)

Acoustic neuroma	Dizziness with unilateral hearing loss is an acoustic neuroma until proven otherwise. If associated skin lesions are present, consider neurofibromatosis.
	Presents insidiously with unilateral hearing loss (sometimes accompanied by dizziness); if untreated, may involve the cerebellopontine angle and affect other cranial nerves, leading to facial numbness/weakness and becoming unresectable.
	Early diagnosis (usually by MRI) to ensure curative surgical resection.
Posterior fossa tumors	Significant involvement of cerebellum is usually necessary for severe loss of function to occur.
	Surgical resection or radiotherapy options depend on histology and staging.
Brainstem ischemia	Diagnosis requires other symptoms of vertebrobasilar insufficiency besides vertigo and disequilibrium, such as diplopia, dysarthria, facial/limb numbness, hemiparesis, ataxia or Horner's syndrome.
	During an acute attack, these additional signs plus vertical or direction-changing nystagmus suggest a brainstem TIA.

(continued)

TABLE 51.3. *(continued)*

Cerebellar stroke	Suggested by new, permanent, severe vertigo and imbalance with a tendency to fall toward affected side, hemiataxia of limbs and multidirectional nystagmus. CT can visualize acute hemorrhage; less adequate in demonstrating posterior fossa infarcts. DWI-MRI has increased sensitivity in detecting acute infarcts. Can be self-limited, but may need to prevent expansion, limit cerebellar edema, and perform surgical decompression.
Cerebellar hemorrhage	May present with or without headache; may not have any nystagmus or limb ataxia, and only physical finding might be truncal or gait ataxia, particularly in paramedian or central hemorrhages. Imperative to elicit ambulation to make this potentially fatal diagnosis, which is confirmed by CT and often requires surgical decompression.
Basilar migraine	Associated with visual disturbances, sensory symptoms, and intense occipital headache; diagnosis of exclusion.
Multiple sclerosis	May present as vertigo or imbalance if demyelinating lesions involve vestibular nuclei or brainstem connections. Diagnosis made by consistent history of varied neurologic deficits with fluctuating temporal course, multiple white matter lesions on CNS imaging, and supporting laboratory data (CFS pleocytosis, elevated CSF γ-globulins with oligoclonal bands, increased CSF myelin basic protein and altered evoked potentials).

Note: CNS, central nervous system; CSF, cerebrospinal fluid; CT, computed tomography; DWI-MRI, diffusion-weighted imaging–magnetic resonance imaging; TIA, transient ischemic attack.

Physical Examination

- Vital signs, including orthostatics
- Inspection of tympanic membranes
- Auditory acuity, Rinne test
- Visual-field testing
- Direction of nystagmus, if present
- Cardiac examination (rhythm, rate, murmurs)
- Full neurologic examination, with particular attention to cranial nerves, sensory function (include Romberg test), cerebellar tests, and gait/balance (tandem)

Provocative Maneuvers

- Designed to replicate the patient's symptoms; may be helpful in obtaining a diagnosis (see Table 51.4).

TABLE 51.4. PROVOCATIVE MANEUVERS

Orthostatics	Supine and standing signs: replication of symptoms and a SBP ↓ more than 20 mm Hg suggest hypovolemia, autonomic dysfunction, or offending meds (BP meds, diuretics, TCAs).
Hyperventilation	Instruct patient to take deep breaths ~every 2 sec for 3 min. If lightheadedness and associated symptoms (circumoral or finger paresthesias, diaphoresis, leg weakness) recur, patient can be reassured and asked to breathe into a paper bag (to prevent hypocarbia) when symptoms recur.
Carotid massage and Valsalva (perform in monitored setting)	Place patient on cardiac mointor with BP cuff, verify absence of carotid bruits; carotid sinus is massaged for ~10 sec without causing occlusion of the artery. In carotid hypersensitivity see bradycardia and an SBP ↓ ~50 mm Hg. Valsalva may cause similar symptoms in other cardiac diseases (AS, hypertrophic obstructive cardiomyopathy) or Chiari malformation.
Positional testing (Dix-Hallpike maneuver)	Rapidly bring patient from sitting to supine position, with head tilted 45 degrees to one side and 45 degrees below the level of examining table; note direction, latency, and duration of nystagmus. A latent period, short duration, rotatory nystagmus with vertical component beating toward patient's forehead, and fatigability suggest benign positional vertigo.

Note: BP, blood pressure; SBP, systolic BP; TCA, tricyclic antidepressant.

Diagnostic Testing

- *Labs:* electrolytes and complete blood cell count; consider thyroid function tests, fasting glucose, vitamin B_{12}, toxicology screen.
- *Electronystagmography* and *rotational vestibular tests:* when vestibular dysfunction is suspected but definite diagnosis cannot be made in the office
- *Audiometry:* hearing loss, tinnitus, or ear fullness
- *Brainstem auditory evoked potentials:* localize auditory pathway damage central to the ear (acoustic neuroma, brainstem tumors, or multiple sclerosis)
- *Magnetic resonance imaging with gadolinium:* when central or cerebellar lesion is suspected.
- *Magnetic resonance angiography (MRA) of the head and neck:* when vascular abnormalities are suspected.
- *Electrocardiogram/Holter monitoring/event loop recorder/echocardiogram:* when suspected symptomatic arrhythmias/structural abnormalities
- *Psychiatric referral* may be useful in the evaluation and management of dizziness (Kroenke et al., 1992).

TREATMENT

Ménière's Syndrome (endolymphatic hydrops)

- Bed rest, symptomatic therapy with vestibular sedative medications (see Table 5) during acute attacks.
- A low-salt diet coupled with a diuretic (thiazide or carbonic anhydrase inhibitors) has been tried; record of success largely anecdotal.
- In severe refractory cases, surgical decompression/excision of the endolymphatic sac can be attempted, with the risk of increased hearing loss.

Benign Positional Vertigo

- Antidizziness medications (see Table 51.5) are seldom beneficial
- Epley maneuver:
  ⇒ Place the patient in supine position with head turned so that affected ear remains inferior.
  ⇒ Shake patient's head carefully and slowly turn it toward unaffected ear, which should now be inferior.
  ⇒ Ask patient to turn on side and face down, continue to shake head; now ask patient to sit up from that position.
  ⇒ Patient should refrain from lying flat for the next 24 to 48 hours, to prevent debris from falling back into the posterior canal.
  ⇒ In good hands, the Epley maneuver is 85% to 94% curative (Lynn et al., 1995; Steenerson and Cronin, 1996; Wolf et al., 1999).
- Brandt-Daroff exercises:
  ⇒ If the Epley maneuver fails, patient can be taught home use of these exercises.
  ⇒ The patient begins in the sitting position and then leans rapidly toward the affected side, placing head on the bed, to replicate vertiginous sensation; remains in position until symptoms subside.
  ⇒ Maneuver repeated toward opposite side, completing 10 to 20 cycles. This maneuver helps patient's vestibular system habituate to the offending stimulus.

Brain Ischemia

- Patients in whom brainstem ischemia is suspected are often anticoagulated until posterior circulation is evaluated by imaging and the heart is assessed for possible embolic sources by echocardiogram.
- If both studies are negative, aspirin or clopidogrel therapy is recommended (Antiplatelet Trialists' Collaboration, 1994).
- Patients with severe vertebrobasilar stenosis or those who continue to have symptoms despite adequate antiplatelet therapy are often placed on oral anticoagulation (without clear evidence).

Medications (Table 51.5)

TABLE 51.5. MEDICATIONS FOR SYMPTOMATIC TREATMENT OF DIZZINESS (ETIOLOGY DEPENDENT)

Medication	Usual Dosage p.o./i.m./i.v./p.r.	Duration of Action
Dimenhydrinate (*Dramamine*)	50 mg q6h	4–6 hr
Diphenhydramine (*Benadryl*)	25–50 mg p.o./i.m./i.v. q6h	4–6 hr
Scopolamine (*Transderm Scop*)	0.5 mg patch	72 hr
Meclizine (*Antivert*)	25 mg p.o. q6-12h	12–24 hr
Promethazine (*Phenergan*)	25–50 mg p.o./i.m./p.r./i.v. q6h	4–6 hr
Hydroxyzine (*Vistaril*)	25–50 mg p.o./i.m. q6h	4–6 hr
Clonazepam (*Klonopin*)	0.25–0.5 mg p.o. q8h	6–12 hr
Lorazepam (*Ativan*)	0.5–2 mg p.o./s.l./i.m./i.v. q8h	6–12 hr
Diazepam (*Valium*)	2–10 mg p.o./i.v. q8h	12–18 hr

Note: i.m., intramuscularly; i.v., intravenously; p.o., orally.

SELECTED REFERENCES

1. Antiplatelet Trialists' Collaboration. Collaborative overview of randomised trials of antiplatelet therapy, I: prevention of death, myocardial infarction, and stroke by prolonged antiplatelet therapy in various categories of patients. *Br Med J* 1994;308:81.
2. Baloh RW. Vertigo. *Lancet* 1998;352:1841–1846.
3. Brandt T, Steddin S, Daroff RB. Therapy for benign paroxysmal positioning vertigo, revisited. *Neurology* 1994;44:796–800.
4. Epley JM. Positional vertigo related to semicircular canalithiasis. *Otolaryngol Head Neck Surg* 1995;112:154–161.
5. Furman JM, Cass SP. Primary care: benign paroxysmal positional vertigo. *N Engl J Med* 1999;341:1590–1596.
6. Halmagyi GM, Cremer PD. Assessment and treatment of dizziness. *J Neurol Neurosurg Psychiatry* 2000;68:129–134.
7. Hoffman RM, Einstadter D, Kroenke K. Evaluating dizziness. *Am J Med* 1999;107:468–478.
8. Kroenke K, Lucas CA, Rosenberg ML, et al. Causes of persistent dizziness: a prospective study of 100 patients in ambulatory care. *Ann Intern Med* 1992;117:898–904.
9. Lynn S, Pool A, Rose D, et al. Randomised trial of the canalith repositioning procedure. *Otolaryngol Head Neck Surg* 1995;113:712–720.
10. Sloane PD. Dizziness in primary care. *J Fam Pract* 1989;29:33–38.
11. Steenerson RL, Cronin GW. Comparison of the canalith repositioning procedure and vestibular habituation training in forty patients with benign paroxysmal positional vertigo. *Otolaryngol Head Neck Surg* 1996;114:61–64.
12. Troost BT, Patton JM. Exercise therapy for positional vertigo. *Neurology* 1992;42:1441–1444.
13. Wolf JS, Boyev KP, Manokey BJ, et al. Success of the modified Epley maneuver in treating benign paroxysmal positional vertigo. *Laryngoscope* 1999;109:900–903.

52

COMMON EYE PROBLEMS

RED EYE

Introduction

- Defined as the engorgement of superficial vessels of conjunctiva, episclera, or sclera; caused by disorders of these structures or adjoining structures (cornea, iris, ciliary body, or adnexa)
- Usually, a benign, self-limited condition (subconjunctival hemorrhage, infectious conjunctivitis)
- More serious conditions (acute angle-closure glaucoma, corneal abrasion) need urgent diagnosis and treatment (see Table 52.1)

TABLE 52.1. DIFFERENTIAL DIAGNOSIS OF RED EYE

Discharge	No discharge: pain
Acute allergic reaction	Abrasion/foreign body
Blepharitis	Acute angle closure glaucoma
Conjunctivitis	Anterior uveitis/iritis/iridocyclitis
	Chemical burn
	Corneal disease and trauma (ulcer, contact lens related)
No discharge: minimal/no pain	Episcleritis
Blepharitis	Foreign body
Conjunctival tumor	Herpes simplex/zoster keratitis
Dry eye syndrome	Hyphema
Pterygium	Keratoconjunctivitis sicca
Subconjunctival hemorrhage	Scleritis
	Secondary to abnormal lid function

Evaluation

History

- Inquire about blurred or decreased vision, pain, photophobia, visual changes (seeing halos, spots), exudate/discharge, itching, foreign body sensation, allergy history, trauma, exposure to people with "pink eye."

Physical Examination

- Check visual acuity, pattern/distribution of redness, characterize any discharge, look for corneal opacities, evaluate for corneal irregularities with penlight, consider fluorescein staining, evaluate pupillary reflex, funduscopic examination.

TABLE 52.2. CLASSIC FINDINGS/TREATMENT OF RED EYE

	Pathogenesis and Symptoms	Treatment
Acute angle-closure glaucoma	• Rapid onset in older age-groups. • Presents with acute eye pain, middilated pupils, "halos around lights," and blurred vision. • Can be precipitated by anticholinergics, stress, and dark rooms (pupils dilate, block aqueous flow).	• Intravenous (I.V.) acetazolamide • Osmotic diuretics • Topical pilocarpine • Topical β-blockers • Laser peripheral iridectomy (treatment of choice)
Anterior uveitis (iritis)	• Can cause nausea/vomiting, headache. • Pain, consensual photophobia, decreased vision w/circumcorneal redness, small pupil (depending on chronicity). • Etiology → idiopathic, trauma, sarcoidosis, urethritis (Reiter's syndrome), IBD, infections (tuberculosis, herpes, syphilis, toxoplasmosis), ankylosing spondylitis, psoriasis, Behçet syndrome. • Check RPR, CXR, tuberculosis skin test, CBC, ACE, ANA, ANCA, HLA—B27, ESR (for chronic or recurrent process).	• Treated by ophthalmologist • Steroids or antibiotics
Chemical burn	• Bright red painful eye after contact with chemical agent	• Institute therapy immediately before testing vision with copious irrigation • Refer to ophthalmologist immediately
Corneal abrasions	• Intense pain, foreign body sensation, tears • Fluorescein +/- short-acting topical anesthetic for examination	• Topical antibiotics • Soft pressure patch • Oral analgesic • Cycloplegic agent for comfort • 24-hr follow-up
Bacterial conjunctivitis	• Purulent discharge • Gram stain hyperpurulent discharge (looking for gonococcus (GC) or *Pseudomonas*) • Usually caused by staphylococcus, streptococcus	• Topical antibiotics • I.V. antibiotics and immediate ophthalmologist referral for GC
Viral conjunctivitis	• Watery discharge • More common in summer • Bilateral with tearing, preauricular adenopathy, and constitutional symptoms • Adenovirus most common	• Cold compresses • Iced artifical tears • Topical nonsteroidal antiinflammatory drug (NSAID) (ketorolac, Acular) • Strict handwashing
Allergic conjunctivitis	• Intense itching • Watery discharge with white stringy mucus • Conjunctival edema	• Cold compresses • Artifical tears • Topical/systemic antihistamines • Patanol (mast cell stabilizer and antihistamine)
Hyphema	• Painful eye with blurred vision • History of trauma • Blood in the anterior chamber	• Refer to ophthalmologist immediately to rule out globe rupture • Place metal shield on eye • Treat with atropine 1% drops three times a day • Avoid aspirin and NSAIDs • Screen for sickle cell disease/trait • Control increased intraocular pressure
Subconjunctival hemorrhage	• Bright red painless eye with normal vision due to rupture of small subconjunctival vessels • Idiopathic, minor trauma, coughing, straining • Rule out hyphema (blood in anterior chamber mandates urgent ophthalmologic referral)	• Reassure • Resolves in 1–2 wk

IBD, inflammatory bowel disease; RPR, rapid plasma reagin, CXR, chest X-ray; CBC, complete blood count, ACE, angiotensin converting enzyme; ANA, antinuclear antibody; ANCA, anti-neutrophil cytoplasmic antibody; HLA, human leucocyte antigen; ESR, erythrocyte sedimentation rate.

Reasons to Refer (Table 52.3)

• Decreased vision
• Corneal ulcer/abrasion that does not heal within 48 hours
• Penetrating trauma
• Chemical burn, motility disorder, orbital cellulitis
• Diabetic retinopathy, macular degeneration
• Corneal ulcer
• Flashes/floaters

TABLE 52.3. WARNING SYMPTOMS FOR REFERRAL

Symptom	Possible Etiology
Painful eye with decreased vision	Acute angle-closure glaucoma
Acute painless loss of vision	Central artery occlusion with cherry red spot on retina
Painful eye in contact lens wearer	Corneal ulcer
Eye pain after eye surgery	
Sore eye with photophobia	Endophthalmitis
"Curtain-like" loss of vision, flashes/floaters	Iritis, anterior uveitis
	Retinal detachment

OTHER COMMON EYE PROBLEMS (TABLES 52.4 THROUGH 52.6)

TABLE 52.4. COMMON EYE PROBLEMS

	Description	Treatment
Cataracts	• Painless blurred vision progressing over months/years due to lens opacities. Most common cause of decreased vision (not correctable with glasses) in the United States • Etiologies: senile (increase with smoking/ultraviolet light exposure), congenital, or steroid-related • Indications for surgery: decrease in vision interfering with daily activities (usually 20/50 or worse vision) • Preoperative workup: medical examination electrocardiogram (if indicated), no food for 8 hrs. prior to procedure. May continue ASA.	• Day surgery, lasting, 1/2–1 hr, local anesthesia • Discharged home within hours of the procedure • Topical antibiotics/steroids for 4–8 wk • Limit lifting/bending 1–3 wk postprocedure
Blepharitis	• Foreign body sensation, burning, mattering of lashes, eyelids sticking together when awakening • Due to chronic lid inflammation affecting eyelash line • May be associated with acne rosacea	• Warm compresses • Cleansing with gentle baby sharmpoo • Topical antibiotics nightly • Doxycycline or minocycline
Dry eyes	• Burning, foreign body/gritty sensation, assoicated with tearing • Associated with aging, medications (antihistamines, diuretics, tricyclics), systemic disease such as sarcoidosis, rheumatoid arthritis, systemic lupus erythematosis, Sjögren disease.	• Artificial tears • Lubricating ointment as is sufficient • Punctal plugs
Keratitis	• Corneal infection (viral or bacterial); can be vision threatening • Caused by viruses, usually herpes simplex virus, bacteria, immunosuppression (including diabetes mellitus)	• Viral: ophthalmology for topical antivirals • Bacterial: ophthalmology for Gram stain and culture, topical quinolone or broad-spectrum antibiotic, disposal of contact lenses
Diabetic retinopathy (please see Chapter 23)	• Ocular complications including cataracts and refractive changes. Most important is diabetic retinopathy, which is the leading cause of new blindness in U.S. patients age 20–65. • Nonproliferative retinopathy: vein dilation, microaneurysms, retinal hemorrhages, retinal edema, cotton wool spots, and hard exudates; vision loss due to capillary nonperfusion or edema of macula/fovea • Proliferative retinopathy: neovascularization, vitreous hemorrhage; proliferation of blood vessels into vitreous leading to tractional retinal detachment.	• Ophthalmology referral at the time of diagnosis and annually • Patients who have been treated with laser surgery/vitrectomy should follow up with ophthalmology
Hypertensive retinopathy	• Hypertension (HTN) causes damage to the retinal vasculature by two mechanisms: (1) elevated blood pressure (BP) and (2) arteriolar sclerosis. • Findings in early hypertensive retinopathy include copper wire arterioles, silver-wire arterioles, anterio-venous (AV) nicking. More severe findings include optic disc swelling, hemorrhages, exudates, and cotton wool spots.	• Adequate systemic BP control • Referral to ophthalmology

(continued)

TABLE 52.4. *(continued)*

	Description	Treatment
Macular degeneration	• Leading cause of legal blindness among people >52 yr • Presents as slow loss of vision, with greater loss of central vision. • Associated with advanced age, white race, female gender, smoking, and family history. • Can be divided into nonexudative and exudative types (this classification has very important treatment implications).	• Ophthalmology if recent onset of decreased vision, distortion of central vision or scotoma or blind spot. • More rapidly progressive exudative type may benefit from laser photocoagulation.
Open-angle glaucoma	• Second most common cause of blindness in the United States. • Gradual loss of peripheral vision due to persistently elevated intraocular pressure. • Risk Factors: Elevated intraocular pressure, African-American race, myopia, diabetes mellitus, age, +family history. • All patients >40 should be screened for glaucoma; every 2 yr between 20–40 yr and every yr >40 yr.	• Topical β-blockers • Adrenergic agonists • Cholinergic agonists • Carbonic anhydrase inhibitor • Prostaglandin analgoues (Xalatan) • Laser or surgery

TABLE 52.5. TOPICAL OPHTHALMIC MEDICATIONS

Allergy medications	Most cell stabilizers: Alomide, Alocril, Crolom; Antihistimine: Livostin; Combination mast cell stabilizer and antihistamine: Patanol, Zaditor
Anesthetics	Proparacaine 0.5% (Ophthaine); to facilitate eye examination
Antibiotics	Ointments: erythromycin, bacitracin, sulfacetamide sodium, gentamicin, tobramycin; Solutions: Ocuflox, Ciloxan, Quixin, sulfacetamide sodium, gentamicin, tobramycin, Polytrim
Antifungal agents	Natamycin, nystatin
Antiviral agents	Idoxuridine (Herplex), trifluridine (Viroptic), vidarabine (Vira-A)
Corticosteroids	Prednisolone (Pred Forte), dexamethasone (Decadron)
Mydriatics/cycloplegics	Tropicamide 0.5% (Mydriacyl); lasts 6 hr Cyclopentolate (Cyclogyl); lasts 2 days
Nonsteroidal antiinflammatory drugs	Diclofenac (Voltaren), ketorolac (Acular)
Vasoconstrictors	Phenylephrine 2.5% (Neo-Synephrine)

	Glaucoma drugs:	pilocarpine (Pilocar), one drop four times a day, 1%, 2%, 4%
	β-blockers:	betaxolol (Betoptic, cardioselective), timolol (Timoptic)
	α-agonists:	Alphagan, Iopidine
	Prostaglandin analogs:	Xalatan, Travatan, Lumigran, Rescula
	Anticholinesterase:	physostigmine, neostigmine
	Sympathomimetics:	epinephrine
	Carbonic anhydrase inhibitors:	acetazolamide (oral), Trusopt (topical), Azopt (topical)

TABLE 52.6. OTHER OPHTHALMIC TERMS

Hordeolum: staphylococcal abscess of the sebaceous gland within upper or lower lid

Stye: same as hordeolum

Chalazion: granulomatous inflammation of Meibomian gland; hard nontender swelling of lid

Entropion: inward turning of (usually) lower lid, seen in the elderly

Ectropion: outward turning in lower lid, also in elderly

Pinguecula: yellow elevated nodule, usually on the nasal side of cornea, common in patients >35 yr

Pterygium: fleshy triangular encroachment of conjuctiva on nasal cornea, associated with wind/sand/dust/sun

Amaurosis fugax: "fleeting blindness" generally due to retinal artery emboli from ipsilateral carotid disease

SELECTED REFERENCES

1. Baum J. Infections of the eye. *CID* 1995;21:479.
2. Bertolini J, Pelucio M. The red eye. *Emerg Med Clin North Am* 1995;13:561.
3. Dahl-Jorgensen K, Brinchmann-Hansen O, Hanssen KF, et al. Rapid tightening of blood glucose control leads to transient deterioration of retinopathy in insulin dependent diabetes mellitus: the Oslo study. *BMJ* 1985;290:811–815.
4. D'Amico DJ. Diseases of the retina. *N Engl J Med* 1994;331:95.
5. Dart JKG. Diseases and risks associated with contact lenses. *Br J Ophthalmol* 1993;77:49.
6. DCCT. The effect of intensive treatment of diabetes on the development and progression of long-term complications in insulin-dependent diabetics. *N Engl J Med* 1993;329:977.
7. The Diabetes Control and Complications Trial Research Group. Early worsening of diabetic retinopathy in the Diabetes Control and Complications Trial. *Arch Ophthalmol* 1998;116:874–886.
8. Freidlander MH. Immunologic aspects of diseases of the eye. *JAMA* 1992;268:2869.
9. Raskin P, Arauz-Pacheco C. The treatment of diabetic retinopathy: a review for the internist. *Ann Intern Med* 1992;117:226.
10. Singer DE. Screening for diabetic retinopathy. *Ann Intern Med* 1992;116:660.
11. Weinstock F, Weinstock MB. Common eye disorders. *Postgrad Med* 1996;99(4):107.
12. Wray S. The management of acute visual failure. *J Neurol Neurosurg Psychiatry* 1993;56:234.

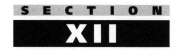

PSYCHOSOCIAL

TOBACCO ABUSE

INTRODUCTION

- The leading preventable cause of death in the United States; 420,000 tobacco-related deaths per year (Centers for Disease Control and Prevention [CDC], *unpublished data*, 1990).
- 24% of U.S. adults smoke; 70% of them want to quit and 30% have made an attempt during the past year.
- 70% of smokers see a physician at least once a year, providing an excellent opportunity for intervention.

PATHOPHYSIOLOGY

- Smoking is an addiction involving physical dependence on nicotine and learned behaviors with complex environmental and emotional cues; most smokers begin during adolescence.
- *Nicotine:* psychoactive substance causing tolerance, physical dependence, and a withdrawal syndrome (nicotine craving, irritability, difficulty concentrating, restlessness, insomnia, depression, anxiety, increased appetite). Most symptoms peak 1 to 2 days after cessation and return to baseline within 3 to 4 weeks.
- *Tobacco smoke* contains nicotine, irritant particulate matter, carbon monoxide, and multiple proven carcinogens, all of which contribute to excess morbidity in smokers.
- *Morbidity:*
  ⇒ *Cancer:* lung, head and neck, esophagus, pancreas, kidney, bladder, cervix
  ⇒ *Pulmonary disease:* major cause of chronic obstructive pulmonary disease (COPD); chronic cough, sputum production, breathlessness, abnormal pulmonary function tests increased in smokers
  ⇒ *Vascular disease:* promotes atherosclerosis; doubles risk of myocardial infarction (MI) and coronary artery disease (CAD); increases risk of cerebrovascular accident
  ⇒ *Pregnancy:* may decrease fertility; increases risk of miscarriage, perinatal death, low birth weight, and sudden infant death syndrome.
  ⇒ *Passive smoking:* increases risk of lung cancer, respiratory infections, asthma, and CAD in nonsmokers. Children of smokers have higher incidence of asthma and acute respiratory infections.

Evaluation

- Screen all patients for smoking, and mark smoking status clearly in the chart.
- Ask about smoking history, history of quit attempts, and smoking-related diseases.
- Assess readiness and counsel smokers to quit at every clinic visit (see Table 53.2).

TREATMENT/INTERVENTION

- Smoking cessation is the ultimate goal (see Table 53.1):
  ⇒ Approximately two thirds of smokers resume within 3 to 6 months; multiple quit attempts (up to five to six over several years) are often required before success.
  ⇒ After 6 months of abstinence, relapse rates are low; half of Americans who ever smoked have quit.

- Benefits to smoking cessation (Department of Health and Human Services, 1990):
  ⇒ *Mortality:* Quitting before age 50 halves the risk of dying over the next 15 years.
  ⇒ *Cancer:* Risk of developing cancer is reduced by 30% to 50% after 10 years of abstinence.
  ⇒ *MI:* Risk is reduced 50% after 1 year; approaches that of nonsmokers after 15 years.
  ⇒ *COPD:* Reduces symptoms of cough, sputum, and wheezing; decreases COPD mortality.
- Give every smoker clear, strong, personalized advice to quit.
- When a patient wants to quit, help him or her set a firm quit date; offer pharmacotherapy and a cessation program.
- Follow up with the patient during the quit attempt by telephone, mail, or in clinic.

TABLE 53.1. SMOKING CESSATION METHODS (2000 PUBLIC HEALTH SERVICE GUIDELINE PANEL CONCLUSIONS)

Effective Methods		Methods without evidence of efficacy	
Pharmacotherapy	Doubles quit rate vs. placebo. First line: nicotine replacement (patch, gum, inhaler, nasal spray), bupropion sustained release (Zyban) Second line: nortriptyline, clonidine	Hypnosis	Little evidence from controlled trials
Behavioral counseling	Individual, group, or by telephone; social support builds confidence	Acupuncture	Ineffective in most randomized trials
Combination	Most effective: amount of counseling determines absolute quit rate, which is doubled with drug therapy	Antidepressants Anxiolytics	Exceptions are buproprion and nortriptyline

Note: Effective treatments exist and should be offered to all smokers. More intensive treatment is more effective, but brief intervention such as that done in office practice works.

- Physician counseling is effective:
  ⇒ Single episode improves quit rates by 2%; multiple episodes improve rates by 5%; counseling patients post-MI improves rates by 36% (Kottke et al., 1988; U.S. Public Services Task Force, 1996; Agency for Health Care Policy and Research, 1996).
  ⇒ Enlist family and friends to assist with quitting when possible.
  ⇒ Advice should be clear, strongly worded, personalized, and reiterated at every visit; Prochazka's "stages of change" model may be used as a guide (see Table 53.2).

TABLE 53.2. RECOMMENDED CLINICAL INTERVENTION, BASED ON A PATIENT'S "STAGE OF CHANGE" (PROCHAZKA AND BOYKO, 1988)

Question	Readiness Stage	Recommended Intervention
1. Do you intend to quit during the next 6 months?	If "no": "Precontemplation" (35% of smokers)	1. Provide nonjudgmental advice. 2. Provide personal reasons to quit. 3. Correct misperceptions about consequences of continued smoking. 4. Offer materials (see below resources).
	If "yes": "Contemplation" (50% of smokers)	1. Provide personal reasons to quit. 2. Assess obstacles to cessation, including role of stress, degree of nicotine addiction, concern about weight gain, smoking triggers, what caused failure of prior quit attempts. 3. Outline a plan to overcome these obstacles. 4. Arrange follow-up discussion.

(continued)

TABLE 53.2. *(continued)*

Question	Readiness Stage	Recommended Intervention
2. Do you intend to quit during the next month?	If "yes": "Preparation" (50% of smokers)	1. Same recommendations as for "Contemplation" stage. 2. Set specific quit date within 4 wk. 3. Offer Zyban or nicotine replacement product (see below). 4. Offer referral to quit smoking program (see below). 5. Provide information materials (see below). 6. Emphasize importance of social support. 7. Arrange follow-up discussion.
3. Have you quit during the past year?	If "yes" and has abstained for <6 mo: "Action"	1. Offer support, boost self-confidence. 2. If slips have occurred, inform patient that slips are common and are part of the learning process. 3. Analyze slips to avoid recurrence.
	If "yes" and has abstained for >6 mo: "Maintenance"	1. Offer congratulations and support. 2. Emphasize positive effects of quitting. 3. Explore ability to refrain in the future.

Behavioral Counseling

- Individual or group counseling by physicians or other healthcare professionals increases quit rates.
- Formal smoking cessation programs are very helpful; often covered by insurance.
- Telephone hotlines and more recently, Web-based support groups can improve cessation rates.

Pharmacotherapy

- Should be made available to all smokers, and offered at initial discussions (Hughes, 1999).
- *Bupropion (Zyban/Wellbutrin SR):*
  ⇒ *Action:* atypical antidepressant with dopaminergic and adrenergic actions
  ⇒ *Evidence:* 7-week quit rates 44.2% for bupropion versus 19% for placebo in nondepressed smokers; 1-year bupropion quit rates 23.1% versus 12.4% for placebo (Hurt et al., 1997). Superior to nicotine replacement in one trial: 1 year quit rates 30% sustained-release bupropion, 16.4% nicotine patch, 15.6% placebo (Jorenby et al., 1999).
  ⇒ *Dosage:* 150 mg daily for 3 days, then 150 mg twice daily for 8 to 12 weeks; start 1 week before preset quit date
  ⇒ *Cost:* $2.50 per day, less than one pack of cigarettes. Zyban occasionally covered by insurance; most will cover Wellbutrin SR.
  ⇒ *Side effects/contraindications:* 0.1% seizure risk; contraindicated in patients with a history of epilepsy, seizure predisposition (head trauma, stroke history, heavy alcohol use), or a history of eating disorders. Mild adverse affects: dry mouth, insomnia, headache.
- Nicotine replacement therapy (NRT) (see Table 53.3):
  ⇒ *Evidence:* NRT (patch, gum, nasal spray, inhaler) approximately doubles quit rates over placebo, yielding 6-month abstinence rates between 9% and 35% (Hughes et al., 1999). Combining a patch with gum increases quit rates and decreases withdrawal symptoms (Fagerstrom, 1994).
  ⇒ *Contraindications:* MI within the last 4 weeks, severe or worsening angina, life-threatening arrhythmia, or pregnancy (although NRT may be preferable to continued smoking in these conditions).

TABLE 53.3. NICOTINE REPLACEMENT THERAPIES

	Availability	Dosing	Side Effects	Comments
Gum	Over the counter	One to two pieces/hr; scheduled dosing more effective than when necessary dosing <25 cigarettes/d: 2-mg dose (max 30 pieces/d) >25 cigarettes/d: 4-mg dose (max 20 pieces/d)	Mouth sores, hiccups, dyspepsia, jaw ache (often alleviated by altering chewing technique). May damage extensive dental work.	May be difficult for denture wearers to use. Six weeks of scheduled dosing, although longer use may be superior.
Patch	16 hr/d over the counter: *Nicoderm* 24 hr/d over the counter: *Nicotrol CQ* Prescription: *Habitrol*	>1/2 PPD: 15-mg dose × 4–12 wk, then 10 mg × 2–4 wk, then 5 mg × 2–4 wk, then 7 mg × 2–4 wk <1/2 PPD, start at 10 mg dose 1–2 PPD: 21-mg dose × 6 wk, then 14 mg × 2–4 wk, then 7 mg × 2–4 wk	Insomnia with 24-hr patch, removal while sleeping may improve symptoms.	No major adverse effects to smoking while on the patch, but patients should be counseled against it (Jimenez-Ruiz et al. 1998).
Nasal spray	Prescription: *Nicotrol nasal spray*	1/2 PPD, start at 14 mg dose step (also with stable angina, patients <100 lb). One to two sprays/hr × 3–6 mo.	Nasal and throat irritation, rhinitis, sneezing, coughing, and watery eyes; tolerance usually occurs after 1 week.	Rapid rise in blood nicotine; may be needed by the most dependent smokers
Inhaler	Prescription	6–18 inhalers/d for 3–6 mo. Nicotine vapor (not smoke) absorbed through the oral mucosa.	Mild coughing and mouth/throat irritation	Resembles a cigarette; provides substitute for hand-to-mouth behavior desired by some quitters

Note: PPD, packs per day.

- *Nortriptyline:*
  ⇒ *Evidence:* cessation rate at 6 months 14% for nortriptyline versus 3% for placebo; small decrease in withdrawal symptoms and quitting-related negative affect (Prochazka, 1998). Efficacy independent of depression history (Hall et al., 1998). No current studies comparing nortriptyline to NRT or Zyban.
  ⇒ *Side effects:* dry mouth (64%), dyspepsia (20%)
- *Clonidine:*
  ⇒ *Action:* central-acting α-agonist; oral and transdermal forms reduce withdrawal symptoms
  ⇒ *Evidence:* approximately double quit rates. Not approved by the Food and Drug Administration for treating smoking
  ⇒ *Side effects:* sedation, hypotension limit clinical use

Barriers to Quitting and How to Overcome Them

- **Weight gain** (average 7 to 12 pounds, <15% gain >25 pounds): Begin an exercise program, consider nicotine gum or bupropion, which appear to blunt weight gain; possible weight gain less detrimental to health than continued smoking.
- **Family or friends smoke:** Ask household members not to smoke in the house during the first month (a "smoke-free" zone of safety for the quitter); consider a formal cessation program for social support.
- **Fear of failure:** Quitting is a learning process, often requiring multiple attempts.
- **Withdrawal symptoms in the past:** Add or increase dose of NRT; add Zyban.
- **"Cigarettes are my friends:"** "Your friends don't kill you." Acknowledge that transient sadness is normal, and screen for depression.
- **Depression on past quit attempts:** Consider treatment with antidepressant before or with quit attempt; follow closely and/or refer to a formal program.

SELECTED REFERENCES

1. Agency for Health Care Policy and Research. Smoking cessation clinical practice guideline. *JAMA* 1996;275:1270–1280.

2. Centers for Disease Control and Prevention. Cigarette smoking–attributable mortality and years of potential life lost—United States, 1990. *MMWR Morb Mortal Wkly Rep* 1993;42:645–649.

3. Department of Health and Human Services. *The health benefits of smoking cessation: a report of the Surgeon General.* Rockville, MD: Department of Health and Human Services; 1990.

4. Fagerstrom K. Combined use of nicotine replacement products. *Health Values* 1994;18:15–20.

5. Hall SM, Reus VI, Munoz RF, et al. Nortriptyline and cognitive-behavioral therapy in the treatment of cigarette smoking. *Arch Gen Psychiatry* 1998;55(8):683–690.

6. Hughes JR. Risk/benefit of nicotine replacement in smoking cessation. *Drug Safety* 1993;8:49–56.

7. Hughes JR. Combining behavioral therapy and pharmacotherapy for smoking cessation: an update. In: Onken LS, et al., eds. *Integrating behavior therapies with medication in the treatment of drug dependence.* Washington, DC: US Government Printing Office; 1995.

8. Hughes JR, Goldstein MG, Hurt RD, et al. Recent advances in the pharmacotherapy of smoking. *JAMA* 1999;281(1):72–76.

9. Hurt RD, Sachs DP, Glover ED, et al. A comparison of sustained-release bupropion and placebo for smoking cessation. *N Engl J Med* 1997;337(17):1195–1202.

10. Jimenez-Ruiz C, Kunze M, Fagerstrom KO, et al. Nicotine replacement: a new approach to reduce tobacco-related harm. *Eur Respir J* 1998;11:473–479.

11. Jorenby DE, Leischow SJ, Nides MA, et al. A controlled trial of sustained-release bupropion, a nicotine patch, or both for smoking cessation. *N Engl J Med* 1999;340(9):685–691.

12. Killen JD, Fortmann SP, Newman B, et al. Evaluation of a treatment approach combining nicotine gum with self-guided behavioral treatments for smoking relapse prevention. *J Consult Clin Psychol* 1990;58:85–92.

13. Kottke TE, Battista RN, DeFriese GH, et al. Attributes of successful smoking cessation interventions in medical practice: a meta-analysis of 39 controlled trials. *JAMA* 1988;259:2882–2889.

14. Prochazka AV, Boyko EJ: How physicians can help their patients quit smoking: a practical guide. *West J Med* 1988;149:188–194.

15. Prochazka AV, Weaver MJ, Keller RT, et al. A randomized trial of nortriptyline for smoking. *Arch Intern Med* 1998;158(18):2035–2039.

16. US Preventive Services Task Force. *Guide to clinical preventive services.* Baltimore: Williams & Wilkins, 1996.

17. US Public Health Service Report. A clinical practice guideline for treating tobacco use and dependence. *JAMA* 2000;283:3244–3254.

ALCOHOL ABUSE

INTRODUCTION

- One "standard drink" = 12 g pure alcohol = 12 oz beer/wine cooler = 5 oz wine = 1.5 oz 80-proof 1 pt = 16 oz; a fifth = 27 oz; a liter = 34 oz; a quart = 32 oz. In general about 100 g of alcohol per day (eight drinks per day) for >1 week is required for clinically significant withdrawal upon stopping.
- 10% of Americans suffer from alcohol dependence or abuse (National Institute on Alcohol Abuse and Alcoholism [NIAAA], *unpublished data*); 15% to 20% of male and 5% to 10% of female patients in the primary care setting suffer from problem drinking; lifetime prevalence may be as high as 36% (Bradley, 1994). It is particularly common in those with co-morbid psychiatric conditions.
- Estimated to cause 100,000 excess deaths annually in the United States; death rates are two to four times greater in people with alcohol dependence than in matched controls.
  - ⇒ Mortality increases for men drinking more than two to three drinks per day (Boffetta and Garfinkel, 1990; Camargo et al., 1997) and women drinking >2.5 drinks per day (Fuchs et al., 1995).
  - ⇒ Drunk driving accounts for >40% of traffic fatalities; two thirds of all drownings are related to alcohol.
- 1995 estimated cost: $167 billion for treatment, drug-associated diseases, crime, perinatal care, maternal abuse/neglect, federal/state benefits, time lost from work.

EVALUATION

- Numerous medical conditions are related to at-risk drinking, dependence, or abuse: hepatitis, cirrhosis, pancreatitis, hypertension, gastritis, gastroesophageal reflux disease, sexual dysfunction, neuropathy, Wernicke encephalopathy, Korsakoff psychosis, depression, sleep disorders, and traumatic injuries.
- Primary care providers are in the ideal position to screen for alcohol abuse and its associated conditions:
  - ⇒ *Screen* all patients for alcohol use.
  - ⇒ Assess *level of problem* (NIAAA or *Diagnostic and Statistical Manual of Mental Disorders* [*DSM*] criteria; CAGE questionnaire).
  - ⇒ Assess *readiness* to reduce consumption (the Prochaska "stages of change" model).
  - ⇒ Conduct 5-minute *brief intervention/motivational interview* (FRAMES mnemonic below).
  - ⇒ Consider pharmacologic intervention (naltrexone is the preferred agent for relapse prevention).
  - ⇒ Consider referral for outpatient counseling or psychosocial treatment.
- Note that many similar considerations apply to substance abuse in general.

Screening

- Ask specific questions to classify patient by NIAAA or *Diagnostic and Statistical Manual of Mental Disorders,* fourth edition (*DSM-IV*), criteria (see Tables 54.1 and 54.2):
  - ⇒ "On average, how many days per week do you drink alcohol?"

⇒ "On a typical day when you drink, how many drinks do you have?"
⇒ "What is the maximum number of drinks you had on any given occasion during the last month?"

TABLE 54.1. NATIONAL INSTITUTE ON ALCOHOL ABUSE AND ALCOHOLISM DEFINITIONS

	Moderate Drinking (Small Mortality Benefit in Adults, [Thun et al., 1997])	*At-Risk Drinking:*
Men	≤2 drinks/d	>14 drinks/wk >4 drinks/occasion
Women	≤1 drink/d	>7 drinks/wk >3 drinks/occasion
Age >65 yr	≤1 drink/d	

TABLE 54.2. *DIAGNOSTIC AND STATISTICAL MANUAL OF MENTAL DISORDERS, FOURTH EDITION,* DIAGNOSTIC CRITERIA

Alcohol abuse
One or more of the following present at any time during the same 12-mo period

- Alcohol use results in failure to fulfill major obligations
- Recurrent use in physically dangerous situations (such as drunk driving)
- Recurrent alcohol-related legal problems
- Continued use despite recurrent social or interpersonal problems
- Has never met criteria for alcohol dependence

Alcohol dependence
Three or more of the following at any time during the same 12-mo period

- Tolerance
- Withdrawal
- Use in larger amounts or for longer periods than intended
- Unsuccessful efforts to cut down or control use
- Significant time spent obtaining alcohol, using, or recovering from alcohol use
- Important activities given up
- Continued use despite knowledge of problems due to alcohol use

- **CAGE** screening questions (see Table 54.3): Two or more positive responses have 60% to 95% sensitivity and 40% to 95% specificity for dependence or abuse (less sensitive for early problem drinking or in patients older than 60 years):

TABLE 54.3. CAGE QUESTIONS

C: Have you ever felt you should **c**ut down on your drinking?
A: Have people **a**nnoyed you by criticizing your drinking?
G: Have you ever felt **g**uilty about your drinking?
E: Have you ever had a drink early in the morning to steady nerves or get rid of a hangover (**e**ye opener)?

- **AUDIT** questionnaire: a ten-item screening instrument developed by the World Health Organization; higher sensitivity and specificity than CAGE for current abuse or dependence (available in the U.S. Preventive Services Task Force Guide [1996]).
- Follow up all screening with a discussion. Those with negative screens should be informed about data regarding safe drinking levels; those with a positive screen require further intervention and treatment.

Assessing Readiness for Change

- Prochaska's six "stages of change" may be helpful (see Table 54.4). A goal of the brief intervention, below, is to help the patient advance to the next stage:

TABLE 54.4. PROCHASKA'S "STAGES OF CHANGE" MODEL AND THE PRACTITIONER'S TASK AT EACH STAGE

Precontemplation: The patient is unaware there is a problem or has no thought of changing behavior.
⇒ *Gather evidence regarding the patient's relationship to the problem. If the patient thinks there is no problem, raise doubts.*
Contemplation: The patient is aware there is a problem but is ambivalent about change.
⇒ *Attempt to tip the balance toward change. Help the patient enumerate reasons to change. Strengthen the patient's self-efficacy.*
Determination: The patient desires change and may be working toward changing behavior but has not yet done so.
⇒ *Help the patient determine the best course of action.*
Action: The patient is actively changing behavior.
⇒ *Help the patient to continue taking the best course.*
Maintenance: The patient has changed behavior patterns and is maintaining the behavior change.
⇒ *Reinforce the change. Help prevent relapse by helping patient delineate coping strategies (e.g., staying away from old haunts, engaging in "replacement" activities such as hobbies).*
Relapse: The patient falls back into old habits.
⇒ *Keep the patient from being hopeless; reduce the patient's shame. Help move toward action again.*

Adapted from: Miller WR, Rollnick S. Motivational interviewing: preparing people to change addictive behavior. New York: Guilford Press, 1991.

TREATMENT

"Brief Intervention" (Motivational Interview)

- 5 minutes of simple advice yields the same results as 20 minutes of counseling: a 17% reduction in daily alcohol consumption after 9 months of follow-up (Barbor, 1996).
  ⇒ A metaanalysis of eight studies calculated a pooled odds ratio of 1.95 for decreased drinking after a brief intervention when compared with no intervention (Wilk et al., 1997).
- The **FRAMES** mnemonic (see Table 54.5) includes key elements of the brief intervention (Bien et al., 1993):

TABLE 54.5. FRAMES BRIEF INTERVENTION MNEMONIC

F:	Provide **f**eedback about the patient's personal risk.
R:	Encourage the patient to take **r**esponsibility for personal change.
A:	Provide clear and direct **a**dvice to change.
M:	Provide a **m**enu of concrete strategies that can be used to facilitate change (e.g., therapy, medications, etc).
E:	Be **e**mpathic.
S:	Communicate optimism or **s**elf-efficacy regarding the possibility of change.

- When a concrete plan is agreed on, consider writing it down with the patient.
- Follow up with a telephone call, note, or appointment.
- Abstinence is the recommendation of choice; there is no convincing evidence that controlled drinking is a predictable or safe strategy in those with a history of losing control of their drinking. However, reduction to a safer level of alcohol consumption is a good harm-reduction strategy.
- Patients with severe and chronic substance dependence often require the help of specialized treatment centers.

Psychotherapy/Recovery Programs

- Counseling and peer support have long been the mainstay of recovery.
- Various levels of care in the different treatment settings: inpatient hospitalization, residential treatment, intensive outpatient treatment (>9 hours per week), and less intensive outpatient treatment. Choose the setting most appropriate for the patient at the time and adjust according to progress.
- Three common psychotherapy modalities: Twelve-Step Facilitation (Alcoholics Anonymous), cognitive behavioral therapy, motivational enhancement therapy. A large NIAAA-sponsored study (Project MATCH, 1997) found that all three increased abstinence levels from 20% of the time to 80% to 90%.

Detoxification

- Symptoms of withdrawal usually begin 6 to 24 hours after reduction or cessation of alcohol use, peak at 24 to 48 hours, and resolve in 4 to 5 days. Withdrawal seizures and delirium tremors (DTs) occur in <5% of patients but may occur up to 7 days after withdrawal starts.
- Withdrawal predictably occurs in patients with prior symptoms of withdrawal.
- *Benzodiazepines* are the drug of choice: Ideally should only be given to inpatients under close supervision. Outpatients should be given sufficient medication for 1 to 2 days at a time with frequent follow-up. Patients must not drive while using benzodiazepines.
  - ⇒ Roughly equivalent doses: Ativan 1 mg orally (p.o.) = Ativan 0.5 mg intravenously (i.v.) = Librium 25 mg p.o. = Valium 5 mg p.o. = Valium 2.5 mg i.v. = Serax 30 mg p.o. = 1.5 to 2 drinks

Pharmacotherapy (Table 54.6)

TABLE 54.6. PHARMACOTHERAPY: RELAPSE PREVENTION AS ADJUNCTS TO PSYCHOTHERAPY

Agent	Considerations
Naltrexone	*Mechanism:* Opioid antagonist. Blunts the pleasurable effects of alcohol, reduces craving. *Evidence:* Reduced risk of relapse to heavy drinking and decreased frequency of drinking compared with placebo; abstinence not substanitially enhanced (Garbutt et al., 1999; Swift, 1999). Limited by nonadherence: ~60% of patients take mediction as prescribed. *Usual dosage:* 50 mg daily, although 100 mg produces blocking effects for 2 days, and 150 mg for 3 days. *Side effects/contraindications:* nausea, headache, dizziness, sedation at higher doses. Larger doses also associated with hepatitis: Monitor liver function tests (LFT) in patients with liver disease.
Disulfiram (Antabuse)	*Mechanism:* Blocks ethanol metabolism, raising acetaldehyde levels and increasing aversive effects. *Evidence:* Placebo-controlled studies mixed and largely inconclusive: Most rigorous trial showed no improvement in abstinence or time to first drink, but mild decrease in drinking frequency (Fuller et al., 1986). Limited by nonadherence, only ~20% of patients take medication as prescribed. *Usual dosage:* 250 mg daily, although clinicians use 25–1,000 mg, based on side effects and response. Some patients use the drug daily, others only when at high risk for relapse. *Side effects/contraindications:* Inhibits metabolism of anticoagulants, phenytoin, and isoniazid. Contraindicated in pregnancy and ischemic heart disease. May cause hepatitis: LFTs should be monitored.
Acamprosate (not currently available in the United States)	*Mechanism:* analogue. Blunts unpleasant symptoms of abstinence, reduces craving. *Evidence:* Reduction in frequency of drinking; influence on abstinence or time to first drink less clear. Longer abstinence periods compared with placebo in one randomized trial (Paille et al., 1995). *Usual dosage:* 2–3 daily in three divided doses. *Side effects/contraindications:* Diarrhea and headache. Renally excreted: Use caution with renal insufficiency.
Selective serotonin reuptake inhibitors (SSRIs)	Insufficient evidence to support use of SSRIs for alchohol dependence, although patients with coexisting psychiatric disorders may benefit.

RESOURCES

- National Library of Medicine: "A guide to Substance Abuse Services for Primary Care Clinicians."
- National Directory of Drug Abuse and Alcoholism Treatment and Prevention Programs: 800-729-6686

SELECTED REFERENCES

1. Barbor, WHO Brief Intervention Study Group. A cross-national trial of brief interventions with heavy drinkers. *Am J Public Health* 1996;86(7):948–955.
2. Bien TH, Miller WR, Tonigan JS. Brief interventions for alcohol problems: a review. *Addiction* 1993;88(3):315–335.
3. Boffetta P, Garfinkel L. Alcohol drinking and mortality among men enrolled in an American Cancer Society prospective study. *Epidemiology* 1990;1(5):342–348.
4. Bradley KA. The primary care provider's role in the prevention and management of alcohol problems. *Alcohol Health Res World* 1994;18:97–104.
5. Camargo CA Jr, Hennekens CH, Gaziano JM, at al. Prospective study of moderate alcohol consumption and mortality in US male physicians. *Arch Intern Med* 1997;157(1):79–85.
6. *Diagnostic and statistical manual of mental disorders,* 4th ed. Washington, DC: American Psychiatric Association, 1994.
7. Fleming MF, Barry KL. The effectiveness of alcoholism screening in an ambulatory care setting. *J Stud Alcohol* 1991;52(1):33–36.
8. Fuchs CS, Stampfer MJ, Colditz GA, et al. Alcohol consumption and mortality among women. *N Engl J Med* 1995;332(19):1245–1250.
9. Fuller RK, Branchey L, Brightwell DR, et al. Disulfiram treatment of alcoholism. *JAMA* 1986;256(11):1449–1455.
10. Garbutt JC, West SL, Carey TS, et al. Pharmacological treatment of alcohol dependence. *JAMA* 1999;281(14):1318–1325.
11. Liskow B, Campbell J, Nickel EJ, et al. Validity of the CAGE questionnaire in screening for alcohol dependence in a walk-in (triage) clinic. *J Stud Alcohol* 1995;56(3):277–281.
12. Paille FM, Guelfi JD, Perkins AC, et al. Doubleblind randomized multicentre trial of acamprosate in maintaining abstinence from alcohol. *Alcohol Alcohol* 1995;30(2);239–247.
13. Prochaska JO, Diclemente CC, Norcross JC, et al. In search of how people change: applications to addictive behaviors. *Am Psychol* 1992;47(9):1102–1114.
14. Project MATCH Research Group. Matching alcoholism treatments to client heterogeneity. *J Stud Alcohol* 1997;58:7–20.
15. Secretary of Health and Human Services. *Special report to the U.S. Congress on alcohol and health.* Washington, DC: National Institute on Alcohol and Alcoholism, 1997.
16. Swift RM. Drug therapy for alcohol dependence. *N Engl J Med* 1999;340(19):1482–1490.
17. Thun MJ, Peto R, Lopez AD, et al. Alcohol consumption and mortality among middle-aged and elderly U.S. adults. *N Engl J Med* 1997;337(24):1705–1714.
18. US Preventive Services Task Force. *Guide to clinical preventive services.* Baltimore: Williams & Wilkins, 1996.
19. Wilk AI, Jensen NM, Haringhurst TC, et al. Meta-analysis of randomized control trials addressing brief interventions in heavy alcohol drinkers. *J Gen Intern Med* 1997;12(1):274–283.

DEPRESSION IN PRIMARY CARE

INTRODUCTION

- Lifetime prevalence of major depression 17%; estimated point prevalence about 5%, with incidence in women twice that in men (Blazer et al., 1994).
- Second leading cause of disability in the United States; up to $43 billion annually in healthcare costs; death rates in patients with mood disorders 1.5 times that of nondepressed individuals (Saz and Dewey, 2001; Vaccarino et al. 2001).
- Half of depressed Americans receive treatment from primary care physicians (Narrow et al., 1993); 20% of primary care patients have clinically significant depressive symptoms (Leon et al., 1995), many of whom remain untreated or undertreated (Hirschfeld et al., 1997).

PATHOPHYSIOLOGY/CLINICAL PRESENTATION

- A constellation of physical and psychological symptoms associated with disordered mood including affective, behavioral, and cognitive symptoms (see Tables 55.1 and 55.2).
- Typical episode lasts 6 to 14 months untreated. Optimal treatment can shorten duration to 4 to 8 weeks.
- Risk of recurrence after one depressive episode is 50%; rises to 80% with two episodes and 90% with three episodes.
- Risk factors: female gender; family/personal history of depression; alcohol or substance abuse; chronic illness; certain personality disorders.

TABLE 55.1. PHYSICAL AND PSYCHOLOGICAL SYMPTOMS OF MOOD AND ANXIETY DISORDERS

Anger attacks	Fatigue	Lack of motivation
Anxiety	Feelings of worthlessness	Loss of interest or pleasure
Backaches	Forgetfulness	Muscle tension
Carbohydrate craving	Headaches	Nervousness
Crying spells	Heart palpitations	Panic attacks
Depressed mood	Heaviness in arms or legs	Psychomotor agitation
Diminished concentration	Hypersomnia	Psychomotor retardation
Distractibility	Hypochondriacal concerns	Recurrent thoughts of death
Dizziness of lightheadedness	Indecisiveness	Suicidal ideation or plan
Excessive guilt	Insomnia	Weight gain or increased appetite
Excessive worrying	Irritable mood	Weight loss or decreased appetite

DIFFERENTIAL DIAGNOSIS

- Several psychiatric and medical disorders may mimic major depressive disorder: the *Diagnostic and Statistical Manual of Mental Disorders,* fourth edition, has specific diagnostic criteria (see Tables 55.2 and 55.3).

TABLE 55.2. *DIAGNOSTIC AND STATISTICAL MANUAL OF MENTAL DISORDERS, FOURTH EDITION:* CRITERIA FOR DEPRESSIVE DISORDERS[a]

Major Depressive Disorder	Dysthymic Disorder
• Depressed mood or markedly diminished interest in almost all activities • Duration at least 2 wk • At least four of the following (*SIG:E CAPS*) ⇒ **S**leep disturbance (decreased or increased sleep) ⇒ **I**nterests decreased (in almost all activities most of the day, nearly everyday) ⇒ **G**uilt or preoccupation of thought ⇒ **E**nergy decreased ⇒ **C**oncentration decreased ⇒ **A**ppetite change (increased or decreased) ⇒ **P**sychomotor agitation or retardation ⇒ **S**uicidal thoughts or recurrent thoughts of death • Symptoms cause significant distress or psychosocial impairment • Symptoms are not better accounted for by bereavement, medical condition, or substance abuse • No history of manic or hypomanic episode • Depressive episode is not superimposed on psychotic disorder and is not better accounted for by schizoaffective disorder	• Depressed mood for most of the day, for more days than not, for at least 2 yr • When depressed, the presence of at least two of the following ⇒ poor appetite or overeating ⇒ insomnia or hypersomnia ⇒ low energy or fatigue ⇒ low self-esteem ⇒ poor concentration or indecisiveness ⇒ feelings of hopelessness • During a 2 yr period, never without depressed mood for more than 2 mo at a time • No evidence of a major depressive episode during the first 2 yr of the disturbance • No history of mania, hypomania, or cyclothymia • Symptoms not caused by medical condition or substance abuse • Symptoms cause clinically significant distress or psychosocial impairment • The disturbance does not occur excessively during psychotic disorders

[a] Depressive disorder not otherwise specified is included as a *Diagnostic and statistical manual of mental disorders*, fourth edition, unipolar depressive disorder and is reserved for disorders with depressive features that do not meet the criteria for major depressive disorder or dysthymic disorder.

TABLE 55.3. DIFFERENTIAL DIAGNOSIS OF UNIPOLAR DEPRESSIVE DISORDERS

Condition	Presentation
Dementia	Patients frequently complain of apathy, poor concentration, and memory difficulties. Unlike demented patients, depressed outpatients rarely score below 23 on Mini-Mental State Examiniation (see Chapter 50).
Bipolar depression	Patients may present with depressive symptoms for the first time. Careful history may reveal prior periods of irritable or expansive mood.
Psychotic disorders	Schizophrenia and other psychotic disorders may be accompanied by depression. Major depressive disorder with catatonic features may be difficult to distinguish from schizophernia.
Premenstrual dysphoric disorder (PDD)	PDD is distinguished from depression by the presence of symptoms only with menses. Because depressed patients may suffer an exacerbation of preexisting symptoms during menses, carefully screen for symptoms between menses.
Anxiety disorders	Irritability, neverousness, insomnia, and impaired concentration characterize many anxiety disorders and may mimic depression.
General medical conditions	Hypo- and hyperthyrodism, hypo- and hyperparathyrodism, hypo- and hyperadrenalism, vitamin B_{12} and folate deficiencies, Parkinson's, hepatitis, systemic lupus erythematosus, rheumatoid arthritis, human immunodeficiency virus infection, and cancer (particularly pancreatic) have been linked with mood disorders.

EVALUATION

Screening

- Recognition of signs and symptoms of depression can be challenging during a routine primary care encounter. Patients, particularly the elderly, tend to discuss physical rather than emotional symptoms, leading clinicians to pursue a medical explanation for symptoms.
- The U.S. Preventive Services Task Force (1996) reports insufficient evidence to recommend for or against the routine use of standardized questionnaires to screen for depression in asymptomatic primary care patients.

⇒ Self-rating scales (e.g., Beck Depression Inventory for primary care) effectively identify depressed patients with high sensitivity and specificity (Steer et al., 1999).

⇒ The SIG: E CAPS mnemonic (see Table 55.2) is a simple screening tool for depression.

- Given the high prevalence of depression in primary care, the following symptoms or historical features should prompt screening (Robinson et al., 1996):

⇒ Physical or emotional symptoms of depression

⇒ Vague somatic complaints, including sleep disorders

⇒ Recent personal loss or stressful situation

⇒ Family or personal history of depression, suicide, substance abuse, or mental illness

⇒ Self-destructive or excessively risky behaviors

⇒ Major medical illness (stroke, heart disease, cancer)

⇒ Recent childbirth

⇒ Chronic pain

⇒ Use of alcohol and nicotine

⇒ Current use of antihypertensives, hormone replacement therapy, histamine (H_2) blockers, anticonvulsants, interferon, metoclopramide, corticosteroids, or levodopa

History

- Psychosocial

⇒ Onset, duration, and course of physical and psychological symptoms; symptom severity, including impact on psychosocial functioning

⇒ Alcohol and/or recreational drug use: Depression may result from psychotropic use or be an attempt at self-medication. Symptoms may improve or even remit with the cessation of substance abuse.

⇒ Psychiatric history, particularly mood disorders (influence prognosis and treatment options); suicidal ideation; any psychotic symptoms

⇒ Recent bereavement; current social support network

- Medical

⇒ Certain medical conditions (see Table 55.3) can mimic or be associated with depression; patients should be screened if there is clinical suspicion and treated if indicated. Occasionally, treating the medical condition (particularly endocrine disorders) ameliorates the depression.

⇒ Certain medications (e.g., propranolol, reserpine, interferon, metoclopramide, corticosteroids, oral contraceptives, and levodopa) may trigger symptoms of depression. If temporally related, medication discontinuation may be warranted.

TREATMENT

Alternatives to Pharmacotherapy

- **Psychotherapy:** cognitive, interpersonal, or behavioral; efficacious treatment option, especially when the patient wishes to avoid medications and side effects (DeRubeis et al., 1999).
- **St. John's Wort:** Herbal preparation widely used in Europe, available over-the-counter in the United States. Appears to have few side effects, but dangerous interactions with antiretroviral drugs and immunosuppressants have been reported; effective in treating mild to moderate depression in European controlled trials (Linde et al., 1996); placebo-controlled, clinical trials underway in the United States.
- **Light therapy:** Used for seasonal depression, or seasonal affective disorder; characterized by recurrent clinical depression in the fall and winter months with resolution in the spring and summer months.
- **Electroconvulsive therapy:** the most effective treatment for depression. Generally reserved for severe depression, those who have failed several trials of antidepressants, or illness marked by delusions.

Pharmacotherapy

- **Choose an appropriate initial medication.**

⇒ *Selective serotonin reuptake inhibitors* and the *atypical antidepressants* (see Tables 55.4 and 55.5): first-line agents given relative safety in overdose and favorable side-effect profile, especially compared with tricyclic antidepressants (TCAs) and monoamine oxidase inhibitors

(MAOIs). Clinicians who choose to use TCAs and MAOIs should be familiar with their side effects and considerable drug interactions.

⇒ All classes have comparable efficacy and similar mechanisms, increasing the concentration of monoamine neurotransmitters (primarily norepinephrine and serotonin) at the neuronal synapse.

- **Use a proper dose for an adequate duration.**
  ⇒ Start at low dose and titrate to the target dose; about 50% of primary care clinicians fail to prescribe antidepressants at recommended doses (Hirschfeld et al., 1997).
  ⇒ 5 to 8 weeks may be necessary before clinical improvement; an adequate trial consists of at least 6 weeks of medication at an appropriate dose.
- **Monitor acute, continuation, and maintenance therapies.**
  ⇒ *Acute therapy:* the first 8 to 12 weeks of treatment, during which the patient's dose is titrated to target. Most patients demonstrate significant clinical improvement, although not full resolution; if no response, alter the treatment plan.
  ⇒ *Continuation therapy:* extending treatment with the same drug at the same dose 6 months or more after resolution of the acute depressive symptoms to maintain remission; indicated in all patients. Depressed outpatients who discontinue therapy within 3 months are about 80% more likely to relapse, compared with patients continuing therapy for >4 months (Melfi et al., 1998).
  ⇒ *Maintenance therapy:* continuation of medication for years or even lifelong; reserved for patients likely to relapse (chronic or severe depression, history of multiple relapses, recent major depressive episode). Combination maintenance therapy and prolonged psychotherapy may be needed in difficult patients (Thase et al., 2000).
- **Conduct follow-up visits and be prepared to change therapy.**
  ⇒ Close follow-up, every 1 to 2 weeks, is necessary during the acute phase of treatment; patients may become paradoxically more likely to commit suicide as apathy improves with treatment. Up to 15% of severely depressed patients may commit suicide (Blair-West and Mellsop, 2001).
  ⇒ After completing 4 weeks on a full dose of a chosen drug, assess for symptom improvement. If no improvement, options include increasing the dose of the current medication, switching to another medication, or adding another agent for combination or augmentation therapy (e.g., lithium, thyroxine, bromocriptine, or psychostimulants).
  ⇒ Optimum treatment strategy after initial failure to respond is unclear: Patient should again be followed closely at 1- to 2-week intervals and reassessed after an additional 4 to 6 weeks for improvement. If there is no significant improvement after an adjustment, referral to a psychiatrist is indicated.
  ⇒ When the decision is made to withdraw treatment, the drug should be slowly tapered (over weeks to months) and the patient should be followed to assess for symptoms of relapse.
- **When to refer to psychiatry:**
  ⇒ Significant suicide risk; disabling depression
  ⇒ History of bipolar disorder; co-morbidities such as substance abuse, anxiety disorder, psychosis, or dementia
  ⇒ The patient is pregnant or plans to become pregnant.
  ⇒ Lack of a social support network
  ⇒ Failure to respond to at least one adequate trial of antidepressant therapy

TABLE 55.4. SELECTIVE SEROTONIN REUPTAKE INHIBITORS (SSRIs)

Generic Name (Commercial Name)	Usual Starting Dose	Target Dose	Side Effects of SSRIs (Class Effects)
Fluoxetine (Prozac)	10–20 mg/d	20–40 mg/d	Nausea, decreased appetite, weight loss, excessive sweating, nervousness, insomnia, sexual dysfunction (delayed ejaculation or no orgasm), sedation. Abrupt cessation may result in lethargy.
Sertraline (Zoloft)	50 mg/d	100–250 mg/d	
Paroxetine (Paxil)	10–20 mg/d	20–60 mg/d	
Fluvoxamine (Luvox)	50–100 mg/d	100–250 mg/d	
Citalopram (Celexa)	10–20 mg/d	20–40 mg/d	
Venlafaxine (Effexor)	37.5 mg twice daily	75–150 mg twice daily	

TABLE 55.5. ATYPICAL ANTIDEPRESSANTS

Generic Name	Usual Starting Dose	Target Dose	Side Effects and Contraindications
Bupropion (Wellbutrin)	150 mg SR q.d. or 75 mg b.i.d.	100–150 mg t.i.d.	Agitation, dry mouth, insomnia, headache, constipation, tremor. **Contraindicated in those with seizure disorders or bulimia.**
Mirtazapine (Remeron)	15 mg q.h.s.	30–45 mg q.h.s.	Sedation, drowsiness, increased appetite, weight gain, dry mouth. **Few drug interactions have been noted; good for combination therapy.**
Nefazodone (Serzone)	100 mg b.i.d.	150–300 mg b.i.d.	Headache, fatigue, orthostatic hypotension, dry mouth, constipation, sedation, blurred vision.
Trazodone (Desyrel)	50–100 mg q.h.s.	200–600 mg/d	Drowsiness, dizziness, headache, orthostatic, hypotension, priapism.

Note: b.i.d., twice daily; q.d., every day; t.i.d., three times a day.

SELECTED REFERENCES

1. Blair-West GW, Mellsop GW. Major depression: does a gender-based down-rating of suicide risk challenge its diagnostic validity? *Aust N Z J Psychiatry* 2001;35:322–328.
2. Blazer DG, Kessler RC, McGonagle KA, et al. The prevalence and distribution of major depression in a national community sample: The National Comorbidity Survey. *Am J Psychiatry* 1994;151:979–986.
3. DeRubeis RJ, Gelfand LA, Tang TZ, et al. Medications versus cognitive behavioral therapy for severely depressed outpatients: meta-analysis of four randomized comparisons. *Am J Psychiatry* 1999;157:1007–1013.
4. *Diagnostic and statistical manual of mental disorders*, 4th ed. Washington, DC: American Psychiatric Association, 1994.
5. Hirschfeld RMA, Keller MB, Panico S, et al. The National Depressive and Manic Depressive Association consensus statement on the under treatment of depression. *JAMA* 1997;277:333–340.
6. Leon AC, Olfson M, Broadhead WE, et al. Prevalence of mental disorders in primary care. Implications for screening. *Arch Fam Med* 1995;4:857–861.
7. Linde K, Ramirez G, Mulrow CD, et al. St. John's Wort for depression: an overview and meta-analysis of randomised clinical trials. *BMJ* 1996;313:253–258.
8. Melfi CA, Chawla AJ, Croghan TW, et al. The effects of adherence to antidepressant treatment guidelines on relapse and recurrence of depression. *Arch Gen Psychiatry* 1998;55:1128–1132.
9. Murphy JM, Monson RR, Olivier DC, et al. Affective disorders and mortality: a general population study. *Arch Gen Psychiatry* 1987;44:473–480.
10. Narrow WE, Reigier DA, Rae DS, et al. Use of services by persons with mental and addictive disorders: findings from the National Institute of Mental Health Epidemiologic Catchment Area Program. *Arch Gen Psychiatry* 1993;50:95–107.
11. Robinson P, Wischman C, Del Vento A. *Treating depression in primary care: a manual for primary care and mental health providers.* Reno, NV: Context Press, 1996.
12. Saz P, Dewey ME. Depression, depressive symptoms and mortality in persons aged 65 and over living in the community: a systematic review of the literature. *Int J Geriatr Psychiatry* 2001;16:622–630.
13. Steer RA, Cavalieri TA, Leonard DM, et al. Use of the Beck Depression Inventory for primary care to screen for major depression disorders. *Gen Hosp Psychiatry* 1999;21:106–111.
14. Thase ME. Treatment of severe depression. *J Clin Psychiatry* 2000;61[Suppl 1]:17–25.
15. US Department of Health and Human Services. *Mental health: a report of the Surgeon General.* Rockville, MD: US Department of Health and Human Services, Substance Abuse and Mental Health Services Administration, Center for Mental Health Services, National Institutes of Health, National Institute of Mental Health; 1999. Available at: www.surgeongeneral.gov/library/mentalhealth/toc.html.
16. US Preventive Services Task Force. *Guide to clinical preventive services*, 2nd ed. Baltimore, MD: Williams & Wilkins, 1996.
17. Vaccarino V, Kasl SV, Abramson J, et al. Depressive symptoms and risk of functional decline and death in patients with heart failure. *J Am Coll Cardiol* 2001;38:199–205.

SLEEP DISORDERS

OBSTRUCTIVE SLEEP APNEA

Introduction

- Defined as repeated episodes of obstructive apnea during sleep (absence of airflow for >10 seconds >5 times per night) and/or hypopnea (reduction in airflow by 30% to 50% >15 times per hour); associated with daytime sleepiness and altered cardiopulmonary dysfunction (>4% drop in oxygen saturation).
- 2% to 4% of all adults suffers from obstructive sleep apnea (OSA). Male-to-female ratio 10 : 1.

Pathophysiology/Clinical Presentation (Table 56.1)

- Three types: *obstructive, central, or mixed*
  - ⇒ Obstructive: absence of airflow in presence of effort to move air into lungs
  - ⇒ Central: absence of respiratory effort, no airflow
  - ⇒ Mixed: begins with a central component, followed by obstructive phenomenon
- Most common etiology: closure of the upper airway at various levels (nasopharynx/oropharynx/hypopharynx)
- Most episodes occur during rapid eye movement (REM) sleep when muscle tone of pharyngeal muscles is decreased; manifested by snoring interrupted by silences (apneic events), followed by gasping or expiratory gruntings. Sleep becomes fragmented.
- Seen in obese patients (>120% ideal body weight); weight gain increases pharyngeal resistance.
- In nonobese patient, tonsillar enlargement or craniofacial abnormalities may play a role.
- Associated complications include cor pulmonale, secondary pulmonary hypertension, focal segmental glomerulosclerosis with nephrotic syndrome, strokes, and heart disease.

TABLE 56.1. DIFFERENTIAL DIAGNOSIS

Acromegaly	Narcolepsy	Chronic obstructive
Amyloidosis	Poliomyelitis	pulmonary disease
Congestive	Primary snoring	Gastroesophageal
heart failure	Upper airway	reflux disease
Hypothyroidism	resistance	Sleep-related
	syndrome	laryngospasm
		Renal failure

Evaluation

History

- Loud snoring, restless sleep, nocturnal choking, flailing movements while sleeping, excessive daytime sleepiness, abnormal mentation, personality changes, morning headaches, impotence

Physical Examination

- Evaluate for retrognathia, tonsillar enlargement, enlarged soft palate, obesity and increased neck circumference, bilateral leg edema, precordial heave, elevated jugular venous pulse or third heart sound (S_3), periorbital swelling.

Diagnostic Tests

- Complete blood cell count (polycythemia), arterial blood gas (hypercarbia/hypoxia)
- Echocardiogram (right heart disfunction)
- Polysomnography is best way to confirm OSA.
  - ⇒ Measures sleep stages (electroencephalogram), heart rate and rhythm (electrocardiogram), oxygen saturation, limb movements (electromyogram), ocular movement (electrooculogram) and respiratory effort.
  - ⇒ Severity graded on apnea-hypopnea index (AHI) and desaturation: mild OSA (AHI 5 to 20, desaturation >85%); moderate OSA (AHI 21 to 50, desaturation 80% to 85%); severe OSA (AHI > 51, desaturation <80%)
- Multiple Sleep Latency Test (MSLT): patient asked to take four naps; time to sleep quantified and averaged. Objective measure of sleepiness, with sleep latency >10 minutes normal, <5 minutes pathologic.
- Epworth sleepiness scale (ESS): eight-item questionnaire. Depending on the total score obtained, a diagnosis of OSA can be made with a value higher than ten.

Treatment

- **Weight loss** (Rubinstein et al., 1988), avoid supine position while sleeping, correct hypothyroidism (Grunstein, 1988), and avoid hypnotic agents, alcohol, and tobacco (Wetter et al., 1994).
- **Medications** for OSA have been largely unsuccessful.
  - ⇒ Medroxyprogesterone increases respiratory drive but is ineffective in improving OSA (Hudgel, 1995).
  - ⇒ Acetazolamide: Low doses (250 mg at bedtime) have some benefit in management of OSA (DeBacker et al., 1995).
  - ⇒ Tricyclic antidepressants: poor results in clinical trials (Brownell et al., 1982).
  - ⇒ Selective serotonin reuptake inhibitors increase upper airway neuron excitation, but studies with disappointing results (Hanzel et al., 1991).
- **Surgery** is reserved for those with specific anatomic abnormalities amenable to correction and those with moderate-severe OSA refusing to take or failing the continuous positive airway pressure (CPAP) test (American Sleep Disorder Association, 1995).
- **Oral appliances** may improve upper airway dimensions by pulling the tongue or moving the mandible forward. They have a role for mild to moderate OSA (Schmidt-Nowara et al., 1995).
- **Nasal CPAP:** Increases intraluminal pressure; generates positive transmural pressure throughout the respiratory cycle keeping pharyngeal cavity open.
  - ⇒ Most effective noninvasive therapy for both central sleep apnea and OSA available (Issa and Sullivan, 1986).
  - ⇒ Side effects include local skin irritation, drying of mucosal membranes, nasal congestion and rhinorrhea.
  - ⇒ Contraindication: bilateral nasal obstruction (American Thoracic Society, 1994)

INSOMNIA

Introduction

- Complaint of unsatisfactory sleep associated with daytime anxiety, mood alterations, or difficulty concentrating.
- Most common of all sleep disorders; 10% to 16% of all adults in the United States report symptoms suggestive of severe or chronic insomnia.
- Two to three times as common in women, two times more common in people older than 65 years (Gillin and Byerley, 1990)

Pathophysiology/Clinical Presentation

- Two types: short term (acute) and chronic (persistent)
- In short-term insomnia, an acute stressor such as job anxiety, pain, stimulants (caffeine, theophylline), drug withdrawal (opiate, benzos, alcohol), or change in schedule (jet-lag syndrome) produces disturbance in sleep that lasts <3 weeks.
- Chronic insomnia, a sleep disturbance lasting >3 weeks, may be caused by multiple disorders:
  ⇒ **Psychiatric:** depression, posttraumatic stress disorder, obsessive-compulsive disorder, schizophrenia
  ⇒ **Neurologic:** stroke (lesions in hypothalamic preoptic nuclei), chronic pain syndrome, Parkinson disease, ALS
  ⇒ **Cardiovascular:** Cheyne-Stokes respiration in congestive heart failure (CHF).
  ⇒ **Toxin related:** chronic alcohol use, withdrawal from benzos/barbiturates/ethanol/opiates, use of amphetamines or other stimulants, including caffeine
- In the absence of the above disorders, primary sleep disorders should be considered:
  ⇒ **Idiopathic insomnia:** lifelong difficulty in initiating or maintaining sleep, resulting in poor daytime functioning; usually begins in childhood
  ⇒ **Inadequate sleep hygiene:** due to consumption of substances known to affect sleep structure (coffee, alcohol, tobacco), erratic work schedules or excessive time spent in bed
  ⇒ **Insufficient sleep syndrome:** most common cause of excessive sleepiness; usually related to lifestyle choices or environmental stimuli
  ⇒ **Restless leg syndrome (RLS):** described as a "creepy crawling" sensation over lower extremities; relieved by leg movement (Walters, 1995); seen in diabetic or uremic neuropathy or iron deficiency anemia
  ⇒ **Periodic limb-movement disorder (PLMD):** characterized by periodically recurring limb movements during non-REM sleep; can lead to arousal and sleep fragmentation (Trenkwalder et al., 1996)

Evaluation

History

- Chronology of symptoms, frequency of nocturnal or early morning awakenings, difficulty initiating or maintaining sleep, any alterations in functional status/mood during daytime
- Evaluate for contributing neurologic, medical, or psychiatric conditions, current use of medications or toxins. Inquire about family history of insomnia.
- Tell patients to keep a sleep log for 2 weeks in which bedtime, rising time, naps, total sleep time, and number of nocturnal awakenings are noted.

Physical Examination

- Focus on signs suggestive of associated organic disorders (e.g., CHF, gastroesophageal reflux disease, Parkinson's disease).

Diagnostic Tests

- Polysomnography: evaluates presence of PLMD/RLS, characterizes complaints suggestive of insomnia once organic causes have been ruled out or after failure of initial treatment.
- MSLT may demonstrate increased sleep latency in cases of idiopathic insomnia.
- Neuroimaging is indicated if H&P suggest presence of organic neurological lesion.

Treatment

- Acute insomnia: Manage by identifying stressor; emphasize sleep hygiene; can use hypnotic agents for short period if symptoms interfere with quality of life.
- Chronic insomnia: Treat associated medical, psychiatric, or neurologic conditions; instruct on avoidance of substances known to produce insomnia. If these measures fail to control symptoms, consider a combination of behavioral and intermittent pharmacologic therapies (Morin et al., 1999).

- Emphasize teaching of sleep hygiene measures, relaxation techniques (meditation, yoga), stimulus control therapy, and sleep restriction therapy (Hohagen, 1996).
- Hypnotics should not be first-line therapy; if used, should be for periods <4 weeks.
- Among hypnotics, short-acting benzodiazepines are preferred (less residual morning somnolence); however, have high risk of rebound insomnia and dependence.
- Antidepressants: have role in treating insomnia with associated depression
- Antihistamines: have sedating properties, but long half-life can result in decreased daytime alertness and sedation.
- Melatonin: advocated for use in treating insomnia but research data are scarce. A study evaluating use in elderly with low melatonin showed some benefit (Haimov et al., 1994).
- PLMD/RLS: dopaminergic agonist (carbidopa-levodopa) first line; benzodiazepines if this fails.
- Cheyne-Stokes breathing in CHF: CPAP may decrease mortality, improve cardiovascular function.

SELECTED REFERENCES

1. American Sleep Disorder Association. Practice parameters for the treatment of snoring and obstructive sleep apnea with oral appliances. *Sleep* 1995;18:511–513.
2. American Thoracic Society. Indications and standards for the use of NCPAP in sleep apnea syndromes. *Am J Respir Crit Care Med* 1994;150:1738–1745.
3. Brownell LG, West P, Sweatman P. Protriptyline in obstructive sleep apnea: a double blind trial. *N Engl J Med* 1982;307:1037–1042.
4. DeBacker WA, Verbraecken J, Willemen M. Central apnea index decreases after prolonged treatment with acetazolamide. *Am J Respir Crit Care Med* 1995;151:87–91.
5. Gillin JC, Byerley WF. Drug Therapy: the diagnosis and management of insomnia. *N Engl J Med* 1990;322:239–248.
6. Grunstein RR, Sullivan CE. Sleep apnea and hypothyroidism: mechanism and management. *Am J Med* 1988;85(6)775–779.
7. Haimov I, Laudon M, Zisapel L. Sleep disorders and melatonin rhythms in elderly people. *BMJ* 1994;309: 167.
8. Hanzel DA, Proia NG, Hudgel DW. Response of obstructive sleep apnea to fluoxetine and protriptyline. *Chest* 1991;100:416–421.
9. Hohagen F. Nonpharmacological treatment of insomnia. *Sleep* 1996;19:S52.
10. Hudgel DW. Pharmacological treatment of obstructive sleep apnea. *J Lab Clin Med* 1995;126:13–18.
11. Issa FG, Sullivan CE. Reversal of central sleep apnea using nasal CPAP. *Chest* 1986;90:165–171.
12. Morin CM, Colecchi C, Stone J. Behavioral and pharmacological therapies for late life insomnia. A randomized controlled trial. *JAMA* 1999;281:991.
13. Rubinstein I, Colapinto N, Rotstein LE. Improvement in upper airway function after weight loss in patients with obstructive sleep apnea. *Am Rev Respir Dis* 1988;138:1192–1195.
14. Schmidt-Nowara W, Lowe A, Wiegland L. Oral appliances for the treatment of snoring and obstructive sleep apnea: a review. *Sleep* 1995;18:501–510.
15. Trenkwalder C, Walters AS, Hening W. Periodic limb movements and restless leg syndrome. *Neurol Clin* 1996;14:629.
16. Walters AS. Toward a better definition of the restless leg syndrome. The International Restless Leg Syndrome Study Group. *Movement Disord* 1995;10:634.
17. Wetter DW, Young TB, Bidwell TR. Smoking as a risk factor for sleep disordered breathing. *Arch Intern Med* 1994;154:2219–2224.

DOMESTIC VIOLENCE

INTRODUCTION

- Defined as a pattern of coercive control exercised by one partner over the other. Abusers use sexual and physical assault, social isolation, economic, emotional, and psychological abuse, threats, and harassment to establish and maintain control over their partners (Eisenstat and Zimmer, 1998)
- 2 million women battered each year in the United States (Gazmararian et al., 1996); leading cause of injuries to U.S. women ages 15 to 44 (Grisso et al., 1991)
- Affects one in five women at some time in their lives (Flitcraft, 1995)
- Up to one in five women experience physical abuse during pregnancy (Gazmararian et al., 1996); women with unplanned pregnancies are at threefold higher risk than those with planned pregnancies (Goodwin et al., 2000).

CLINICAL PRESENTATION (TABLE 57.1)

TABLE 57.1. CLINICAL PRESENTATION OF ABUSE: IT MAY BE OBVIOUS OR SUBTLE (EISENSTAT AND BANCROFT, 1999)

Physical trauma	Psychological
Head and neck injuries, including dental trauma	Depression, suicidal ideation
Central distribution of injuries	Anxiety including hyperventilation and panic attacks
Multiple areas of injuries	Eating disorders
Forearm injuries from self-defense (blocking face)	Substance abuse
Bruises in various stages of healing	Evidence of psychological trauma: dissociation, vigilance, psychic numbing, and instrusive thoughts
Inconsistent explanation for injury	
Sexual assault	
Neurologic symptoms (headache, numbeness/tingling)	
Partner behavior	Presenting behavior
Overly solicitous, refuses to leave the examining room	Evasiveness and vague symptom history
Aggressive behavior toward patient or staff	Repeated visits to the emergency ward or clinic
	Poor adherence with medical regimens
Chronic pain syndromes	Delay in seeking medical treatment
Headaches, chest pain, abdominal and pelvic pain	Pediatric presentation
Choking sensation or hyperventilation	In many cases of child physical/sexual abuse, mothers are also being abused
Fatigue and insomnia	
Palpitations of unclear etiology	

EVALUATION

- Occurs in all racial, educational, geographic, and socioeconomic groups (Flitcraft, 1995).
- Biggest risk factor is being a woman; pregnant women are at high risk. Risk factors in male abusers include alcohol or cocaine use, (recent) unemployment, less than a high school education, and being a former husband/boyfriend (Kyriacou et al., 1999).

- Domestic violence (DV) in gay and lesbian relationships is as common as it is in heterosexual relationships (Renzetti and Miley, 1996).

Screening

- Routine screening must be a regular part of preventive care.
  ⇒ Screening only those patients considered "high risk" will miss a substantial number of cases.
  ⇒ Emergency department studies reveal that victims are willing to disclose abuse if they are asked (Hayden et al., 1997).
- Routine screening does not need to be time consuming; simple direct questions are sensitive for DV (Feldhaus et al., 1997).
  ⇒ Partner violence screen: three questions about DV and perceived safety; 71% sensitive, 84% specific for DV

1. Have you been hit, kicked, punched, or otherwise hurt by someone within the past year? By whom?
2. Do you feel safe in your current relationship?
3. Is there a partner from a previous relationship who is making you feel unsafe now?

Implementing Routine Screening

- **Starting the interview** (Eisenstat and Zimmer, 1998)
  ⇒ Ensure confidentiality; always interview the patient alone.
  ⇒ Reassure the patient that the environment is safe.
  ⇒ Do not disclose the results of the screening questions to the partner.
  ⇒ Always use a professional interpreter (not family or friends) when language is a barrier.
- **Framing the question** (Eisenstat and Bancroft, 1999)
  ⇒ Generalize the question to make the patient more comfortable: "We're concerned about the health effects of partner abuse, so we now ask a few questions of all our patients."
- **Suggested routine screening questions**
  ⇒ Do you ever feel unsafe at home or in your relationship?
  ⇒ Has anyone at home hit you or tried to injure you in any way?
  ⇒ Has anyone ever threatened you or tried to control you?
  ⇒ Have you ever felt afraid of your partner?

TREATMENT
What to Do if Screening is Positive for Domestic Violence

- Obtain more information about the incident (Eisenstat and Bancroft, 1999):
  ⇒ Date and time of the event, where, how?
  ⇒ History of previous assaults?
  ⇒ Worst incident?
  ⇒ Associated trauma?
- Acknowledge and affirm the patient's statements.
- Obtain a full medical history, including pregnancy and immunization status.
- Clearly document the event in the medical record: details, diagrams, pictures of injuries (photographs can only be used with written patient consent).
- For sexual assault, use the state sexual assault protocol.
- Protect the chart for confidentiality; discuss nothing with the partner.
- Avoid labels such as battered, abused, DV; validate and support the patient.
- Leave the door open for future discussions if the patient is not yet ready to discuss it.

Recommended Interventions When You Have Identified Current Episodes of Abuse

- If patient reports DV and requests intervention:
  ⇒ Assess for patient safety to leave the clinical setting (emergency ward, clinic).
  ⇒ Assess for safety of children in the home.
  ⇒ Contact local shelters/social services for further action and safety planning.

- If patient reports DV and declines intervention:
  ⇒ Acknowledge patient's disclosure.
  ⇒ Validate and support the patient.
  ⇒ Assess for patient safety to leave the clinical setting (emergency ward, clinic).
  ⇒ Assess for safety of children in the home.
  ⇒ Offer services and information to the patient, including number for the National Domestic Violence Hotline (800-799-SAFE).
  ⇒ Document in chart.
- When there is a concern for patient or staff safety, call police/security immediately.
  ⇒ Leaving an abuser is often the most dangerous time for an abused woman; leaving before she is ready may further increase the danger.
  ⇒ Ask if abuser is here or if patient anticipates abuser arriving.
  ⇒ Do not attempt to manage aggressive behavior alone.
  ⇒ Ask if patient feels safe leaving the hospital. Arrange for safe exit from healthcare facility if abuser is present.
  ⇒ Ask if abuser has access to weapons. Ask if children are safe.
  ⇒ Not mandatory to report adult abuse in most states; reporting abuse could be dangerous to the patient.

SELECTED REFERENCES

1. Eisenstat S, Bancroft L. Domestic violence. *N Engl J Med* 1999;341:886–892.
2. Eisenstat S, Zimmer B. Providing medical care and advocacy for survivors of domestic violence. J Clin Outcomes Manage 1998;5(5):54–65.
3. Feldhaus KM, Koziol-McLain J, Amsbury HL, et al. Accuracy of 3 brief screening questions for detecting partner violence in the emergency department. *JAMA* 1997;277:1357–1361.
4. Ferris LE, Norton PG, Dunn EV, et al. Guidelines for managing domestic abuse when male and female partners are patients of the same physician. *JAMA* 1997;278(10):851–857.
5. Flitcraft A. From public health to personal health: violence against women across the life span. *Ann Intern Med* 1995;123:800–802.
6. Flitcraft A. Learning from the paradoxes of domestic violence [Editorial]. *JAMA* 1997;277(17):1400–1401.
7. Gazmararian JA, Lazorick S, Spitz AM, et al. Prevalence of violence against pregnant women. *JAMA* 1996;275:1915–1920.
8. Goodwin MM, Gazmararian JA, Johnson Ch, et al. Pregnancy intendedness and physical abuse around the time of pregnancy: findings from the pregnancy risk assessment monitoring system, 1996–1997. PRAMS working group. *Matern Child Health J* 2000;4:85.
9. Grisso JA, Wishner AR, Shwartz DF, et al. A population-based study of injuries in inner-city women. *Am J Epidemiol* 1991;134:59.
10. Hayden SR, Barton ED, Hayden M. Domestic violence in the emergency department: how do women prefer to disclose and discuss the issues? *J Emerg Med* 1997;15:447–451.
11. Kyriacou DN, Anglin D, Taliaferro E, et al. Risk factors for injuries from domestic violence. *N Engl J Med* 1999;341:1892–1898.
12. McCauley J, Kern DE, Kolodner K, et al. The "battering syndrome": prevalence and clinical characteristics of domestic violence in primary care internal medicine practices. *Ann Intern Med* 1995;123:737–746.
13. Rand M. *Violence-related injuries treated in hospital emergency departments.* Special Report. Bureau of Justice Statistics. Washington, DC: US Department of Justice, 1997.
14. Renzetti CM, Miley Ch, eds. *Violence in gay and lesbian domestic partnerships.* New York: Haworth, 1996.

CHRONIC NONMALIGNANT PAIN

INTRODUCTION

- Chronic pain affects up to 50 million Americans; costs >$79 billion per year (American Academy of Pain Medicine, 2001).
- The International Association for the Study of Pain defines pain as "an unpleasant sensory and emotional experience arising from actual or potential tissue damage." Patients describe pain in various ways, ascribing to it qualities that are often culturally rooted.
- Pain is the fifth vital sign; 2001 to 2010 declared the "Decade of Pain Control and Research" by the U.S. government.
- Chronic nonmalignant pain may or may not have an identifiable biologic stimulus, is by definition not self-limited, has psychosocial underpinnings, and is less amenable to pure pharmacologic intervention.

PATHOPHYSIOLOGY

- **Acute pain** is classified into two types:
  ⇒ *Nociceptive pain:* actual or potential tissue damage. Somatic nociceptive pain, attributable to specific anatomic areas or structures, is well localized and stabbing, throbbing, or achy. Visceral nociceptive pain is less well localized, dull, and crampy.
  ⇒ *Neuropathic pain:* derives from direct nerve stimulation. Burning, tingling or lancinating pain, often in a dermatomal distribution, may be associated with sensory deficit. Includes post–herpetic neuralgia, diabetic neuropathy, sciatica, reflex sympathetic dystrophy, and phantom limb pain.
- **Chronic pain** is less well understood. May have only a minor biologic stimulus or even no organic component; psychosocial factors play a large role in modulating and perpetuating the perception of pain.
  ⇒ *Psychological components:* modulate the perception of pain; may be classified as cause or effect of chronic pain. Major depression, anxiety and personality disorders, or substance abuse problems may all heighten awareness of somatic sensations and create a charged emotional state. A charged emotional state sensitizes nociceptive fibers to stimuli, leading to an enhanced conscious perception of pain.
  ⇒ *Social contributors:* home, leisure, and work environments. Secondary gain (family sympathy, ongoing litigation, worker's compensation) may drive the chronic nature of pain.

DIFFERENTIAL DIAGNOSIS

- Chronic pain frequently localizes to five areas: head/face, nonaxial musculoskeletal structures, low back, abdomen/pelvis, and peripheral nerves. See Table 58.1 for potentially reversible etiologies.

TABLE 58.1. DIFFERENTIAL DIAGNOSES OF CHRONIC PAIN BASED ON LOCATION

Location	Differential of Reversible Etiologies		
Headache/facial	Tension headache	Sinusitis	Trigeminal neuralgia
	Migraine headache	Medication	Postconcussive
	Chronic otitis	Chronic meningitis	Glaucoma
	Cluster headache	Abscess	Bruxism
	Temporal arteritis	Subdural	Sialadenitis
	Large arteriovenous	Tumor	Glaucoma
	malformation	TMJ	Dentalgia
	Hypertension		
Musculoskeletal	Fibromyalgia	Rheumatoid arthrtitis	Paget's disease
	Polymyalgia rheumatica	Osteoarthritis	Tumor
	Polymyositis	Gout/pseudogout	Cramps
	Dermatomyositis	Systemic lupus erythematosis	Bursitis/tendonitis
	Drug myositis	Osteomyelitis	Reflex symptoms dystrophy
	Hypothyroidism	Trichinella	Sickle cell disease
	Trauma	Lyme disease	Syphilis
Low back	Chronic disc disease	Osteoporotic fracture	Tumor (bone/retroperitoneum)
	Sciatica	Spinal stenosis	Seronegative
	Vertebral osteomyelitis	Epidural abscess	spondyloarthropathy
Abdominal/pelvic	Irritable bowel syndrome	Inflammatory bowel disease	Kidney stones
	Biliary colic	Diverticulitis	Chronic pyelonephritis
	Esophagitis	Gastritis/PUD	Polycystic kidney disease
	Pancreatitis	Hepatitis	Endometriosis
	Parasitosis	Tumor	Ovarian cysts
	Aortic aneurysm	(gastrointestinal/gastrourinary/	Pelvic inflammatory
	Sickle cell	gynecologic)	disease/tuboovarian abscess
	Medicines	Abdominal angina	Familial mediterranean fever
		Poisoning (e.g., lead)	Porphyria
		Internal hernias	
Peripheral nerve	Diabetic neuropathy	Vitamin B_{12} deficiency	Charcot-Marie-Tooth disease
	Human immunodeficiency virus	Connective tissue disease	Hypothyroidism
	neuropathy	Renal failure	Poisoning (ethanol, isoniazid)
	Paraneoplastic		

EVALUATION

- Think of chronic pain as a chronic problem requiring continuous therapy, such as diabetes or hypertension.
- Document the nine cardinal features of pain: *onset/duration, quality/severity, location/spread, alleviating/aggravating factors, and associated symptoms*
- Remember that patients describe pain qualitatively based on their cultural background. Pain severity scales are valid regardless of culture and are useful in tracking an individual's pain over time.
- Treatment goals should be improvement in quality of life and function, rather than complete elimination of the patient's pain.
- Consider the role of psychosocial factors in the patient's experience of pain (see Table 58.2).

TABLE 58.2. CLUES THAT PSYCHOSOCIAL FACTORS ARE PREDOMINANT IN A PATIENT'S CHRONIC PAIN

- *Depression* or *anxiety* that pre-date the pain
- Pain began in adolescence or at time of trauma (suggests *pain disorder* or posttraumatic stress disorders)
- History of *substance abuse*
- Multiple, unrelated sites of pain over time (suggests *somatization disorder*)
- No demonstrable pathophysiologic mechanism to explain the physical symptoms
- History of difficult social interactions suggesting *personality disorder*
- Evidence of physical, sexual, or emotional *abuse*
- Potential for or history of the patient pursuing secondary gain (litigation, workman's compensation) suggests malingering

TREATMENT

- Systematic, stepwise, multifactorial approach is crucial to achieving a successful outcome. One approach is the **five A's:**
  - ⇒ **Agree** on expectations based on quality of life and function.
  - ⇒ **Address** biologic and psychological components concurrently. Assuring the patient that the validity of the complaint is not in question improves compliance with psychiatric referrals.
  - ⇒ **Anticipate** needs for psychiatry and/or pain specialists and refer early.
  - ⇒ **Analgesic** ladder: Progress in a stepwise fashion through the various agents (see below).
  - ⇒ **Alternative** approaches: Pharmacologic, psychological, and surgical methods, along with complementary techniques, may need to be combined for maximal relief.

Nociceptive Pain

- **Nonopiate analgesics**
  - ⇒ *Acetaminophen:* 1,000 mg four times a day as effective as nonsteroidal antiinflammatory drugs (NSAIDs); safe for patients without known hepatic dysfunction who drink more than five alcoholic beverages per day
  - ⇒ *NSAIDs:* the next step for diseases with a prominent inflammatory component
  - ⇒ *Tramadol:* centrally acting analgesic with dual effects. Primary effect is as a monoamine reuptake inhibitor, blocking pain transmission in the spinal cord. It also targets central nervous system micro-opioid receptors and should not be given to opiate abusers.
- **Opiates**
  - ⇒ The gold standard of analgesia; however, a difficult balance between treating pain and creating addiction in a patient population
  - ⇒ There is a recent trend toward prescribing opiates for patients with chronic nonmalignant pain who meet basic criteria (see Table 58.3), following certain general principles (see Table 58.4). The Appendix contains a sample opioid use contract that helps limit addictive behavior.

TABLE 58.3. CRITERIA FOR GIVING A PATIENT OPIATES FOR CHRONIC NONMALIGNANT PAIN

- Subjective chronic pain on more than one occasion, consistently reported.
- Pain inhibits function and decreases quality of life.
- Reversible etiologies have been addressed.
- Other measures have been tried with inadequate response.
- The patient does not meet formal criteria for substance abuse or a primary psychiatric disorder.
- No other contraindications to opiates (liver disease, operating heavy machinery, drug tested at work).
- The patient is capable of adhering to a simple contract about appropriate follow-up and opiate use.

TABLE 58.4. GENERAL PRINCIPLES TO FOLLOW WHEN PRESCRIBING NARCOTICS FOR CHRONIC PAIN

- Keep the patient to a simple *contract* with a "two strikes and you're tapered to zero" approach; stick to all the terms of the contract tightly.
- Treat pain *proactively* before chronic patterns and secondary psychiatric comorbidities become ingrained.
- Use *long-acting agents* as round-the-clock treatment (fentanyl patch), avoiding short-acting medications for long-term use; use the same medication in short-acting formulation during the initial titration phase and for occasional breakthroughs (e.g., OxyContin plus oxycodone).
- Maintain close *follow-up*.

APPENDIX

Neuropathic Pain

- Typically more resistant to pharmacologic interventions than nociceptive pain.
- **Antidepressants**
  ⇒ *Tricyclic antidepressants*
  1. Demonstrate analgesia for post–herpetic neuralgia, diabetic neuropathy, tension and migraine headaches, rheumatoid arthritis, and low back pain in controlled trials.
  2. Potentiate opioid analgesics; use selectively in nociceptive pain situations.
  3. Analgesic effect may occur at much lower doses than those required for affective disorders.
  ⇒ Selective serotonin reuptake inhibitors: not yet fully evaluated for most chronic pain syndromes.
- **Anticonvulsants**
  ⇒ *Gabapentin:* the agent of choice for most neuropathic pain, especially the lancinating types (e.g., sciatica). Titrate up from low doses to avoid oversedation.
  ⇒ *Baclofen:* a well-tolerated gabapentin agonist used primarily for painful spasticity (e.g., with spinal cord–injured patients)
  ⇒ *Phenytoin and carbamazepine:* shown to relieve pain associated with trigeminal neuralgia
- **Topical agents**
  ⇒ *Capsaicin cream:* useful for low back pain, arthritis, post–herpetic syndromes, and diabetic neuropathy
  ⇒ *Lidocaine:* 5% patch good for post–herpetic neuralgia; EMLA (lidocaine + prilocaine) comes in a disk or as a cream, which should be covered with an occlusive dressing.

Other Modalities

- **Acupuncture:** possible adjunctive therapy for chronic pain due to fibromyalgia, myofacial pain, and osteoarthritis
- **Behavioral approaches:** useful adjuvants that patients rely on to gain control of their pain:
  - ⇒ Relaxation
  - ⇒ Hypnosis
  - ⇒ Cognitive-behavioral therapy
  - ⇒ Biofeedback
- **Invasive techniques,** initially used to treat patients with terminal cancer, are now being extrapolated for use in the patient with chronic nonmalignant pain. Most pain specialists will have access to these techniques.
  - ⇒ *Local anesthetics*
  - ⇒ *Sympathetic or neurolytic blocks*
  - ⇒ *Long-term spinal opioids*

RESOURCES

- Pain specialists may be located via The American Pain Society (847-375-4715) or the American Academy of Pain Medicine (www.painmed.org).
- Many physicians have been trained in acupuncture (www.medicalacupuncture.org).

SELECTED REFERENCES

1. American Academy of Pain Medicine. Available at: www.painmed.org/faws/pain_faqs.html 4/30/01.
2. Anonymous. NIH Consensus Conference: acupuncture. *JAMA* 1998;280(17):1518–1524.
3. Anonymous. NIH panel. Integration of behavioral and relaxation approaches into the treatment of chronic pain and insomnia. *JAMA* 1996;276(4):313–318.
4. Backonja MB, Beydoun A, Edwards KR, et al. Gabapentin for the symptomatic treatment of painful neuropathy in patients with diabetes mellitus. *JAMA* 1998;280(21):1831–1836.
5. Burchman SL, Pagel PS. Implementation of a formal treatment agreement for outpatient management of chronic nonmalignant pain with opioid analgesics. *J Pain Symptom Manage* 1995;10(7):556–561.
6. Grant DJ, Bishop-Miller J, Winchester DM, et al. A randomized comparative trial of acupuncture vs. TENS for chronic back pain in the elderly. *Pain* 1999;82(1):9–13.
7. Jung AC, Staiger T, Sullivan M. SSRI's for the management of chronic pain. *J Gen Intern Med* 1997; 12(6):384–389.
8. Katz WA. Pharmacology and clinical experience with tramadol in OA. *Drugs* 1996;52S:39–47.
9. Portenoy RK. Opioid therapy for chronic nonmalignant pain: a review of the critical issues. *J Pain Symptom Manage* 1996;11(4):203–217.
10. Shekelle PG, Adams AH, Chassin MR, et al. Spinal manipulation for low back pain. *Ann Intern Med* 1992; 117(7):590–598.
11. Silverstein FE, Faich G, Goldstein JL, et al. Gastrointestinal toxicity with celecoxib versus NSAIDs for osteoarthritis and rheumatoid arthritis: the CLASS study. *JAMA* 2000;284(10):1247–1255.
12. Smith GR. The epidemiology and treatment of depression when it coexists with somatoform disorders, somatization or pain. *Gen Hosp Psychiatry* 1992;14:265–272.
13. Tannenbaum H, Davis P, Rusell AS, et al. An evidence-based approach to prescribing NSAIDs in musculoskeletal disease: a Canadian consensus. *CMAJ* 1996;155(1):77–88.
14. Turk DC, Brody MC, Okifuji EA. Physicians' attitudes and practices regarding the long-term prescribing of opioids for non-cancer pain. *Pain* 1994;59:201–208.
15. Zenz M, Donner B, Strumpf M, et al. Role of invasive methods in the treatment of chronic pain. *Acta Anesth Scand* 1997;111[Suppl]:181–183.

SUBJECT INDEX

A